PSYCHOPHARMACOLOGY
PROBLEM SOLVING

PSYCHOPHARMACOLOGY PROBLEM SOLVING

Principles and Practices to Get It Right

F. SCOTT KRALY

W. W. Norton & Company

New York • London

For information about permission to reproduce selections from this book, write to
Permissions, W. W. Norton & Company, Inc., 500 Fifth Avenue, New York, NY 10110

For information about special discounts for bulk purchases, please contact W. W. Norton
Special Sales at specialsales@wwnorton.com or 800-233-4830

Manufacturing by R.R. Donnelley, Harrisonburg
Production manager: Leeann Graham

Library of Congress Cataloging-in-Publication Data

Kraly, F. Scott, author.
    Psychopharmacology problem solving : principles and practices to get it
right / F. Scott Kraly. — First edition.
        p. ; cm.
    "Norton professional book."
    Includes bibliographical references and index.
    ISBN 978-0-393-70875-2 (hardcover)
    I. Title.
    [DNLM: 1. Psychotropic Drugs—therapeutic use.   2. Problem Solving.
QV 77.2]
    RM315
    615.7'88—dc23
                                        2014001248

ISBN: 978-0-393-70875-2

W. W. Norton & Company, Inc., 500 Fifth Avenue, New York, N.Y. 10110
www.wwnorton.com
W. W. Norton & Company Ltd., Castle House, 75/76 Wells Street, London W1T 3QT

1 2 3 4 5 6 7 8 9 0

To Ellen, Marjorie, Ruth, Mary, Irene, Susan, Sandra, and Charlie
for their strength, grace, and determination
in the face of significant challenges.

Contents

Acknowledgments

Deborah Malmud, director of Norton Professional Books, offered valuable criticism that helped me to more clearly conceptualize this project. Her excellent advice and subsequent gift of turning me loose to write are much appreciated. Others on the Norton staff provided excellent assistance, including Andrea Costella Dawson, Kevin Olsen, and Sophie Hagen. Thanks to copyeditor Trish Watson as well. James Kraly of the Department of Chemistry at Keene State College and Geoff Kraly read early drafts of several chapters and offered thoughtful criticism that had a continuing impact on my writing and revising. Noongar artist Sandra Hill and Koori elder Julie Freeman from Wreck Bay generously shared their experiences and wisdom. Finally, Colgate University and the Charles A. Dana Foundation provided resources necessary to write this book. Colgate has consistently supported my development as a scientist and teacher, providing resources and encouragement to take risks when attempting new academic endeavors.

Preface

The use of drugs to treat psychopathology has experienced success beyond reason—and that is the problem. Our current use of psychotropic medication demands a hard look at the extraordinary and increasing trust that clinicians, patients, and families of patients appear to place in the use of these drugs. The trust is excessive because the successful use of psychotropic drugs occurs in the face of significant problems that the drugs present. These problems concern more than merely unwanted drug-induced side effects—they include the use of medication that is not supported by scientific evidence, especially: the increasing use of psychotropic drugs to treat children and adolescents; the use of medication in situations that might better benefit from nondrug therapy; and the unresponsiveness of some patients to psychotropic medication. In short, some of the use of psychotropic medication is not judicious, not carefully considered, and likely not serving the best interests of the patient.

The solution to this problem is not to stop medicating for psychopathology. Psychotropic medications are good and useful clinical tools. But, it is the right time to consider what it means to be medicating judiciously, because it appears that the use of psychotropic medication is approaching its zenith, if it hasn't already reached it. It is time to slow down, pause, maybe back up a bit, and then proceed more cautiously doing the business of psychopharmacology for mental health.

The goal of this book is to encourage more judicious, cautious, better-informed, and more appropriate use of psychotropic medication—to encourage use that is more respectful of the strengths and the limitations of these drugs. I work toward this goal by presenting some fundamental principles of pharmacology as they apply to clinical treatment of patients and by offering some broad recommendations for making decisions about the use of drugs as therapy. This is a book that encourages the use of psychotropic medication as a useful tool—one of a number of useful options in the toolkit for treating patients having psychological disorders. I hope that you find it informative, useful, and a friendly read.

F. Scott Kraly
Hamilton, NY

Introduction

"What's the harm in taking a little pill every day? Everyone's doing it, and it helps, so let's get this thing done! A drug will be good for Robert—he'll do better in school. So let's just have you write the prescription for our son, okay? It will help him sit still and concentrate better. He needs to have the best grades to get into medical school some day."

The justification is weak—a 10-year old boy already committed to becoming a physician, if only he performs better in grammar school? The only nearly respectable reason to prescribe methylphenidate is the parents' sketchy description of symptoms of attention deficit and hyperactivity. But there are a dozen good reasons to consider not writing that prescription—reasons based on guidelines for making an appropriate diagnosis, the clinical scientific evidence, knowledge of principles of pharmacology, and the exercise of due caution. Unfortunately, Robert's parents are not really open to having a conversation that permits making an informed, judicious decision about what would be best for their child—about whether or not prescribing a drug is a good thing for Robert, whether or not the benefits outweigh the risks.

A psychoactive drug can be a useful tool. A drug can alter the chemistry of the brain, and the chemistry of the brain contributes in significant ways to our behavior, thoughts, and emotions. These are undeniable facts revealed by research in animals and humans. Our growing understanding of the role of the brain's chemical messengers for human behavior provides knowledge that convincingly supports the rationale for the use of drugs as a therapeutic tool for psychopathology.

The use of psychoactive or psychotropic drugs as treatment for psychopathology began to realize its heyday only in the 1950s (Gerard, 1957), when most notably the neuroleptic drug chlorpromazine, the antidepressant imipramine, and the mood stabilizer lithium carbonate entered the clinical arena (Ban, 2001; Jacobsen, 1986). The subsequent 50 years saw great advances in the discovery of drugs having clinical utility for treating each and every diagnosable psychopathology. Today, any psychological problem that comes your way will find an appropriate recommended psychotropic medication.

This recent 50-year period of drug discovery and implementation of therapeutic psychopharmacology is marked by trends for increased use (Frank, Conti, & Goldman, 2005; Pincus et al., 1998) and increased spending (Mark, Kassed, Levit, & Vandivort-Warren, 2012; Zuvekas, 2005) on psychotropic medications. The successful use of these drugs has improved access to treatment for many patients, has facilitated the development of newer drugs that are equally or more effective while accompanied by fewer side effects, and has diminished costs and improved the overall quality of care for people with psychological illness (Frank et al., 2005). So what's not to like about psychotropic medications?

Pharmacotherapy for psychopathology has become increasingly commonplace over the past half century, bringing new problems to confront patients and clinicians. One new problem is that the much heralded successful use of pharmacotherapy has encouraged the increased use of drugs as therapy instead of using equally effective, or sometimes more effective, nondrug therapies—various methods of behavior therapy or psychotherapy, in particular (Chisolm, 2011; Mojtabai & Olfson, 2008; specifically for treatment of depression, see Marcus & Olfson, 2010). There certainly are advantages of drug therapy over psychotherapy, such as its privacy, its minimal demand upon the patient's time, its reduced expense, its constant availability on the medicine shelf, and the presumption of more pronounced and more rapid improvement. These positive attributes encourage considering the use of a drug therapy as the first, presumably best option. So attractive are the positive attributes of pharmacotherapy that the incidence of psychotropic polypharmacy—the simultaneous use of several drugs to treat a single disorder or several disorders—has become more common despite limited published evidence supporting the benefits of specific combinations of drugs for treating patients who are not responsive to a single therapeutic drug (Mojtabai & Olfson, 2010).

A second new problem nurtured by the successful use of drugs as therapy is the increased influence of the perspective that all forms of psychopathology represent nothing more than problems in the functioning of the brain's chemistry and that a drug-induced correction in a specific target in brain chemistry will remove the underlying cause of the psychopathology. This perspective is tantalizing for its simplicity, supporting the bias that the most effective way to remedy abnormal behavior is to use a drug that will return brain chemistry to normal—a maneuver that may produce a full remission of symptoms. One difficulty with this perspective is that using a drug may not be the only way to make adjustments in brain chemistry; the drug may represent the most direct and most efficient way, but the use of a drug comes at the cost of drug-induced adverse effects. A second difficulty with the perspective is its implicit assumption that drug therapy represents the single best way to improve the quality of life for the patient. This assumption is contrary to a *biopsychosocial* medical model (Engel, 1977) of disease—a model that perhaps best serves contemporary medicine and clinical psychology (Adler, 2009; Alvarez, Pagani, & Meucci, 2012), a model that encourages a multidimensional therapeutic program that makes adjustments in the brain, in behavior, and in relevant social factors.

A third new problem accompanying the success of psychopharmacology is the simple fact that, as the years have gone by, many, many more drugs have been introduced that have psychoactive properties and are useful medications. As a single case in point, R. M. Julien's *A Primer of Drug Action*, in its 12th edition (Julien, Advocat, & Comaty, 2010), has more than twice the number of pages as the first edition, published in 1975. A book such as Julien's must grow over subsequent editions owing to the appearance of new drugs on the market. These more recently developed drugs, however new and improved and useful they may be, rarely put to pasture the older drug options. For example, the vintage tricyclic antidepressants (e.g., imipramine), the vintage antianxiety agents (e.g., diazepam, chlordiazepoxide), and the vintage antipsychotic drugs (e.g., chlorpromazine, haloperidol) remain useful options despite the development of newer-generation drugs in each category. And in some situations, a vintage drug may provide the best option for a particular client. We are now virtually buried in facts about psychopharmacology, and there seems to be no end to the continuing accumulation of information relevant for making good decisions about the use of psychotropic medications.

Considering these three problems together, we are currently in the situation of having a continually growing, immense catalogue of older and newer pharmacological options for treating a variety of psychopathological conditions, and the use of these options is strongly encouraged by numerous tales of success found in the professional literature and in multimedia advertisements. But not one of these drug options represents the holy grail of treatments for any psychopathology—none of the drug options provides a risk-free cure for a diagnosable problem. Therefore, novel drugs will continue to be developed for both their clinical and market potentials, and these new drugs will further lengthen the list of options.

The problem that now faces the clinician and the patient is the need to sort through the continually growing set of options working toward a judicious choice of therapeutic drug, and then to decide how to use the drug as one component of a treatment program. How does one sort through the immense amount of information about options and be confident that the best decisions are being made?

It is fairly impossible for clinicians to have in their heads a complete command of all there is to know about all psychoactive medications. And even if someone had it, such knowledge would require tweaking each time a new drug enters the list of clinically useful tools—because the careful consideration of the utility of a new drug demands a comparison of the new drug (its benefits and its risks) with each and every one of the older drugs that have been used to treat that specific disorder. So what is one to do? How do clinicians and patients deal with the facts about pharmacology as those facts continue to increase in number and complexity, making it seem as if a judicious decision is becoming more and more difficult to make?

Increasing one's memory storage capacity in order to better hold and integrate the details of pharmacology is not the answer. A more useful tactic is to develop a *working knowledge* of some fundamental principles of pharmacology, together with an understanding of important factors that determine the availability and effectiveness of drugs used as medications. A working knowledge of fundamental principles and important factors provides a helpful framework or a remindful set of guidelines and recommendations to facilitate approaching a new problem. The new problem is tackled by using a framework or checklist based on useful principles learned when solving previous, related problems. For example, developing solutions for difficulties encountered when treating depression with a particular frequently prescribed drug may prove to be useful when anticipating similar difficulties using a new drug to treat depression or to treat anxiety or bulimia. A working knowledge of psychopharmacology establishes an approach for solving a *category* of problems—an approach that makes it possible to confront new problems regarding making decisions about using drugs as therapy.

Part I of this book offers a set of principles, recommendations, or guidelines to keep in mind when working toward making judicious decisions regarding using a drug as therapy for psychopathology. Part II uses select examples of behavioral problems and psychological disorders to illustrate how research findings in humans (and sometimes animals) support the significance of the principles or recommendations presented in Part I. The Conclusion briefly considers persistent problems and challenges to progress for current and future use of psychotropic medications. All the while, this book attempts to demonstrate that, although the facts of psychopharmacology are numerous and the complexity is daunting, it is possible to develop an approach to problem solving in psychopharmacology that serves the goal of bringing to the patient realistic expectations for drug therapy having greater benefits and fewer risks.

What is the best way to use a psychotropic mediation to achieve greater benefit with fewer risks? We first must acknowledge that each individual patient presents a relatively unique puzzle. We also must understand that each individual drug is an imperfect tool that will function best when judiciously applied to solve that unique puzzle. Judicious use of the pharmacological tool within the context of a multifaceted treatment program, together with the cooperation of the patient and a little luck, should maximize the tool's capacity for helping while minimizing the tool's potential for harm—to get it right.

PSYCHOPHARMACOLOGY PROBLEM SOLVING

PART I

Fundamental Principles and Recommendations

Part I offers a set of principles, guidelines, recommendations, or reminders useful for taking on the complicated task of deciding how a psychotropic medication can best be employed as an important part of a therapeutic program. The goal of Part I is to help the reader become thoughtful, thorough, and respectfully cautious when recommending or when accepting psychotropic medication. This goal is contrary to facilitating the development of the cowboy psychopharmacologist who is the quickest on the draw in prescribing the use of a drug as therapy, and this goal also is contrary to urging the patient to always accept that magic bullet. Citations in the published scientific literature are intended to provide places for the reader to turn for illustrative examples or for further reading on topics that may be important or appealing.

CHAPTER ONE

Cardinal Rules of Pharmacology

Grace is realistic about her situation. She knows that her depression will come and go; she has been debilitated by depression before, and she will be again. She knows this newer antidepressant drug may or may not be of help. The side effects will be unpredictable—there surely will be some, but with any luck they will be tolerable. She knows that finding an effective and acceptable dosage might take a bit of trial and error that could take months. And she hopes that her inability to stop smoking does not present a problem for the ability of this new drug to help her. Despite all this uncertainty, she is optimistic, because her psychiatrist understands her concerns and is open to discussing their shared approach to solving her problem.

A drug is not a familiar friend to the brain and its chemical processes—a drug is a foreign substance to a brain and a body. A drug is a chemical with a three-dimensional configuration that is placed into one or another type of vehicle to facilitate insertion into the body of a human or animal. The vehicle is most often a capsule or a solution used to facilitate getting a swallowed, injected, infused, or absorbed substance situated so as to gain access to the target tissue that will mediate the drug's action upon the organism. Psychoactive drugs—drugs that alter psychological processes and behavior—are generally assumed to achieve most of their psychoactivity by interacting with targets in the brain. But *how* drugs do this is not so simple, because the brain is a chemically very complex organ, and because the brain's complexity is rather poorly understood.

The *endogenous* chemical complexity of the brain presents a somewhat awkward interface for an *exogenous*—ingested or injected—drug. In other words, whoever or whatever designed the brain did not deliberately plan for it to comfortably interact with each and every drug that could possibly be invented, manufactured, and ingested by humans. The brain must therefore do the best that it can when interacting with a drug, attempting to accommodate the drug's intended purpose. This awkward interface between brain chemistry and drug chemistry presents several important problems for the use of a psychotropic medication as therapy. The principal problem is that an ingested drug always has multiple consequences.

NO DRUG HAS ONLY ONE EFFECT

Ask a pharmacologist for the single most important principle of pharmacology to keep in mind as one begins to think about using a drug for any purpose—as medication or recreational device or research tool. The pharmacologist will answer with the principle that *no drug can have only one effect*. What is the scientific basis for this principle, and why is it so important when considering the use of a drug in a clinical setting?

Let's begin with the assumption that *ideally* a drug is used in a clinical setting to elicit only *one* outcome—the so-called main effect. Getting the main effect of a drug is the top priority for the patient. The main effect is the benefit of the drug: diminished anxiety, elevated mood, or decreased incidence of binging and purging in bulimia, for example. But the principle that *no drug can have only one effect* declares that the desired (main) effect inevitably will be accompanied by undesired (side) effects. This assertion is certainly a curse for the use of any drug as therapy, because it promises that there will be some physiological and/or behavioral price to pay when experiencing the benefit of a drug. The specific currency (e.g., headache, rash, or tremor) of the price to pay may be somewhat unpredictable, and the amount (the intensity, duration) of the price to pay also may be unpredictable. Despite the unpredictability, the patient using a drug can expect to get some bad with the good.

Why is there such certainty associated with this principle—that the benefit of a drug must be accompanied by some risk, harm, or inconvenience? Consider the rationale for using a drug as therapy for psychopathology, where the goal is for the drug to change a psychological process and some behavior. The rationale in its simplest form is that the drug will alter some endogenous chemical process (likely in the brain), and this chemical intervention will produce the desired behavioral outcome. For a drug to do that, it must in some way intervene in a process that is endogenous or natural to the brain. But an intervention by a foreign object or substance—whether it is with a scalpel, drill bit, screw, or drug—is a deviant act, insofar as normal brain chemistry is concerned. The pharmacological intervention is an intrusion into the normal functioning of the brain.

Here are four ways in which the administration of a drug represents an intrusion or an insult to the normal functioning of the brain:

- A drug is not *of* the brain. A drug is not synthesized within a person's brain; it does not originate within the brain. A drug is synthesized (or perhaps extracted from organ tissue) on a workbench in a laboratory. A drug is moved from the workbench into a delivery device (e.g., a syringe, a capsule) that will place it into the brain. Because it is exogenous to the brain, a drug enters the brain as a foreign object, and therefore a drug should be expected to have effects that are somewhat different from the effects of chemicals that are endogenous to the brain (e.g., neurotransmitters).
- A drug is highly unlikely to have the identical chemical structure or configuration as that of an endogenous chemical. If the exogenous chemical is dissimilar to any endogenous chemical, then the exogenous drug will interact with the brain's chemistry in a manner that does *not mimic* normal endogenous chemical processes.
- A drug makes its entry in an unusual manner. A psychoactive drug's site of action is likely in the brain, but the drug's point of origin in the body usually is outside the brain. A drug is more likely to enter the body through the mouth or the lungs, or into a vein or a muscle, or beneath the skin. Unlike an endogenous chemical synthesized and released in the vicinity of its target site in the brain, the exogenous drug enters a site at some distance from its ultimate target site in the brain. The exogenous drug must work its way to the site. Along the way, the drug must survive obstacles (e.g., digestion, metabolism) that tend to degrade its effectiveness. And as a drug meets various organs on its way to the target site, it may affect those organs in a way that produces undesired effects—side effects.
- The mode of delivery of a drug does not reproduce the manner in which an endogenous chemical makes its appearance at its target site in the brain. A drug is often administered as a bolus or as a continuous slow infusion; neither mode of delivery is likely to enable a drug to mimic the natural rise and decline of an endogenous chemical at its target site.

Each of these issues emphasizes that a drug should not be expected to precisely mimic the effects of an endogenous chemical, essentially because a drug is not a natural chemical in the brain, and because a drug gets to a target in the brain through a somewhat unusual route and at a somewhat unusual rate. These facts decrease the likelihood that a drug will have effects that are identical to those of an endogenous chemical. An endogenous chemical essentially has assigned effects and functions that are customary to the brain, whereas an intrusive drug does not.

Failure to embody the effects of an endogenous chemical in the brain is not the only reason that some of the effects of a drug can be somewhat surprising and undesirable. Another reason is that the effects of a drug on the chemistry of the brain cannot be fully known and predictable. This is because the study of brain is a frontier science in which much is known, but even more is unknown, about brain chemistry and its functions (Iversen, Iversen, Bloom, & Roth, 2009). Moreover, it is difficult to *thoroughly* measure the effects of a drug on brain chemistry.

To explore these ideas further, consider that only a fraction, certainly less than half, of the chemicals in the brain have been identified. The aspects of the brain's chemistry that *have* been identified usually can be measured (and manipulated). The point here is that (a) if you can see something and you know where to find it, you probably can measure that something and also manipulate it; and (b) if you cannot see something, or do not know where to find it, or do not possess a tool that will measure that particular something, then you cannot measure it and cannot manipulate it with any precision.

Precise manipulation and measurement represent the fundamental business of experimental science. So, if we want to find out in an experiment what a drug can do to the chemistry of the brain, we can learn the effects of the drug on *only those processes that we know exist and that we can measure*. As a hypothetical case in point, we can measure that a drug has an effect on processes related to the chemical dopamine in the brain, and at the same time we can measure that the same drug has no measurable effect on processes related to the chemical serotonin in the brain. But, we cannot say with any degree of certainty that the drug has no effect whatsoever upon other chemical processes in the brain that have not yet been identified, or for which no one has the technical skills to measure. In summary, we can be fairly certain that a drug induces those changes that we can measure, but we cannot be at all certain that the drug does absolutely nothing else.

Now let's consider this issue as it applies in a clinical setting. For most of the psychotropic medications that are used clinically, there is published evidence that each drug alters some specific, measurable chemical process (or multiple measurable processes) in the brain. There is usually also evidence that the same drug appears to have no measurable effects on one or several other measurable chemical processes in the brain. It is also possible to speculate with confidence that this same drug is very likely to have undetermined effects on other chemical processes—processes that are unidentified and therefore not measurable, or identified but not readily measurable. In a case like this, the state-of-the-art assessment would be that the drug has an identified *presumed* mechanism of action (to produce its main effect) through one or another measured chemical process, and that the drug has *no other currently known* measurable effects on other chemical processes. This interpretation does not rule out the possibility that the drug is in fact directly or indirectly altering some chemical processes other than its stated and presumed mechanism of action. And it is entirely possible that these currently unmeasurable effects on known or unknown chemicals are responsible for some of the drug's undesired side effects, and they may even contribute to some of the drug's desired main effect.

This thicket of thoughts about pharmacology may benefit from a more explicit example of a psychotropic medication and its presumed mechanism of action. The older, first-generation antipsychotic drugs—the neuroleptics—are known to block some of the effects of the neurochemical dopamine in the brain. This dopamine blockade is understood to be the mechanism by which drugs in this class improve symptoms of schizophrenia. But drugs known to block the activity of *nondopamine* chemical processes, such as a drug that inhibits the effects of endogenous acetylcholine, can diminish some of the side effects of these dopamine-antagonizing neuroleptic drugs. Thus, the main effect of a neuroleptic drug may be due to its effect on dopamine transmission, whereas one or more of the side effects of a neuroleptic drug may be due to its secondary effect on acetylcholine transmission.

Undesired side effects can also be attributed to the fact that many drugs alter chemical systems in the brain that are massive systems serving multiple brain areas (Figure 1.1). For example, a drug may have its main effect by altering dopamine function in the frontal cortex, but the drug's simultaneous alteration of dopamine function in the caudate nucleus may explain the side effect of involuntary facial tics. Moreover, while the target for the main effect of a drug may be in the brain, the drug may also have effects on chemical processes outside the brain—in the peripheral nervous system. Some of these peripheral effects of the drug, when interpreted by the patient as undesirable, would be identified as side effects. Here are two examples of the effects of drugs on multiple sites in the brain and nervous system:

- Atomoxetine is a relatively newer drug useful for treating attention deficit hyperactivity disorder (ADHD). The ability of atomoxetine to improve symptoms of ADHD is understood to be due to the drug's ability to selectively enhance activity of norepinephrine in the brain. But the most common side effects reported in clinical trials include gastrointestinal distress and nausea, presumably at-

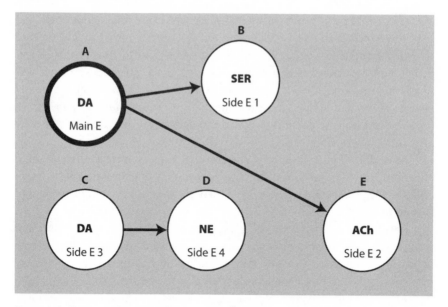

Figure 1.1. Diagram depicting (a) a hypothetical functional relation among four neurochemical systems served by the neurotransmitters dopamine (DA), norepinephrine
(NE), serotonin (SER), and acetylcholine (ACh) in the brain, and (b) the multiple
direct and indirect effects of an ingested medication that will have access to the entire brain. The five circles (A, B, C, D, and E) each represent a target site for one of
the identified endogenous neurochemicals, that is, a site in the brain that has synapses for one of these neurotransmitters. This schematic depicts a main effect and side
effects for a drug that is ingested with the goal of targeting a single site in the brain for
the purpose of obtaining a main effect. Site A for DA is the single intended target for
the psychotropic medication; drug-induced activation of DA receptors in site A
should produce a main effect (Main E): relief of symptoms of a psychopathology.
Secondary, indirect consequences of drug-induced activation of DA receptors in site
A will include the activation of SER synapses in site B, inducing a SER-mediated side
effect (Side E 1), and activation of ACh synapses in site E, inducing an ACh-mediated
side effect (Side E 2). This is due to direct neuroanatomical connections (arrows)
between sites A and B and between sites A and E. Ingestion of that same medication
will also activate DA receptors in target site C; the direct consequence of activating
site C will be a DA-mediated side effect (Side E 3). Secondary to drug-induced activation of site C will be indirect activation of NE synapses in site D, through a neuroanatomical connection between sites C and D (arrow), inducing an NE-mediated
side effect (Side E 4). Taken together, this scenario depicts the potential for a psychotropic medication that ideally would specifically target DA synapses in one DA receptor site in the brain to elicit one main effect for relief of symptoms and four side effects
mediated by the medication's combined direct effects upon DA synapses and indirect
effects upon NE, SER, and ACh synapses.

tributable to atomoxetine's effects outside of the brain in the peripheral autonomic nervous system.

- The antidepressant properties of fluoxetine—a drug that enhances serotonin transmission in the brain—may be primarily attributable to fluoxetine's effect on serotonin in the cortex and subcortical limbic system of the brain. But fluoxetine's ability to induce sedation may be due to its effect on serotonin in the brainstem.

Main effects or undesired side effects can also be attributed to the fact that many drugs directly alter chemical systems in the brain, and these direct alterations have secondary or indirect consequences in *other* chemical systems in the brain. For example, a drug may have its main effect (or a portion of its main effect) by altering dopamine function in the frontal cortex, and this alteration of dopamine function in turn may cause an alteration of serotonin function in frontal cortex that can explain a particular side effect or an additional portion of the drug's main effect (Figure 1.1).

In summary, there are a variety of explanations for why any drug would be expected to always have more than one effect on chemical processes in the brain. The expectation that a drug will always have more than one effect has important implications for patients and clinician having a realistic set of expectations for the success or failure of pharmacotherapy.

COMPROMISE ON BENEFITS AND RISKS IS A REALISTIC GOAL FOR PHARMACOTHERAPY

His symptoms of bipolar disorder are now mostly absent, but his fellow musicians know that Jon is not the same player that he was before he became ill. Jon also knows this to be true, and he knows why it is so. The use of chlorpromazine to treat his symptoms has not provided Jon a reasonable compromise between the drug's benefits and risks—surely the mood swings have been smoothed out, but one side effect that lingers is simply intolerable. The drug-induced tremor in his fingers has reduced this world-class performer on his stringed instrument to just another player. His fellow musicians hear the difference—the decline in prowess—but it affects them less than it troubles Jon. He cannot accept the fact. He has decided to no longer comply with instructions to continue his use of chlorpromazine. He would rather be manic or depressed than be second-rate.

If the expectations for successful drug therapy are to be realistic, those expectations must acknowledge the fact that each and every drug will bring, at best, positive and negative consequences. A realistic expectation, or a reasonable goal for drug therapy, should include meaningful benefit together with a degree of risk or discomfort that the patient, ideally, would be willing to accept as part of the cost for the benefit. In other words, the patient should know, at the point that drug therapy is initiated, that pharmacotherapy will be considered to be successful when the patient can say, "I am willing to tolerate this much discomfort in order to feel that much better."

A set of specific expectations for this benefit/risk compromise should be discussed and agreed upon by clinician and patient in advance of initiating drug therapy, including each time a new drug is introduced to the patient and each time there is a prescribed change in dosage. This dialogue is most useful when it requires the patient to identify the most troubling symptoms and prioritize among the most desired benefits of pharmacotherapy, and when it requires the clinician to enumerate the potential impact on symptoms, as well as the probable side effects. When both the patient and the clinician bring to the conversation their experiences, expertise, and expectations, the two parties will more likely reach mutual understanding toward a reasonable compromise set of goals (Tasman, Riba, & Silk, 2000). If it can be identified in advance, a compromise set of goals for therapy should facilitate the patient having at the outset of treatment the following prospects:

- A conservative degree of hopefulness for improvement
- A realistic expectation that improvement will be accompanied by some degree of discomfort
- A personal investment in the commitment to follow the prescribed regimen of pharmacotherapy
- A conscientious self-assessment of changes in symptoms and appearance of side effects
- A diminished expectation of a drug-induced miracle cure
- A willingness to engage in thoughtful consideration of using non-drug treatment in combination with drug therapy

The quality of a successful end point for pharmacotherapy is likely to vary for individual patients with the same diagnosis, and it could also differ within the same patient, depending upon that patient's history with the disorder and its treatment. The patient with a history of pharmacological treatment for the disorder can have the advantage of being able to draw upon personal experience to anticipate which side effects need to be avoided, which side effects can be tolerated, and which symptoms must be improved and to what degree.

Finally, when articulating a realistic set of expectations regarding successful pharmacotherapy as being a compromise between benefit and risk, it also should be clear to the patient that a complete remission of symptoms, or a more sustained duration of improvement, might be more likely when drug therapy is employed as one therapeutic tool among several. For example, the role of nondrug therapeutic approaches such as counseling, psychotherapy, establishing lifestyle changes, and so forth, may acquire greater value when the patient realistically faces the limitations of drug therapy alone.

DESIRED EFFECTS AND UNWANTED EFFECTS ARE RELATED TO DOSAGE

The insomnia that accompanies the lifting of his depression is tolerable during the summer but not during the school year—his teaching and coaching responsibilities require a good night's sleep, every night. So Robin has requested a smaller dose of fluoxetine to use during the school year, trusting that the smaller dose will not make sleeping difficult but still will have some ability to treat his depression. He is willing to risk having diminished relief of his depression as long as he can continue to have the energy he needs to get his work done. He loves working with the kids, and perhaps being with them will lift his mood enough to compensate for the smaller amount of assistance he'll be getting from the smaller amount of fluoxetine. That seems like a reasonable compromise—a risk he is willing to take.

Despite the somewhat inseparable relation between main effect and side effects, it is worth considering how to attempt to maximize the good while minimizing the bad consequences of drug therapy. Separating the impact of a drug upon main effect and side effects can be difficult to accomplish because, generally speaking, the magnitude of a main effect increases as dose increases, and side effects also increase as dose increases. But reasonable hope for separation of the influence of a drug on main and side effects can be found in the knowledge that *each effect of a drug can have a different dose-response relation.*

First consider the simple fact that any one effect of a drug can be described by an empirically determined dose-response relation (or curve). A dose-response relation describes the association between individual doses of a drug (ranging from small to large doses) and the magnitude of an effect. Usually, but not in all cases, larger doses produce greater magnitude effects. In addition, various characteristics of a dose-response curve can be different for each main effect and each side effect (Figure 1.2). For example, the threshold dose for an effect (i.e., the smallest dose that will have a measurable effect) may be different for the main effect and side effects (Figure 1.2). If the thresh-

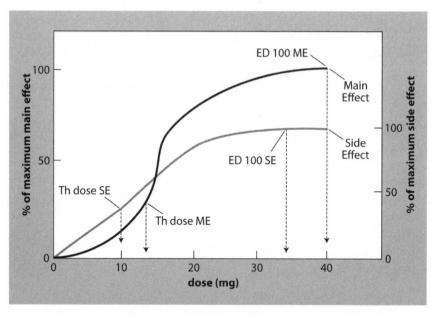

Figure 1.2. Dose-response curves for a main effect and a side effect for a single drug. The scenario is one in which the threshold dose for a side effect (Th dose SE) is smaller than the threshold dose for a main effect (Th dose ME); on average, 10 mg of the drug is the lowest dose capable of eliciting a side effect, while at least approximately 13 mg of the drug is necessary for eliciting the main effect. This situation predicts that a therapeutically effective low dose of the drug will inevitably produce a side effect. At the other end of each dose-response curve is depicted the dose that will produce a maximum magnitude of main effect (ED 100 ME), which is approximately 40 mg, and the maximum dose for achieving a maximum-size side effect (ED 100 SE), which is approximately 34 mg. This situation predicts that, although the drug will likely produce a side effect regardless of dosage used, the magnitude of the side effect will not increase above its maximum when the therapeutic dosage is raised from approximately 34 to 40 mg.

old dose for the main effect is smaller than the threshold dose for each of the side effects, then it is theoretically possible to use a low enough therapeutic dose of a drug that accomplishes some degree of the main effect and at the same time has minimal risk of side effects. On the other hand, if the threshold dose for the main effect is larger than the threshold dose for one or more potential side effects, then the likelihood of one or more side effects is substantial when the threshold dose for the main effect of that drug is administered (Figure 1.2). In that particular situation, one or several side effects are quite likely to occur coincident with any main effect (even for small doses). Here are two examples of dose-related main and side effects:

- Most people using imipramine for treatment of depression experience dry mouth as a side effect regardless of dosage. The fact that this side effect is virtually inescapable suggests that the threshold doses for the main effect and this particular side effect are likely to be similar.
- A more alarming example is provided by clozapine, one of the newer-generation antipsychotic drugs: For some individuals, the threshold dose for inducing a seizure is lower than the threshold dose for clozapine's ability to improve symptoms of schizophrenia!

A dose-response relation or curve(s) can also identify the doses that elicit the maximum main effect response and the maximum magnitude of each side effect (Figure 1.2). Doses between the threshold dose and the dose that elicits the maximum effect (whether for main or side effects) are also likely to be clinically meaningful doses. A complete knowledge of the effects of a variety of doses is important, especially if it is difficult to predict which dose (at which particular place on the dose-response curve) will be the most effective at eliciting the main effect for each individual patient. Unfortunately, it is difficult to successfully select the ideal dosage when initiating drug therapy— the ideal dosage being an amount and regimen of drug that elicits a maximal benefit while eliciting few, if any, intolerable adverse effects.

To determine such an ideal dosage at the time a prescription is first written would require having thorough knowledge of the dose-response relations for the main effect, as well as all potential side effects. Such detailed knowledge is almost never available, and even if it were, it still would be difficult to predict whether or not an individual patient would demonstrate the effects predicted from data obtained from studies in other people.

Given these uncertainties, the most practical way to initiate treatment is with a small dose. A small dose might run some risk of being below the threshold for a main effect, but it also has the advantage of sometimes being below several different threshold doses for various side effects. Gradually increasing the dose until some main effect is achieved permits an assessment of (a) whether or not the relief of symptoms caused by a small dose is sufficient, and if it is, (b) whether or not the side effects caused by that small dose are tolerable for that individual patient. This cautious approach amounts to a systematic trial-and-error methodology performed upon a client. As long as the trial-and-error approach begins at the low end of the range of clinically useful doses, it is a conservative approach that may help to select a dosage regimen that maximizes benefit while minimizing drug-induced side effects.

In contrast, the least conservative treatment approach would be to begin drug therapy with a dosage regimen reputed to elicit the maximal main effect.

The problem with this approach, intended to aggressively reduce symptoms of the disorder, is that the dosage likely to produce the maximal main effect is also more likely to maximize the potential for side effects (Figure 1.2). There are clinical situations in which that aggressive approach may be warranted (e.g., when suicidal ideation is one of the symptoms), but generally speaking, it is an approach that maximizes potential for harm while attempting to maximize helping.

DRUG INTERACTIONS CAN BE POTENT AND UNPREDICTABLE

> No one has asked Paul whether or not he smokes weed, and even if they do ask, he will lie and say "no." And although he was warned at some annoying and forgettable anti-drug forum to not combine the use of marijuana and alcohol—that the combination can produce extraordinary negative consequences on motor control—he does not realize that the alprazolam prescribed to treat his generalized anxiety symptoms will act in much the same way as alcohol when combined with marijuana.

The task of minimizing drug-induced risks is further complicated when a patient is being medicated with more than one drug. Even with complete knowledge of the current use of drugs by a patient, it can be difficult to predict the effect of a drug on the main effect and side effects. The magnitude and complexity of this problem increase in some proportion to the number of prescriptions being used by an individual patient, the patient's concurrent use of herbal remedies or dietary supplements, and the patient's use of drugs for recreational purposes.

On the other hand, some drug interactions can be expected based on knowledge of each of the drugs' mechanisms of action. For example, someone who has been prescribed a benzodiazepine drug to alleviate symptoms of anxiety would be advised to anticipate that the concurrent use of alcohol would very likely enhance both the main and side effects of the antianxiety agent. This is because the benzodiazepine drugs and ethanol share the ability to enhance activation of specific receptors for the endogenous neurotransmitter gamma-aminobutyric acid (GABA) in the brain. This sort of knowledge is readily available for some but not all drugs. Less readily available is knowledge regarding the potential for interaction between two drugs that do not share the same mechanism of action.

A major reason for the relative lack of information regarding drug-drug interactions is the fact that most clinical trials assessing a drug's effectiveness are structured in such a way as to avoid the possibility of drug interactions. For example, in many clinical drug evaluation trials, one explicit exclusion factor is likely to be the use of another drug(s) for clinical or recreational purposes; a candidate subject for a study can be excluded from the study when identified as using another drug. Therefore, when subjects using a drug that is not under direct examination in the current study are removed from clinical trials in the interest of having the study measure a "pure" effect of the one drug targeted by the study, then the ability to assess for the interaction of the study drug and another drug is eliminated. There can be no information collected on drug interaction in a study that by design removes the possibility of drug-drug interactions! In such a study, there has been a reasonable trade-off of information that can be collected: information about an interaction between drugs is lost at the expense of having a clinical trial in which the drug manipulation is well controlled, and the drug's effects can be measured and interpreted for only the drug that is the target of the study.

Being aware and wary about drug-drug interactions is of growing importance given the increasing trend to combine drugs to treat a disorder, in particular depression or schizophrenia (Mojtabai & Olfson, 2010). This increased use of psychotropic medication polypharmacy is particularly worrisome given the limited research demonstrating better therapeutic effectiveness of drug combinations, despite evidence for increased side effects of drug combinations (Mojtabai & Olfson, 2010).

SUMMARY AND PERSPECTIVE

A realistic goal for successful drug therapy is a compromise between the benefits and risks associated with a particular drug being given to an individual patient. This compromise is as good an outcome as can be expected given that all drugs will have more than one effect, and given that it is reasonable to expect that some number of side effects will accompany a main effect in all circumstances. This compromise is further complicated by the fact that the main effect and side effects can have different dose-response relations, which can make it difficult to select a therapeutic dosage that both is maximally effective and has the lowest risk. Moreover, the ability of prescribed drugs to interact with other drugs used therapeutically or recreationally further complicates the selection of drugs and their ideal dosages. These realities suggest the following tactics pertaining to the selection of drug and dosage:

- When possible, select a therapeutic drug with an identified mechanism of action. This should facilitate anticipating at least some of the potential for drug-drug interactions.
- When possible, select a drug based on published evidence for its effectiveness, along with published evidence for its potential for eliciting side effects. Selecting a drug with a known mechanism of action, and with a documented history of successful use, frequently favors the selection of a reputable older drug rather than a newer drug for which relatively less is known.
- Begin treatment using the smallest dose that, based on the published evidence and clinical experience, is likely to elicit a main effect.
- Consider the patient's use of all other pharmaceuticals, herbal remedies, dietary supplements, and recreational drugs in order to better anticipate potential for drug-drug interactions.
- Recognize that each time a dosage of a drug is prescribed, the exercise is essentially a test trial on a patient to determine whether or not the drug will be effective with that dosage. Regularly assess for effectiveness and tolerability, and change dosage or switch drugs when necessary.
- When a drug offers insufficient relief of symptoms, and it is not prudent to further increase the dose, and it is not realistic to switch to another drug, consider adding (or increasing) nondrug therapy to the treatment program.

In conclusion, these guidelines for judiciously selecting a drug and a dosage are also useful when choosing and using a drug in a research project or when using a drug recreationally. Using a drug recreationally can carry different risks (e.g., legal, moral, toxicity) than using a drug as therapy, but the fundamental principles of pharmacology discussed in this chapter are as meaningful and relevant for drugs used as therapy, drugs used for pleasure, and drugs used as tools for research.

THIS CHAPTER REDUCED TO A SENTENCE

A psychotropic medication at best can achieve a favorable balance between helping and harming; use the smallest dose possible, attempt to avoid the risks of polypharmacy, and, when appropriate, combine with nondrug treatment.

CHAPTER TWO

Each Patient Is a Unique Case
for Pharmacotherapy

Paul's anxiety is at times overwhelming. On some days he cannot overcome his fear of the terrible things that may happen if he is foolish enough to attempt to retrieve the mail from the mailbox located only 40 feet from the house. But if he acknowledges openly that he needs help—needs a therapist—well, that will be interpreted by his family as a sign of weakness. "Be a man!" his father will say. Paul has tried previously to evade that particular embarrassment by asking his physician to prescribe an antianxiety drug, but the imipramine ended up being more of a problem than a solution. Even a small dose of the drug effectively terminated his ability to have sex, which so stunned him that the suggestion of switching to a different medication seemed to offer only further potential for humiliation. He is now beginning to appreciate that his situation is complicated, perhaps too complicated for a quick, private remedy by medication. There is all this machismo in his immediate family, and they and he for many years have heavily used alcohol. Being told to curtail his drinking behavior has gone nowhere in the past, and stopping his drinking is not a change in lifestyle that he can embrace. His appetite for alcohol is as great as is his anxiety. And he cannot imagine telling his brothers and father that he will not be drinking with them.

Each individual patient presents a unique set of characteristics and circumstances to the prospect of using medication to treat a diagnosed psychopathology. This certainty, coupled with the knowledge that each psychoactive medication is a chemical substance that is foreign to the brain and body, brings into sharp focus the difficulty of making a judicious choice of an appropriate therapeutic drug for an individual patient: The task is not simply choosing a drug best suited to treat a named disorder. The task is to choose the best drug to fit the relatively unique situation of a particular patient who happens to fit the diagnostic criteria for a disorder. Taken seriously, that task is an *original* assignment for each and every individual facing treatment. Responsibly taking on that assignment requires consideration of individual differences or idiosyncrasies in physiology, history of drug use, habits, social circumstances, ethnicity, and cultural expectations or biases.

Some of the individual characteristics that must be considered are simply features of a person's anatomy and physiology, for example, age, sex, genetics, and functional capacity of organ systems. Other individual characteristics to consider are products or consequences of that individual's behavior over the years, for example, previous use of therapeutic or recreational drugs, and the person's habits and attitudes. Other characteristics important to the individual represent the impact that other people and organizations have upon that individual, for example, implementation of diagnostic criteria, one's ethnicity, expectations and biases held by family and community, and religious beliefs. All of these characteristics can in one way or another influence not only the decision of whether or not to accept a drug as therapy but also the degree of effectiveness that a therapeutic drug ultimately may have upon the person's malady.

SENSITIVITY TO A DRUG VARIES FROM ONE INDIVIDUAL TO ANOTHER

The magnitude of response to a drug will vary among people. Any study conducted to determine the dose-response relation between a range of doses of a drug and the magnitude of the drug's main effect will reveal for each dose a single data point representing the magnitude of the main effect for each individual in the group of human subjects in that study (Figure 2.1). The dose-response curve for the study will incorporate each of those individual data points to obtain the *average* magnitude of response for the entire group of people. Closer examination of the raw data for the study—a look at each of the responses for each of the individual subjects—will reveal that some people have a smaller than average response and some people have a larger than average response; this will be the case for each dose used in the study (Figure 2.1). In other words, for some people, the drug will appear to be less potent for

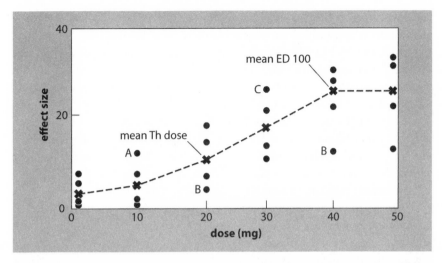

Figure 2.1. Hypothetical dose-response curve for a main effect for a drug administered to four human subjects. The raw data point for each subject for each of six doses is indicated by a black circle. The mean response for the group of four subjects is indicated by an x for each of six doses. The dashed line connects this average response for each dose, establishing the dose-response curve for the experiment. The average lowest dose that elicits a statistically significant increase (for the group of subjects) compared with the zero dose is the threshold dose (mean Th dose)—20 mg. The smallest average dose that elicits the average maximum attainable main effect (mean ED 100) is 40 mg. Note that subject A appears to be quite sensitive to the effect of the drug, showing the largest response to the subthreshold 10 mg dose; in fact, subject A's response to 10 mg is greater than the group's average response to 20 mg. Note that subject B appears to be the least sensitive to the effects of the drug; in fact, subject B is the least responsive of the group to the 20 and 40 mg doses, and the average threshold dose of 20 mg is apparently ineffective in this subject. Subject C appears to be the most sensitive to the effects of the drug, for example, showing the largest response to the 30 mg dose; in fact, subject C's response to 30 mg is slightly greater than the average group response to the mean ED 100 dose.

producing the main effect, and for other people the drug will seem to be more potent.

Recognizing the difference between the raw data for individual subjects and the average for a group of subjects reveals several important issues related to an individual's sensitivity to a drug's effects. Consider first the threshold dose determined from such a study. Assume that a threshold dose is identified from a study in a *group* of people as the smallest dose that produces a statistically significant increase of the main effect above the effect produced by a zero dose (i.e., above *baseline*). This threshold dose is actually the *average* smallest dose that produces a significant increase above baseline. Thus, some of the people in the study would have responded to a lower dose than this average smallest effective dose, and some other people in the study would not have responded to the average dose at all but would have responded to a dose slightly larger than the average threshold dose (Figure 2.1).

The results of such a study will also reveal the average dose able to elicit the maximum main effect in this group of people. For some of the people in the study, a dose smaller than this average maximally effective dose would be sufficient for producing a maximum effect; other people in the study would need a larger dose than the average maximally effective dose (Figure 2.1).

Thus, people will exhibit different sensitivities to a drug's effects (whether it is a main effect or a side effect). This fact makes it difficult to predict (from the results of a dose-response study reporting only *average* effective doses for a group of subjects) how an *individual patient* will respond to the doses used in the study. Moreover, these facts about individual differences can help to explain why a specific dose of a drug might elicit a particular side effect in one patient but not in another.

Does any of this consideration of data in dose-response studies lead to a guiding principle regarding the selection of proper dosage for an individual patient? Perhaps the most useful relevant tactic is the general advice to initiate drug therapy with a smaller dose than the average threshold dose. Beginning with a smaller dose is a more conservative approach and is reasonable because it assumes that there are some people who *will* benefit (main effect) or be bothered (side effects) by doses lower than the average threshold dose. This broad advice will not be useful, of course, in situations where a therapeutic response must be had as soon as possible, regardless of the risk of untoward effects.

SEX, AGE, AND GENETICS CAN DETERMINE THE MAGNITUDE OF EFFECTS OF A DRUG

"Take my worry pill, Mom. It's the same pill that he gave you a few years ago. Here, take mine—it will save you a trip to see the doctor."

Well, taking that 10 mg tablet twice a day, rather than the 2 mg dose that Mom's physician had prescribed for her 15 years ago when she was only 65 years old, ended up sending her to the doctor anyway, complaining of frightening dizzy spells. Fortunately, Mom is an experienced and avid complainer, and this situation gives her something interesting to do on Tuesday and talk to her friends about for the rest of the week.

Why are different people more or less sensitive to the effects of a drug? Why do women and men respond differently to the effects of some drugs? Why do the elderly respond differently to some drugs than do younger adults or children? How does one's genetics determine responsiveness to some drugs? Some of the answers to these questions can be found by considering the impact of a drug upon organs and organ systems in the body.

Ingestion of a drug presents an immediate challenge to a person's physiology. Organ systems in the body act upon the foreign substance in a variety of ways that essentially represent what are referred to as *pharmacokinetics*. The pharmacokinetics of a drug ultimately determines the magnitude of the impact that drug will have upon the drug's target site(s), where the drug produces its effect(s). Most drugs arrive at their ultimate target site as they are carried in the circulating blood. The amount of drug circulating in blood can be taken as a measure of the drug's *bioavailability*—the amount of drug available for having an impact on biological functions, both physiological and behavioral.

The bioavailability of a drug is determined not simply by the amount of drug injected or ingested, because the total administered amount of drug is not likely to reach the drug's ultimate target. Some fraction of the entire ingested amount will be degraded by activity of enzymes (e.g., in the stomach or liver). Some fraction will be removed from the blood (e.g., by the kidneys) and eliminated from the body through excretory processes. Some fraction may be sequestered (e.g., in fat or bound to protein) and therefore made not readily available. The degree to which an ingested drug is metabolized, excreted, or sequestered can vary from person to person, male to female, and young to elderly and as determined by genetics.

Let's take a look at the pharmacokinetics related to ingested alcohol as a case study to elucidate some of the issues. Drinking an alcoholic beverage immediately exposes the ingested alcohol to gastric alcohol dehydrogenase in the stomach. This enzyme metabolizes a fraction of the ingested alcohol, such that less alcohol appears in the circulating blood than if there had been no metabolism of alcohol in the stomach. The availability of gastric alcohol dehydrogenase is different for young adult men and women; on average, women have less of the enzyme in the stomach than do men (Frezza et al., 1990; Parlesak, Billinger, Bode, & Bode, 2002; Seitz et al., 1993). Thus, the capacity for the stomach to metabolize alcohol is lower for young adult women than for young adult men. This means that for the same amount of alcohol consumed, a greater proportion of the alcohol ingested will reach the blood of a young adult woman compared with a young adult man. In other words, the bioavailability of alcohol on average will be greater in the woman than in the man for the same dose of alcohol.

This difference in gastric alcohol dehydrogenase between women and men also is age related. Gastric alcohol dehydrogenase declines in men as they age, but apparently it does not decline as women age (Parlesak et al., 2002; Seitz et al., 1993). Therefore, generally speaking, for people over 55 years of age, men and women come to have similar amounts of gastric alcohol dehydrogenase. Thus, across ages spanning roughly 20 to 80 years, men, but not women, have diminishing capacity for metabolizing alcohol in the stomach. As men age, generally speaking, a decreasing amount of alcohol is required to achieve any of alcohol's effects.

These differences between men and women are primarily for Caucasians and may not be representative of the situation in non-Caucasian men and women. For example, there appear to be genetic or ethnic differences in gastric alcohol dehydrogenase activity: Japanese show lower gastric alcohol dehydrogenase activity than do Caucasians, but Japanese appear to have a greater capacity for metabolism of alcohol in the liver (Dohmen et al., 1996).

If these circumstances of gastric alcohol dehydrogenase and the pharmacokinetics of ingested alcohol can be considered to be exemplary, how do these facts represent what might be expected generally regarding the effects of other psychoactive drugs? What guideline principles are worth keeping in mind related to the broad issue of individual differences in pharmacokinetics?

- The bioavailability of an administered drug can be different for women and men.
- The bioavailability of a drug can depend upon the age of the patient.
- The magnitude of difference in bioavailability between women and men can depend upon age.
- The bioavailability of a drug can depend upon the ethnicity (and sex, and age) of the patient.
- Age, sex, and ethnicity should be taken into account when selecting a drug and when determining the dosage of psychoactive medication.

The pharmacokinetics of psychoactive drugs concern more than metabolism by enzymes. Pharmacokinetics pertinent to a drug can also include absorption, metabolism, rate of excretion, sequestration, and body weight, fat, and water content. Regarding these physiological processes and parameters, there are a variety of differences in pharmacokinetics between men and women (Beierle, Meibohm, & Derendorf, 1999; Yonkers, Kando, Cole, & Blumenthal, 1992), between young adults and the elderly (Hilmer, McLachlan, & Le Couteur, 2007; McLean & Le Couteur, 2004), and between different ethnic groups (Johnson, 1997; Lin, Anderson, & Poland, 1995). These various differences in pharmacokinetics undoubtedly have an impact on the effectiveness of psychoactive drugs, and therefore upon decisions regarding selection and proper use of psychotropic medication. When they are available regarding the pharmacokinetics of a specific psychotropic medication, published findings should be consulted when selecting a drug and determining a dosage regimen for an individual patient. Generally speaking, more will be known and published on the pharmacokinetics of older drugs compared with newer drugs.

The impact of age upon pharmacokinetics and upon a drug's effects (i.e., the drug's pharmacodynamics) deserves further attention, particularly as it concerns the use of psychotropic medications in the elderly. Psychotropic medications are an important component of care for the elderly, a large proportion of whom (a) are prescribed psychotropic drugs, (b) exhibit comorbidity for psychiatric and medical disorders, (c) are using more than one psychotropic medication, and (d) generally are highly vulnerable to adverse effects of a drug and combinations of medications (Lindsey, 2009). Thus, the use of pharmacotherapy in the elderly is characterized by several concerns (Aparasu, Mort, & Sitzman, 1998; Lindsey, 2009; McLean & Le Couteur, 2004):

- The aging person experiences numerous changes in pharmacokinetics (Hilmer et al., 2007) related to the body and to the brain, generally resulting in increased apparent sensitivity to the positive and the negative effects of psychotropic drugs. For example, elderly patients can be expected to show greater sensitivity to the effects of benzodiazepine anxiolytics, antipsychotics, antidepressants, and lithium (Trifiro & Spina, 2011); this generally predicts that lower doses will be more effective in the elderly than in younger adults. Despite the lack of published evidence that convincingly demonstrates the need for always using lower doses of psychotropic medications in the elderly, the use of lower doses appears to be the best choice (Le Couteur et al., 2004) based on demonstrated differences in pharmacokinetics.
- Relatively little research examines the effectiveness and side effects of psychotropic medications in the elderly, because elderly subjects are inadequately represented in clinical trials (Le Couteur et al., 2004).
- Many psychotropic drugs commonly used in younger adults are considered to be inappropriate for use in the elderly (e.g., diazepam, chlordiazepoxide, meprobamate, flurazepam, amitriptyline),

principally owing to the greater likelihood of untoward side effects in the elderly (Lindsey, 2009). Moreover, psychoactive medications—in particular, benzodiazepines and antipsychotics, but not antidepressants (Landi et al., 2005)—increase the likelihood of catastrophic falling in the elderly (Leipzig, Cumming, & Tinetti, 1999).

- There is evidence for neurochemical abnormalities in the aging human brain, for example, decreased neurochemical receptor numbers for the chemical transmitters dopamine, norepinephrine, serotonin, and acetylcholine (Meltzer, Becker, Price, & Moses-Kolko, 2003); this evidence alone is not helpful for establishing guidelines for determination of dosages of psychoactive medications in the elderly.

- Comorbidity of psychiatric conditions is relatively more common in the elderly, complicating the determination of a therapeutic regimen and increasing the likelihood of imprudent use of psychotropic polypharmacy (Aparasu et al., 1998).

- Many prescriptions for psychotropic drugs for the elderly are written without formal diagnosis of a psychiatric disorder (Aparasu et al., 1998).

One of these concerns for treating the elderly—the lack of published research from clinical trials supporting the effectiveness and safety of psychotropic medications in the elderly—presents an even greater problem for the use of psychotropic drugs in the treatment of children and adolescents. Despite this lack of published evidence, the trends of increasing use of psychotropic medications in children and adolescents (Jensen et al., 1999) raise serious concern for several reasons:

- Lack of research in children and adolescents creates uncertainty regarding how differences in pharmacokinetics related to the effects of psychoactive drugs in the young are to be compensated for when selecting drugs and dosages.

- Because the vast majority of approved psychotropic medications have been approved by the U.S. Food and Drug Administration (FDA) for use in adults (based on results of clinical trials in adults), the use of these drugs in children and adolescents constitutes off-label use (Novak & Allen, 2007), that is, use that is not evidence based.

- Based largely upon the success of off-label, trial-and-error use of psychotropic medications in children and adolescents, the trend for psychotropic polypharmacy in children and adolescents is increasing, including the combined use of medications for ADHD and antipsychotic drugs (Comer, Olfson, & Mojtabai, 2010), and the use of second-generation antipsychotic drugs to treat depression, bipolar disorder, anxiety, behavior disorders, and psychosis in children and adolescents (Aparasu & Bhatara, 2007; Olfson, Blanco, Liu, Moreno, & Laje, 2006a).

- Structural and functional development is occurring in the brains of children and adolescents. Exposing these immature brains to psychotropic medications may have consequences that alter the course of maturation of the brain. Using psychotropic medications in children and adolescents, especially when lacking published evidence supporting effectiveness and relative safety, is a gamble of significant proportion (Andersen, 2003; Andersen & Navalta, 2004). The difficult question facing the clinician and the family is, "Under what circumstances is that a gamble worth taking?"

In summary, it is no simple matter to consider and accommodate what is known and what remains unknown regarding individual differences in pharmacokinetics and pharmacodynamics in men versus women, young versus mature versus elderly, and Caucasian versus nonwhite patients when one is tasked with the problem of selecting an appropriate psychotropic medication and dosage regimen. But it is possible to contemplate several helpful steps for a course of action when treating children, adolescents, or the elderly:

- First consider whether nondrug options for therapy might be useful, especially when there is little published evidence to support the use of psychoactive drug therapy.
- When psychoactive drug therapy appears to be the most suitable option (either alone or as adjunctive therapy), attempt to choose a drug for which there is published evidence regarding its effectiveness and relative safety.
- Attempt to use the published literature from clinical trials to select a dosage regimen.
- Use the lowest effective doses possible for children, adolescents, and the elderly, and attempt to minimize the duration of drug therapy.
- Examine the published literature for information on the effects of ethnicity on pharmacokinetics or pharmacodynamics for a non-Caucasian patient.
- Communicate with the patient at the outset regarding the pa-

tient's views (and the family's views) on the use of psychotropic medication. Be willing to adjust the use of the drug to accommodate beliefs or biases that could lead to noncompliance for proper use of medication.

- Be vigilant regarding the use of other medications, psychoactive drugs, herbal remedies, and dietary supplements in an elderly patient.
- Be vigilant and actively probing regarding assessment of adverse effects in children, adolescents, and the elderly.
- Avoid polypharmacy if at all possible.
- Avoid using a drug to diminish a side effect induced by another drug.

A PERSON'S DRUG HISTORY CAN AFFECT A DRUG'S EFFECTIVENESS

The first time it happened, Charlie was frightened by the experience. But by now he has learned to sit back and enjoy it. It seems as if his history of prodigious use of LSD has set the stage for the flashbacks induced by marijuana. It's as if the memories of those acid-induced visual hallucinations are being summoned by simply smoking a little weed. Seems like a great bargain! He now needs only the marijuana, without the LSD, to get the hallucinations—two psychedelic experiences for the price of one. He does wonder, however, how those two drugs have changed his brain to enable this phenomenon to happen. He also worries about how else those drugs might have changed his brain, and whether those changes will spell more trouble for him down the road.

The task of selecting an appropriate dosage regimen must also take into account a person's history of use of drugs. Previous use of a drug can influence the effectiveness of that same drug or other drugs. This can be illustrated by exploring further the case of gastric alcohol dehydrogenase.

The availability of gastric alcohol dehydrogenase appears to be diminished by the chronic consumption of alcohol. There are two components to the evidence supporting this idea: (a) a correlation between increased consumption of alcohol and decreased metabolism of alcohol by gastric alcohol dehydrogenase in Caucasian men (Parlesak et al., 2002; Seitz et al., 1993) and women (Frezza et al., 1990) and (b) decreased gastric alcohol dehydrogenase activity in male alcoholics returning to normal following several weeks of abstinence from alcohol (Seitz et al., 1993). Thus, the chronic consumption of alcohol apparently reduces the capacity to metabolize ingested alcohol, which means that relatively more alcohol is able to reach the circulating blood in a person with a history of prodigious alcohol consumption. This means that the same volume of alcohol consumed will now have greater bioavailability (i.e., more will reach the circulating blood), which should lower the threshold dose of consumed alcohol for all of alcohol's physiological and behavioral effects, including its ability to contribute to development of addiction. This is a clear example of how previous use of a drug alters pharmacokinetics related to that drug in a manner that then alters the effectiveness of future use of the drug.

Here is another example of how previous use of alcohol can alter the pharmacokinetics related to that drug: Repeated ingestion of alcohol leads to development of tolerance to the acute effects of alcohol, such that it becomes necessary to ingest a larger dose of alcohol to achieve the same effect that a person was previously able to achieve with a smaller dose of alcohol. A physiological explanation for this tolerance is that chronic ingestion of alcohol increases the capacity of the liver's enzymes to metabolize ingested alcohol. The increased metabolism diminishes the bioavailability of the ingested alcohol, so more alcohol now needs to be ingested, to "overcome" the enhanced capacity for metabolism by the liver, to get the desired acute effect.

A related example, this one of past use of one drug altering the present effect of a second drug, is found in the phenomenon of cross-tolerance—the previous use of one drug producing apparent tolerance to a different drug. For example, a chronic user of alcohol will require a larger dose of a benzodiazepine drug (e.g., diazepam) to relieve anxiety than would a person who previously had used alcohol infrequently or never. This drug-induced tolerance to a drug that has never been used can have an important impact on choice of drug and its dosage for therapeutic purposes.

In summary, a patient's candid account of current and recent use of any medications or chemical supplements can provide information that is useful for determining a choice of psychotropic medication and its appropriate dosage. Such information should also be useful for advising patients regarding their continuing use of other chemicals once the new psychotropic medication is prescribed.

CULTURE AND COMMUNITY CAN AFFECT THE UTILITY OF PHARMACOTHERAPY

Julie knows that she is ill because the land is suffering. She and the land will have to get better together for her to feel well again. She also knows that her doctor, who practices "Western medicine," will want to make a formal diagnosis to label her, offer her a prescription medication for her disturbed mood, and probably recommend that she speak with a clinical psychologist. This worries Julie, because she is certain the drug will not make the land well—it will not fix the prolonged drought, and it will not fix other troubles in the lives of her extended family that weigh heavily upon her. And she knows that the clinical psychologist, who is located a 60-kilometer bus ride from her home village, is reputed to not be respectful of Aboriginal views on disturbed mood. The psychologist's tendency is to see people like Julie and others as having a diagnosable mental or emotional disorder. But Julie knows that the only way to understand and to deal with her situation is from the perspective that treatment will need to address the totality of her emotional and social well-being. A successful treatment will need to incorporate not only the connection between her illness and the drought but also the particulars of her place in her extended family and in her community.

Individual differences in physiology are not the only factors that can have an impact on the effectiveness of pharmacotherapy. A person's behaviors, whether normal or pathological, are not simply a product of underlying brain chemistry. Each individual behaves in a social context. Behaviors may be motivated toward achieving short-term or long-term goals in a person's local environment. Behaviors may be features of interactions between that person and others. A person's behavior may be influenced by the surprising actions of another person. And a person's behavior may be the product of the social and cultural context in which they were educated and in which they currently are attempting to fit.

This broader perspective holds that an individual's behavior at a single point in time is likely to have something to do with brain chemistry *and also* with experiences that occurred long ago, with goals that are immediate or far into the future, and with influences from the biases, beliefs, and expectations of other people. Likewise, the behaviors indicative of psychopathology also can be considered as not only products of brain processes and brain chemistry but also products of a personal history and a sociocultural context. This biopsychosocial perspective holds that the therapeutic effectiveness of a drug will depend upon more than that drug's pharmacokinetic and pharmacodynamic profiles—it will also be influenced by social and cultural factors.

The perspective that pathological behavior is partially attributable to social and cultural factors does not always sit comfortably with the practice of Western medicine (Adler, 2009; Alvarez et al., 2012), despite the influence of the biopsychosocial perspective (Gerard, 1957). The dominant perspective within Western medicine encourages a search for underlying organ dysfunction to explain symptoms—most likely dysfunctional brain chemical processes, when behavior is disordered. The most direct tactic for restoring normal functioning to dysfunctional brain chemistry is to pharmacologically manipulate the brain. This simplistic chemical model serves reasonably well because it supports a therapeutic approach that to some degree *can* be effective: Drug therapy alone can be a successful treatment in some situations. But a one-dimensional pharmacological approach, even when it appears to be effective, disregards two aspects of psychopathology: that some factors external to the person (a) are likely to contribute to that person's illness, can continue to be present despite successful drug therapy (e.g., a stressful relationship with a member of the family), and can contribute to relapse; and (b) may counteract efforts toward successful pharmacotherapy (e.g., a cultural bias against the use of drugs as therapy).

Let's take a look at a case in point that can serve to more vividly illustrate some of the issues raised above: the case of social and emotional well-being of Aboriginal and Torres Strait Islander Australians. Aboriginal Australian people know that they have come from the land and are one with the land. Their extended family and community on their home land have a history that is important to the present. Elders in the community ensure the memory of the past, and they expect to be respectfully consulted on important matters. Symbols offer important meanings. Spirits and animals convey important messages. It is understood that all of these aspects of society—land, people, animals, spirits—influence an individual's thinking, emotions, and behavior in meaningful ways. The acceptance of these various forces acting within the community presents difficulty for accepting the notion that an Aboriginal person showing signs of depression, anxiety, psychosis, or substance abuse has a mental illness. Conceptualizing these behavioral problems as reflecting mental illness suggests that there is principally something wrong with the mind—with that individual's thinking. This discomfort with the concept of mental illness has encouraged an alternative characterization: to see an individual's "mental illness" as instead a challenge to that individual's "social and emotional well-being" (Vicary & Westerman, 2004). The perspective that such behavioral signs as depression, anxiety, psychosis, and substance abuse are problems of social and emotional well-being emphasizes that the nature of the problem is that of *a person with a brain behaving in a social context*. This perspective encourages the selection of therapeutic treatment options that address social context and relationships primarily and brain chemistry secondarily. Moreover, this perspective may explain reluctance to use psychotropic medication as a treatment option.

Consider some characteristics about Aboriginal Australian culture and values that may diminish the value and potential effectiveness of drug therapy for psychopathology:

- There is a tendency to not seek professional help for behavioral problems (Isaacs, Pyett, Oakley-Browne, Gruis, & Waples-Crowe, 2010). The label of having a diagnosed psychiatric condition is perceived as identifying persons as candidates to be removed from their home community (Vicary & Westerman, 2004). This is due in part to the use of psychiatric diagnosis to facilitate removal of Aboriginal children from their parents during the period of the Stolen Generations (1930s–1960s) in Australia (Parker, 2010). In addition, an Aboriginal person removed from the community for treatment can return to the community seeming to be a "changed person." This perceived outcome can engender distrust of Western medical practices, contributing to nonadherence to prescribed medication regimen (Vicary & Westerman, 2004).
- Pharmacotherapy is viewed as being of lesser importance as a treatment option (Parker, 2010), diminishing the likelihood that a client will accept drug therapy.
- A pharmacist can play a key role in the Aboriginal community. The pharmacist's effectiveness is enhanced by knowledge of Aboriginal culture—a knowledge that earns respect within the community (Hamrosi, Taylor, & Aslani, 2006). Compliance with instructions for properly using medication is likely to increase with increased trust of the pharmacist.
- Active engagement in caring for the land is viewed as an important aspect of social and emotional well-being (Rigby, Rosen, Berry, & Hart, 2011). No psychotropic drugs are reputed to facilitate active engagement in caring for the land.
- The limited number of health workers of Aboriginal ethnicity weakens the impact that health workers can have in Indigenous communities, because non-Aboriginal health workers often lack credibility in those communities (Isaacs et al., 2010; Vicary & Westerman, 2004).
- Access to health workers can be severely limited for people living in rural areas. The increased effort required to see a practitioner or to consult a pharmacist can diminish the likelihood that drug therapy will be available and used effectively (Isaacs et al., 2010).
- Mainstream (i.e., Western) health care workers are more effective when they have been educated regarding Aboriginal culture. A culturally informed health care worker can better anticipate the

obstacles to successful pharmacotherapy (Isaacs et al., 2010). Moreover, the effectiveness of mainstream mental health professionals is enhanced if someone in the Aboriginal community can vouch for them (Vicary & Westerman, 2004). Again, the issue is trust; a solid reputation in the community engenders trust, increasing the likelihood of compliance to the recommended treatment.

- It is important for Aboriginal patients to be able to tell their full story to the health practitioner—it is important that they be heard (Nagel, Robinson, Condon, & Trauer, 2009). The significance of meaningful dialogue between client and practitioner suggests that conversation builds trust and that trust increases the likelihood of compliance and the client's confidence that drug therapy can be effective. In addition, an Aboriginal patient is likely to prefer no separation between the personal and the professional in a relationship with a clinician (Vicary & Westerman, 2004). A client who knows the therapist personally (not just professionally) will be more likely to trust the therapist and will likely be more amenable to considering therapeutic options.
- It is often the case that illness is attributed to sorcery (Chenhall & Senior, 2009). Could a belief in sorcery *increase* the likelihood that a drug potion would be a successful therapy?

It should be apparent from the issues outlined above that drug therapy is likely to be successful in an Aboriginal patient *only when* it is combined with counseling or psychotherapy in an approach that is mindful of the traditions, beliefs, and biases of the Aboriginal community.

If the context for considering the use of psychotropic medication for treating Aboriginal Australians is in some measure representative of the kinds of issues a clinician faces when treating a patient of other non-Western or non-Caucasian Western ethnicities, then there should be some apparent similarities between other ethnic groups and the case outlined above for Aboriginal Australian people. Here are some findings selected from published reports regarding Asian, African-American, and Hispanic ethnicities:

- The stigma of diagnosis appears to be greater for African-Americans than for Caucasian Americans (Givens, Katz, Bellamy, & Holmes, 2007). Worry over stigma can reduce likelihood of seeking treatment.
- African-Americans and Hispanics are less likely to be diagnosed with depression than are Caucasians (Sclar et al., 2012).

- African-Americans are more likely to be diagnosed with psychosis than are Caucasians (Baker & Bell, 1999; Rey, 2006), and those diagnosed African-Americans are more likely to be prescribed antipsychotic medication (Rey, 2006).
- Asians require lower doses of haloperidol for optimal relief of symptoms of schizophrenia than do Caucasians (Lin et al., 1989). This difference appears to be attributable to differences in the effectiveness of haloperidol and not to differences in the drug's access to target sites in the brain.
- Ethnicities differ regarding the effectiveness of placebo in double-blind clinical trials studying the effects of anxiolytic drugs, apparently revealing the significance of cultural processes (Moerman, 2000).
- There are differences among ethnic groups in the acceptability of treatments for depression (Comas-Diaz, 2012); for example, Caucasians report greater stigma associated with all treatment modalities than do African-Americans, and African-Americans report lesser willingness to accept prescription drugs but greater willingness to accept spiritual counseling (Givens et al., 2007). African-Americans and Hispanics report less acceptance for drug therapies than do Caucasians (Cooper et al., 2003).
- Reporting of use of drugs and side effects of drugs varies across ethnic groups, and is sensitive to the beliefs and expectations for that culture (Comas-Diaz, 2012; Rey, 2006). For example, Asian patients frequently combine herbal remedies with prescription medications (Comas-Diaz, 2012) but tend to report use of herbals or dietary supplements only upon being asked questions intended specifically to elicit such information (Lin & Cheung, 1999).
- Adherence to a prescribed drug regimen is to some extent determined by the beliefs and expectations of a culture (Diaz, Woods, & Rosenheck, 2005) and is also affected by the perceived diminished value of drug therapy versus counseling (Rey, 2006). Latinos appear to have difficulty waiting for the long-latency effects of drugs such as antidepressants, leading to failure to comply with the recommended medication regimen (Comas-Diaz, 2012).
- In Hispanic and Asian cultures, members of a patient's family can influence the patient's choice of therapy and compliance with psychotropic drug regimen (Rey, 2006).

In conclusion, ethnicity is a important factor for determining the likelihood of seeking help and obtaining a diagnosis, selection of a specific mode of treatment, adherence to the prescribed drug regimen, and reporting of adverse effects of medication. In addition, there are differences among ethnic groups in pharmacokinetics (Johnson, 1997; Lin et al., 1995) and pharmacodynamics (Lin et al., 1995) that can have an impact on the effectiveness of specific psychoactive drugs. Ideally these factors should be considered when selecting an appropriate psychoactive medication and a dosage regimen, but there is little published evidence to provide useful guidelines. Moreover, ethnically appropriate decisions about medication made for the young adult patient may not apply to the choice of drug and dosage for the elderly patient (Akincigil et al., 2012). Finally, while decisions regarding psychoactive medication for treating various ethnicities must be culturally appropriate (Chaudhry, Neelam, Duddu, & Husain, 2008), so also must the selection of method of psychotherapy (Tseng, 2004).

Here is a course of action of general applicability when considering psychotropic medication for non-Caucasian ethnicities:

- First attempt to understand the significance of the individual patient's relationship with family and community, in particular the beliefs and biases that could affect the choice and effectiveness of psychotropic medication.
- Next consider whether or not some form of counseling or psychotherapy will be required to enable pharmacotherapy to be effective, in particular to increase the likelihood of adherence to a drug regimen.
- Consult the published literature for any available information regarding selection of drug and dosage.
- When the published literature provides little or no guidance for treating a patient of a specific ethnicity, assume that the patient's sensitivity to a drug will likely be increased compared with Caucasians. Choose a lower dose to initiate pharmacotherapy than what would be recommended for a Caucasian, and increase the dose cautiously.
- Frequently inquire whether the patient is using the drug as prescribed, and ask specific questions regarding the use of herbal remedies or dietary supplements and regarding the appearance of side effects.

SUMMARY AND PERSPECTIVE

Various factors can influence an individual's response to a therapeutic drug, including physiology of organs, sex, age, a person's previous history of drug use, and the social and cultural context facing the individual. Altogether, this essentially means that each individual presents a unique case for considering therapeutic options and the proper role of psychotropic medication.

Guidelines for selection of appropriate drug and dosage are difficult to construct, because the majority of useful published information that comes from scientific inquiry is pertinent mainly to adult Caucasian subjects. Recognition of important differences in pharmacokinetics, pharmacodynamics, beliefs, biases, dietary habits, and expectations between Caucasian and other ethnicities begs for more research on these topics and for more clinical trials that use as subjects a greater number of people of color, including children, adolescents, and the elderly. The use of psychotropic medications in children, adolescents, and the elderly poses somewhat unique problems, because the still developing brains of children and adolescents and the more fragile bodies and brains of the elderly are more vulnerable to the deleterious effects of psychotropic drugs.

Finally, serious consideration of the significant role for community and culture in the enabling of the success (or failure) of pharmacotherapy is consistent with a biopsychosocial model of medical and psychiatric disorders. That model encourages the consideration of some combination of counseling or psychotherapy together with pharmacotherapy as being in the patient's best interests.

THIS CHAPTER REDUCED TO A SENTENCE

Consider each patient's age, sex, ethnicity, drug history, biases, and family and social context and the presence of comorbidity; use a drug that treats part of the unique biopsychosocial problem that the patient presents and, when appropriate, combine with nondrug treatment.

CHAPTER THREE

Drugs Can Change the Brain

Caleb did not want to hear that it could be two weeks before his mood was lifted by fluoxetine. He also did not want to hear that this anticipated delay means that he is strongly advised to engage immediately in psychotherapy. The psychotherapy will begin now rather than later because he has admitted to thoughts of suicide. He has agreed to meet with a therapist, but ultimately he wants to rely more upon the drug than the talk. Taking the drug would be a private matter, and he will not hazard the chance that someone might see him entering a shrink's office for psychotherapy. What will people think of him if they know he needs psychotherapy? On the other hand, his degree of comfort with drug therapy is challenged by his physician's view that the drug gradually will re-organize the chemistry of Caleb's brain, and that is why it will require weeks before the drug becomes effective for relieving his depression. Caleb worries about the implications of this. If the drug permanently relieves his depression by reorganizing the chemistry of his brain, does that mean that the drug is giving Caleb a different brain—making him a different person?

Drugs can have short-term and long-term effects on the brain and nervous system. The short-term, acute effects of a drug are observed to occur in seconds, minutes, or several hours after the administration of a drug. The long-term effects, appearing days, weeks, or months after initiating chronic administration of a drug, are no less meaningful than the acute effects, can be very powerful, and can sometimes be enduring. Drugs having *psychoactive* properties, evident in their ability to change behavior and psychological processes, can produce their effects in the short or long run. Thus, the acute and the long-term effects of a psychoactive drug can represent an immediate interaction between the exogenous chemical and endogenous chemical processes and a chronic-drug-induced reorganization of the brain's chemical processes, respectively. For example, the mild euphoria induced by a small dose of alcohol can occur while the first glass of wine is still being consumed. In contrast, the ability of chronic ingestion of alcohol to produce the behavioral and psychological characteristics of addiction is a long-term consequence of sustained use of alcohol.

THE BRAIN IS A CHEMICAL PLAYGROUND FOR AN INTRUDER DRUG

A drug enters the brain as an intruder bearing chemical properties. These properties provide a drug with opportunities to alter chemical processes in the brain in ways that cause changes in physiology and behavior. The chemical structures of some drugs permit those drugs to nearly mimic the effects of chemicals that are natural to the brain. Other drugs, unable to imitate, may enhance or may interfere with normal chemical processes in the brain. Drugs having psychoactive or psychotropic properties, whether they imitate, enhance, or interfere with normal brain chemical events, can alter psychological processes and behaviors. How do they do this?

Among all of the brain's biological properties and chemistry can be found a variety of targets for drugs of various kinds. Some drugs can alter physical properties of cells, some can alter properties of blood vessels, some can alter synthesis of chemicals in cells, and some can alter chemical interactions that are important for the transmission of information. The drugs that alter transmission of information likely have direct or indirect effects on chemical processes in synapses between neurons in the brain. The assumption is that most psychoactive drugs have their effects on behaviors and psychological processes by intervening in chemical processes in synapses. A reasonable working hypothesis is that synapses are somewhat specialized for transmitting information that is important for the brain's ability to organize physiological and behavioral functions. Let's briefly look at how the brain is equipped to do this, with a focus on how drugs alter specific chemical processes in synapses in the brain.

The brain can be conceptualized as a complex organ composed of many types of cells. Some of these cells—neurons—are specialized for communication: they have structures and properties that permit transmission of information. Neurons in the mammalian brain are in close proximity to one another. In fact, they nearly touch at the synapse—the gap between the sending end of one neuron and the receiving end of another neuron (see Figure 3.1). The sending end of a neuron, the *presynaptic* axon terminal, releases molecules of one or more chemical neurotransmitters into a synapse, where the neurotransmitter(s) interacts with chemical *postsynaptic* receptors on the neurons receiving the message. *The neurochemistry of the synapse is presumed to be the core target for most psychoactive drugs.* There are many demonstrations of psychoactive drugs directly or indirectly altering the neurochemistry of synapses, thereby producing changes in behaviors and psychological processes.

There are so many neurons, synapses, and neurochemicals in the brain that it is reasonable to view the brain as a rather tangled mess of billions of neurons, with trillions of synapses served by thousands of neurotransmitters (and other neurochemicals). But this apparently tangled mess of neurons in a chemical soup has levels of organization that are fairly well understood. This understanding comes from the study of the anatomy, physiology, and chemis-

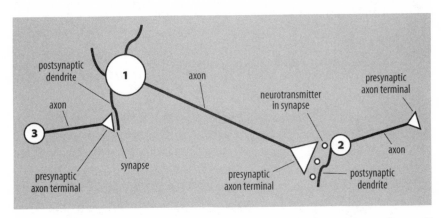

Figure 3.1. Schematic of a neuroanatomical relation among three neurons whose cell bodies are labeled 1, 2, and 3. Neuron 1 sends an axon, ending in a presynaptic axon terminal, to a synapse adjacent to a postsynaptic dendrite on neuron 2. The presynaptic axon terminal of neuron 1 releases neurotransmitter into the synapse between neuron 1 and the postsynaptic dendrite of neuron 2. In a similar manner, neuron 3 can release neurotransmitter into the synapse between the presynaptic axon terminal of neuron 3 and the postsynaptic dendrite of neuron 1. Now imagine that these three neurons are among the billions communicating with one another in the human brain, and imagine further that these three neurons are likely to also be communicating directly with many hundreds of other neurons that are not depicted in this drawing.

try of animal brains and human brains (e.g., Iversen et al., 2009) and can be summarized as having five elements:

- *Neurons are organized in systems.* Bundles of neurons run together from one destination to others in systems that are distinguishable (Figure 3.2). This organizational property of the brain is essentially the brain's *neuroanatomy.* In addition, the various places in the brain that are the origins and destinations of groups of neurons have identified functions. For example, it is possible to identify those neurons that take information from a specific site below the cortex to a specific site within the cortex that is known to receive visual information. This essentially describes one aspect of the brain's *functional neuroanatomy*—specific sites and systems of the brain have relatively specific functions.

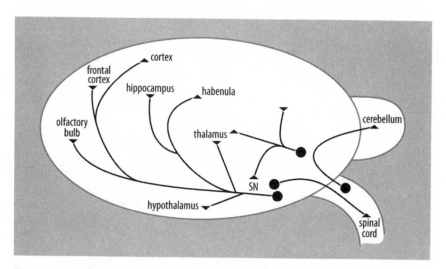

Figure 3.2. Diagram of a system in the brain served by a single neurotransmitter. This is a view from the left side of a brain, with the system of neurons depicted for only the left half (hemisphere) of the brain. The sites of cell bodies for neurons are identified by four black circles at the base of the brain and spinal cord. Emanating from these cell bodies are axons (curved black lines), some short and others very long, destined for different sites in the brain, in this case including hypothalamus, frontal cortex, hippocampus, thalamus, cerebellum, substantia nigra (SN), and others. At these various destinations, the axons end in axon terminals (black triangles), where neurotransmitter is released into synapses. In this drawing, the circles, lines, and triangles represent thousands of cell bodies, axons, and synapses for a single neurotransmitter system (e.g., serotonin) that is massive in its distribution within the brain.

- *The brain's neuroanatomy has a neurochemistry.* Neurons and groups of neurons synthesize and release specific chemical transmitters. These neurotransmitters can be found in particular regions within the brain (Figure 3.2) and can be identified as serving specific functions. Thus, the brain has a *functional neurochemistry*.
- *The functional neurochemistry uses chemicals to communicate in synapses.* The chemical transmission in synapses can be very complex: Numerous chemicals (e.g., neurotransmitters, neuromodulators) in a synapse can interact with numerous chemical receptors (Figure 3.3).
- *The locations and density of receptors for neurotransmitters can be identified in the brain.* This is important because it is assumed that receptors determine the functions of endogenous neurochemicals, and the availability of receptors can be altered by psychoactive drugs. In fact, receptors in synapses are considered to be the most significant targets for psychoactive medications.

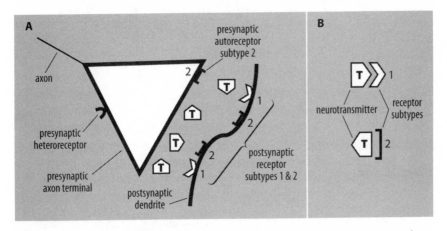

Figure 3.3. (A) Greater detail of Figure 3.1: an axon, presynaptic axon terminal, released neurotransmitter in a synapse, and a variety of receptors in various locations. The postsynaptic dendrite has two subtypes of receptors (labeled 1 and 2); each of which can bind to neurotransmitter T. The presynaptic axon terminal has one subtype 2 presynaptic autoreceptor (binding neurotransmitter T) and a presynaptic heteroreceptor (binding a different neurotransmitter). Imagine that the presynaptic subtype 2 autoreceptor, activated by neurotransmitter T, regulates synthesis of neurotransmitter T within the neuron. Also imagine that the presynaptic heteroreceptor, activated by a different released endogenous neurochemical (not depicted), functions to modulate the amount of neurotransmitter T released by the presynaptic axon terminal. (B) Visual representation of the capability for a single neurotransmitter to have a structure that can bind to and activate two different subtypes of receptors.

- *Groups of neurons using different neurotransmitters to communicate interact with one another* (Figure 3.4). For example, pharmacologically altering the functioning of neurons that use dopamine as a neurotransmitter in synapses can in turn alter the functioning of neurons that use serotonin as a neurotransmitter.

To summarize, the brain offers a variety of sites and interacting neurochemical systems. These systems communicate at synapses between neurons, where receptors interact with endogenous neurotransmitters. These neurotransmitter-receptor interactions function in the control of physiology and behavior and can be altered by drugs. Drug-induced alterations of synaptic

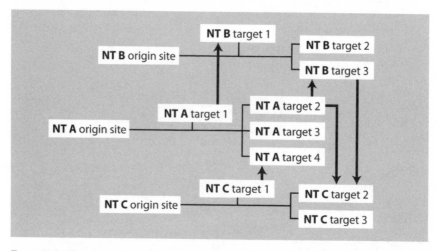

Figure 3.4. The manner in which three distinct neurotransmitter systems, such as the one depicted in Figure 3.2, can interact. The site of origin for each of the neurotransmitter systems (NT A, NT B, and NT C) is at the far left. Each system can affect multiple sites in the brain. For example, activation of the NT A origin site subsequently activates NT A targets 1, 2, 3, and 4. Note that activation of the NT A origin site, which then activates NT A target 1, can in turn directly (arrow) alter NT B target 1. Similarly, NT C target 1 can directly (arrow) alter NT A target 4. In short, three chemically distinct systems can interact to affect one another. For example, a psychotropic drug that affects the NT A origin site not only can directly affect NT A neurotransmission at multiple sites in brain but also can indirectly alter NT B and NT C neurotransmission at multiple sites. Each of these neurochemical systems (e.g., dopamine, serotonin, and norepinephrine) has a massive distribution in the brain (see Figure 3.2), and they can interact with other massive neurochemical systems in complex ways. So, if someone asks you, "Will a psychoactive drug that selectively activates a subtype of receptor for dopamine affect *only* dopamine neurotransmission?" you know the answer is "no."

processes can enhance, diminish, or prevent synaptic chemical transmission of information between neurons.

SOME DRUGS CAN IMITATE ENDOGENOUS NEUROCHEMICALS

The methadone that Connie uses daily seems as if it is producing part of the feeling that she gets when using heroin. There is some experience of euphoria from her methadone medication, but it is much less intense. There is enough pleasure there to encourage her to make the trip to the clinic to get her dose of methadone, and just enough pleasure in taking it to prevent her from seeking heroin. Her daily use of methadone appears to be taking the edge off of her former compulsive use of heroin, and she is thankful for that. She acknowledges that methadone's partial mimicry of heroin has probably saved her life.

The most direct way that a drug can intervene in the synaptic neurotransmitter-receptor interaction is when the exogenous drug essentially imitates or approximates what the endogenous neurotransmitter does at its receptors. This attempted mimicry usually requires some portion of the drug's chemical conformation to resemble or be functionally similar to that of the endogenous neurotransmitter. This similarity of drug and neurotransmitter permits the drug to effectively replace the activity of the neurotransmitter at the receptor. The ability of the drug to replace the activity of the neurotransmitter requires that the drug (a) be available at the synaptic site in sufficient quantity and (b) have sufficient affinity for the relevant receptors so as to win the competition between drug and neurotransmitter for access to the receptors. A drug that acts at the receptor in this manner is called an *agonist* for that receptor type.

A drug can be an agonist for one or several *subtypes* of receptors for a specific neurotransmitter. An endogenous neurotransmitter typically has the capacity to bind to and activate multiple subtypes of receptors for that neurotransmitter (see Figure 3.5A). For example, the endogenous neurotransmitter dopamine binds to each one of the subtypes of dopamine receptors, D1, D2, D3, and so on; the D1 *subtype* of receptor is a dopamine *type* of receptor. An agonist drug that binds to all identified subtypes of receptors for a single neurotransmitter would be said to be *nonselective* with regard to activating receptor subtypes for that neurotransmitter. In contrast, a drug that binds to only one of the numerous subtypes of receptors for that neurotransmitter would be a *selective agonist* for only that particular receptor subtype (Figure 3.5B). If a selective agonist drug fully replicates the effectiveness of the en-

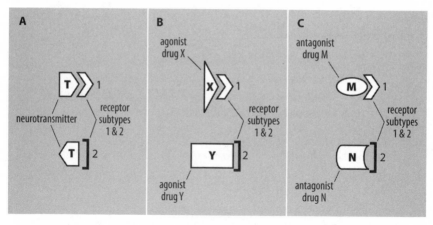

Figure 3.5. (A) The ability of neurotransmitter T to bind to and activate two subtypes (1 and 2) of receptors. (B) Pharmacological selectivity of two receptor agonist drugs. Agonist drug X is capable of binding to and activating receptor subtype 1, but not receptor subtype 2, for neurotransmitter T. In a complementary manner, agonist drug Y is capable of binding to and activating receptor subtype 2, but not receptor subtype 1, for neurotransmitter T. (C) Pharmacological selectivity of two receptor antagonist drugs. Antagonist drug M can selectively bind to receptor subtype 1 for neurotransmitter T, but is not a good enough chemical "fit" to activate the receptor, and does not bind to receptor subtype 2. In a complementary manner, antagonist drug N can selectively bind to receptor subtype 2 for neurotransmitter T, but does not activate the receptor, and does not bind to receptor subtype 1. When antagonist drug M binds to receptor subtype 1, the receptor is occupied, but not activated—this prevents neurotransmitter T from binding to and activating receptor subtype 1. The same can be said for the effect of antagonist drug N upon receptor subtype 2.

dogenous neurotransmitter at that receptor subtype, the selective agonist drug would be identified as a *full agonist*. If a selective agonist drug reproduces only a fraction of the effectiveness of the endogenous neurotransmitter at that receptor subtype, the selective agonist drug would be referred to as a *partial agonist*.

Selectivity of agonist drugs is a characteristic that is highly prized. It is reasonable to assume that the more selective an agonist drug is, the more selective it is for binding and activating *only one subtype* of receptor—the more likely it is that the drug will have a very focused desired effect and have relatively fewer undesired effects. Therefore, in theory, a highly selective agonist drug might produce a main effect with fewer side effects than a drug that was nonselective in its agonist activity. It is worth keeping in mind, however, that receptors for a single neurotransmitter are likely located in various sites in the brain (see Figure 3.2). Let's consider a hypothetical case relevant to these issues: It is possible that symptoms of some behavioral disorder are due princi-pally to a malfunction related to receptor subtype X located in brain region A. A receptor agonist drug that selectively activates receptor subtype X in brain region A may repair the neurochemical malfunction, thereby produc-ing the desired main effect on behavior. At the same time, however, the ago-nist drug very likely will have access to receptor subtype X in brain regions B and C, and by virtue of activating those receptors at those other two sites, the drug may produce undesired side effects (see Figure 1.1).

Here are examples of maladies for which psychotropic receptor agonist drugs have therapeutic utility or potential for treating:

- *Alcohol addiction.* Baclofen is a selective agonist for the B subtype of the GABA receptor. Baclofen has been investigated in clinical trials for its therapeutic potential for treating alcoholism and au-tism. Its utility for treatment of alcoholism is due to baclofen's re-ported ability to diminish craving for alcohol (Addolorato et al., 2002), presumably because baclofen activates the GABA-B sub-type of receptor (Ross & Peselow, 2009).

- *Opioid addiction.* Buprenorphine is characterized as a partial selec-tive agonist for mu-opioid receptors. It has been investigated in clinical trials for its therapeutic potential for treating addiction to opioid drugs such as heroin and prescription opioid analgesics. Bu-prenorphine's partial agonist activity apparently permits its ability to partially mimic the effect of a drug such as heroin. For example, when administered during abstinence from heroin, buprenorphine can mimic the effect of heroin sufficiently to forestall withdrawal symptoms and diminish craving, without mimicking heroin's abil-ity to induce intense euphoria. This mu-opioid receptor-mediated partial mimicry presumably establishes the therapeutic potential of buprenorphine for treating addiction for heroin and other drugs that activate mu-opioid receptors (O'Brien, 2005; Ross & Peselow, 2009).

- *Obesity.* Lorcaserin is a selective agonist for 5HT-2C subtype of serotonin receptor. It is one of the newer, FDA-approved pharma-cological options for reducing food intake and body weight (Heal, Gosden, & Smith, 2009).

- *Schizophrenia.* Aripiprazole is relatively new to the treatment of schizophrenia. Among the older- and newer-generation drugs having antipsychotic properties, aripiprazole is unique in having combined partial agonist properties for both dopamine D2 and serotonin 5HT-1A subtypes of receptors. Presumably this combined agonist activity diminishes the likelihood of drug-induced side effects related to movement disorders that emerge when using neuroleptic antipsychotic medications (Tamminga, 2009).

- *Anxiety.* Agomelatine potentially offers a novel approach for treating anxiety in patients who fail to respond to traditional anxiolytic medications (Levitan, Papelbaum, & Nardi, 2012). Agomelatine appears to be an agonist for MT1/MT2 melatonin receptor subtypes and also is able to block 5HT-1A receptors for serotonin, which presumably accounts for agomelatine's antidepressant properties.

- *Depression.* Vilazodone may present a novel approach for the treatment of major depression (Reinhold, Mandos, Lohoff, & Rickels, 2012). Vilazodone combines effects as an agonist for 5HT-1A serotonin receptors with inhibition of reuptake of serotonin.

Note that both aripiprazole and agomelatine described in this list have combined effects on two neurotransmitter systems, yet their effects are upon specific subtypes of receptors. Drugs with these kinds of combined properties are of particular interest for having the potential to maximize clinical effectiveness in a single drug by incorporating the clinically effective pharmacological properties of two different drugs.

The direct activation of receptors is not the only way in which a drug can activate or heighten activity of a neurotransmitter system. Drugs that enhance synthesis or release of a neurotransmitter, which may have therapeutic value (Langer, 2008), can be characterized as having agonist-like properties. In addition, drugs that inhibit the removal of a neurotransmitter from a synapse, thereby permitting the neurotransmitter released into the synapse to linger and have more prolonged effects on receptors, can be characterized as having agonist-like properties. One of the better-known examples of this latter category of drug is the group of antidepressant medications known as selective serotonin reuptake inhibitor (SSRI) drugs. SSRI drugs prevent the transport of released serotonin back into the axon terminal of the neuron that released it. This effect permits the released serotonin to linger in the synapse to have a prolonged effect on *all* available subtypes of serotonin receptors; this mechanism is presumably the means by which SSRI pharmacotherapy diminishes symptoms of depression (Berman, Kuczenski, McCracken, & London, 2009).

Here are examples of maladies for which drugs that inhibit reuptake of released neurotransmitters (i.e., inhibit presynaptic transport) have clinical utility:

- *Bulimia nervosa.* Fluoxetine, perhaps the best-known SSRI, is useful for improving symptoms of bulimia nervosa, although cognitive behavioral therapy is generally considered to be the treatment of choice for bulimia (Kaye, Strober, & Jimerson, 2009).
- *Attention deficit hyperactivity disorder (ADHD).* Atomoxetine selectively inhibits the reuptake of norepinephrine and is perhaps the best-known nonstimulant medication for treatment of ADHD.
- *Anxiety.* Venlafaxine is an inhibitor of reuptake of both serotonin and norepinephrine (SNRI). It is approved for treatment of generalized anxiety disorder, panic disorder, and social anxiety disorder (Mathew, Hoffman, & Charney, 2009).
- *Obesity.* Tesofensine is being developed as a drug for suppression of appetite and reduction of body weight. It appears to inhibit the reuptake of serotonin, norepinephrine, and dopamine (Heal et al., 2009).

In summary, the imitation of endogenous neurotransmitter effects on receptors, or the drug-induced enhancement of endogenous neurotransmission, can have clinical utility for the treatment of a variety of behavioral and psychological disorders.

OTHER DRUGS CAN BLOCK EFFECTS OF ENDOGENOUS NEUROCHEMICALS

When David takes his naltrexone in the morning, injecting heroin in the afternoon does not induce the rush that he expects. It is obvious to David that the naltrexone blocks that effect of heroin. That kind of day represents a great waste of the time and expense that it costs David to obtain his heroin. This places him squarely in a dilemma: "Do I take my naltrexone today or not? No, not if I expect to use heroin."

Just as some psychotropic drugs can bind to and activate receptors for endogenous neurotransmitters, other drugs can bind to receptors but not activate them. Such drugs are identified as *receptor antagonist* drugs. A receptor antagonist drug can be more or less selective for different subtypes of receptors for a neurotransmitter (Figure 3.5C). Selectivity of an antagonist drug for one (or few) subtype of receptor is a highly prized characteristic. As described above for receptor agonist drugs, the assumption is that the more selective an antagonist drug is for one subtype of receptor, the more likely it is that the drug will have a very focused desired effect and relatively fewer undesired effects. Therefore, in theory, a highly selective antagonist drug might produce a main effect with fewer side effects than a drug that is nonselective in its antagonist activity. But just as an agonist drug can simultaneously bind to and activate receptors in multiple sites in the brain, an antagonist drug can also simultaneously block receptors at multiple sites in the brain. This lack of site specificity, regarding the locations in the brain of an antagonist drug's effects, increases the likelihood that the drug may have undesired side effects.

Here are examples of maladies for which receptor antagonist drugs have therapeutic utility or potential:

- *Schizophrenia*. Chlorpromazine is perhaps the first receptor antagonist drug to demonstrate its utility as a psychotropic clinical tool (Jacobsen, 1986). Chlorpromazine can improve symptoms of schizophrenia. The presumed mechanism of action for this effect is its ability to block the D2 dopamine receptor subtype (Lehmann & Ban, 1997). D2 receptors that have already bound to chlorpromazine cannot bind endogenous dopamine; this prevents them from being activated. Although chlorpromazine is not highly selective for only binding to D2 dopamine receptors, other drugs (e.g., haloperidol) with antipsychotic properties also have the ability to act as D2 receptor antagonists.

- *Alcohol addiction*. Naltrexone is a receptor antagonist with a fairly wide spectrum of antagonist activity upon three subtypes of receptors for endogenous opioids. Some or all of the receptor-mediated (blockade) effects are presumably the mechanism by which naltrexone has its clinical effect of reducing the craving for alcohol. This naltrexone-induced reduction can diminish the likelihood of relapse of alcoholism (Ross & Peselow, 2009).

- *Obesity*. Rimonabant, a selective CB1 cannabinoid receptor antagonist, can inhibit eating and produce weight loss, but its development for the treatment of obesity has stalled owing to concern about psychiatric side effects (Heal et al., 2009). Rimonabant also has shown potential for prevention of relapse for addiction to cocaine or nicotine (O'Brien, 2005; Ross & Peselow, 2009).

- *Depression*. Ketamine is a selective antagonist for the N-methyl-D-aspartate (NMDA) receptor for the neurotransmitter glutamate. Ketamine has been studied for its potential utility for the treatment of major depression and bipolar disorder, especially in patients who are less responsive to traditional antidepressant medications

(Machado-Vieira, Ibrahim, Henter, & Zarate, 2012; Mathew, Manji, & Charney, 2008; Owen, 2012).

Drug-induced blockade of receptors for endogenous neurotransmitters can have clinical utility in the treatment of various behavioral and psychological disorders. The use of some receptor antagonist drugs has revealed the extraordinary potency and potential for harm that can attend the chronic use of some drugs. For example, the vintage antipsychotic dopamine D2 receptor antagonist drugs (chlorpromazine and haloperidol) can induce tardive dyskinesia—a long-lasting involuntary movement disorder that reflects drug-induced changes in brain neurochemistry and behavior that persist despite discontinuation of the medication. Fortunately, tardive dyskinesia usually can be avoided with the use of newer-generation antipsychotic medications (Casey, 2004).

PHARMACOLOGICAL EFFECTS ON BRAIN NEUROCHEMISTRY CAN BE ENDURING

Brian had never craved anything but the occasional piece of chocolate—usually within one hour after eating a meal. But this new feeling is different. He is experiencing more than simply "wanting" something—he really is obsessed with the thought of getting his nose on some cocaine. He cannot stop thinking about wanting it; the craving is intense and it lingers. The craving does not stop until he is able to use the drug. What perplexes him the most about this new aspect of his life is that he has never before so intensely desired a drug despite his occasional use of a variety of recreational drugs. But he now craves cocaine, and the craving began after no more than 10 episodes of using it. Whatever cocaine has done to him has changed his life dramatically.

A drug repeatedly introduced into the neurochemical workings of the brain has entered into a dynamic system that can react to the acute effects of the drug and also adapt to the chronic presentation of a potent exogenous pharmacological agent. Chronic administration of a drug can produce *neuroadaptations* in the brain—changes in the functional neurochemistry of the brain. These neuroadaptations represent a reorganization of neuronal communication serving physiological, behavioral, and psychological processes. Some of these drug-induced changes appear to provide the mechanism for the therapeutic effects of some drugs. And some of these neuroadaptations explain the appearance of drug-induced side effects.

One of the earliest examples of apparent drug-induced neuroadaptation associated with behavioral consequences is the appearance of tardive dyskinesia following a regimen of treatment with neuroleptic antipsychotic drugs in some schizophrenics. The involuntary movements of tongue, lips, jaw, and face can appear some weeks or months following initiation of neuroleptic therapy—apparently not an acute effect of the drug but, rather, a consequence of sustained exposure of the brain to the drug. Even more surprising is the paradoxical fact that the drug-induced symptoms of tardive dyskinesia can be diminished by increasing the dose of the very drug responsible for inducing the symptoms. Moreover, termination of neuroleptic drug therapy is followed by persistence of the tardive dyskinesia. What does it mean that a therapeutic-drug-induced movement disorder can persist long after use of the therapeutic drug is discontinued? The most reasonable explanation, requiring no stretch of the imagination, is that the chronic neuroleptic drug-induced blockade of D2 receptors for dopamine induces a long-lasting or permanent reorganization of brain neurochemistry, with the consequence that the altered brain produces bizarre movements of the tongue, lips, jaw, and face. Some research using animal models supports the hypothesis that the permanent change may be due to a neuroleptic-drug-induced increase in the number of D2 dopamine receptors in the brain (Casey, 2000, 2004).

Drug-induced changes in brain neurochemistry can take multiple forms (Iversen et al., 2009). One example is that chronic exposure of receptors in synapses to agonist drugs can induce *downregulation* of receptors. Downregulation of receptors is a reduction in number and/or density of receptors in synapses that have experienced excessive exposure to neurotransmitter or to drug. Downregulation can be conceptualized as an adaptation to this overstimulation: When a postsynaptic neuron faces overstimulation at its receptors, one way to adapt would be to reduce (e.g., by inhibiting synthesis) the number of receptors being exposed. The neuroadaptation of receptor downregulation can explain development of tolerance to some drugs (Meyer & Quenzer, 2013).

The *upregulation* of receptors is an increase in the number and/or density of receptors in response to the lack of their being activated. Upregulation can be conceptualized as an adaptation to understimulation: When a postsynaptic neuron faces lack of activation of its receptors, one way to adapt would be to increase the number of receptors (e.g., by increasing synthesis), thereby increasing the potential for receptors being activated by whatever limited amount of neurotransmitter is available in the synapse. The neuroadaptation of receptor upregulation can explain the development of hypersensitivity or supersensitivity to some drugs (Meyer & Quenzer, 2013).

Other neuroadaptations to chronic exposure to drugs include decrease (or destruction) of presynaptic transport resulting in decreased reuptake of released synaptic neurotransmitter, decrease or increase in synthesis of neurotransmitter, and decrease or increase in enzymatic degradation of neurotransmitter. Some of these neuroadaptations in the functional neurochemistry of the brain are likely to explain behavioral phenomena characteristic of addiction (Zahm, 2010). For example, drug-induced downregulation of dopamine receptors may establish the psychological phenomenon of craving (Volkow et al., 2006b).

Here are some clinically relevant examples of neuroadaptations in response to psychotropic drugs:

- Downregulation of the beta-adrenergic subtype of norepinephrine receptor is hypothesized to explain the effects of some antidepressant medications, specifically drugs that inhibit reuptake of norepinephrine. The time course of such downregulation in animal models of depression may explain the delayed latency for therapeutic response to antidepressant medication in humans (Dunlop, Garlow, & Nemeroff, 2009).

- Chronic stimulation by the pharmacologically active constituent of marijuana, delta-9-tetrahydrocannabinol, elicits downregulation and desensitization of the CB1 cannabinol receptor subtype (Sim-Selley, 2003); these effects occur with a time course consistent with the development of tolerance.

- Chronic stimulation by cocaine in animals induces downregulation of D2 dopamine receptors; this receptor neuroadaptation persists during abstinence from cocaine, and the rate of recovery of receptor number is related to previous duration of exposure to stimulation by cocaine (Seger, 2010).

- MDMA (3,4-methylenedioxymethamphetamine or "ecstasy") stimulation in animals and humans induces downregulation of 5HT-2A receptors for serotonin. Repeated administration of large doses of MDMA appears to have neurotoxic effects on serotonin neurons in animals (Seger, 2010).

- Ingestion of alcohol can induce long-lasting sensitization to the effects of the locomotor stimulant properties of alcohol in animals. This alcohol-induced sensitization is a neuroadaptation apparently mediated by D1 receptors for dopamine (Camarini, Marcourakis, Teodorov, Yonamine, & Calil, 2011).

- Chronic exposure of adolescent rats to methylphenidate, the most frequently prescribed stimulant medication for ADHD, produces a variety of neural and behavioral adaptations that endure into adulthood, including hyperactivity of dopamine neurotransmission (Marco et al., 2011).

In summary, psychotropic drugs used therapeutically or recreationally are capable of producing long-lasting changes in behavior and in the brain that endure beyond the cessation of use of a drug. These drug-induced changes in behavior are readily observable and quantifiable, but the changes in the brain are much more difficult to detect and measure in humans. Current research focuses on understanding the functional relation between enduring psychotropic-drug-induced neuroadaptations in the brain and concurrent changes in behavior. Much of this work explores these issues for drugs of addiction and abuse (Luscher & Malenka, 2011; Russo et al., 2010; Seger, 2010).

DRUGS DIFFER IN THEIR POTENTIAL FOR ADDICTION

Roscoe loves the small town, neighborhood bar nightlife. He enjoys seeing his friends, watches ball games on the televisions above the bar, and engages in the banter about pretty much any topic. And he also enjoys the drinking and the smoking, despite the bother of needing to light up on the quiet downtown street outside the bar. He is at his favorite spot every night, nearly without fail. That means he is consuming alcohol and nicotine every day. Roscoe does have self-control. He avoids becoming intoxicated, and he consumes what he considers to be moderate amounts of drinks and cigarettes. But gradually some things have changed. He can go days without consuming alcohol and not much notice that he has been abstaining. At the same time, he cannot abstain from smoking—every 20 minutes he seems to need a cigarette. It is clear to Roscoe that he is addicted to nicotine, but perhaps not addicted to alcohol.

The development of addiction to a drug essentially requires initiation of drug use followed by regular and sustained use. The use of a therapeutic or a recreational drug having addictive potential will result in addiction or dependence as determined by the factors that characterize addiction as a biopsychosocial problem:

- The genetic and physiological characteristics of the user that establish the person's physiological and psychological vulnerability to addiction
- The frequency of use of the addictive drug
- The size of the doses used of the addictive drug
- The addictive potential of the drug being used

- The magnitude of the reinforcing effects of the drug that define the individual user's appetite, drug-seeking behaviors, and consumption
- The social context in which the drug user is living: the availability of the drug and associates who either facilitate or discourage use

Considering the six features listed above, a person's behavior can maximize the likelihood of drug addiction or dependence when the user chooses a drug having maximum potential for addiction, uses large doses of that drug as frequently as possible, lives in a social environment that facilitates getting access to that drug and encourages recreational drug use, and caves in to all appetitive thoughts and emotions that encourage the user to seek out and use the drug. On the other hand, if one chooses to use a potentially addictive drug (for therapeutic or recreational purposes) but wants to minimize the likelihood of drug addiction or dependence, the user should choose friends and a social context in which to live that discourage recreational drug use and make it difficult to obtain addictive drugs, choose a drug that has relatively low potential for addiction, use small doses of that drug as infrequently as possible, and exert some self-control when one feels the urge to use the drug. How do these issues apply to the use of psychotropic medications?

- The genetic and physiological characteristics of the user contribute to the person's vulnerability to addiction, but the patient is using the therapeutic drug in a context in which the principal expectation is the relief of symptoms and not the induction of euphoria. The context in which an addictive drug is used is an important determinant of continuing use in humans and animals (Badiani & Robinson, 2004; Caprioli et al., 2009), and use that is *not* motivated by the reinforcing properties of drug-induced euphoria is less likely to lead to addiction (Goldstein, 2001).
- The frequency of use and the magnitude of the doses used of the potentially addictive therapeutic drug are decided by the prescribing professional, and appropriate use depends upon the patient's willingness to adhere to the recommended drug regimen. A drug regimen that minimizes the dose, frequency, and duration of use of an addictive substance is in the best interests of the patient.
- The relative addictive potential of the drug being used can be approximately known by the prescribing professional and the patient.
- The magnitude of the reinforcing effects of the drug that determine the individual user's appetite, drug-seeking behaviors, and

consumption are relevant to therapeutic use, but the medical context of proper use (i.e., absent drug-induced euphoria) is likely to diminish the reinforcing effects of the prescribed drug and therefore not encourage use beyond its therapeutic utility (Goldstein, 2001).

- The social context in which the drug user is living, and the availability of the drug and associates who facilitate or discourage use, can support the patient's adhering to the prescribed therapeutic drug regimen.

How does a clinician or a patient know whether or not a drug has lower, medium, or higher potential for addiction? Information on incidence of addiction to specific drugs, estimates of number of failed attempts to abstain from using an addictive drug, and data for frequency of relapse of addiction following a period of abstinence together help estimate the addictive potential of drugs used recreationally and drugs used therapeutically. Drugs having addictive potential can be grouped into three *loosely defined* categories of lower, medium, and higher potential for addiction (based on Nutt, King, Phillips, and Independent Scientific Committee on Drugs, 2010):

- Higher potential for addiction: crack cocaine, heroin, methamphetamine, nicotine, oxycodone
- Medium potential for addiction: alcohol, amphetamine, barbiturates, benzodiazepines, cannabis, ketamine, buprenorphine, mephedrone, methadone
- Lower potential for addiction: caffeine, ecstasy, khat, LSD, mushrooms, steroids, antidepressants, antipsychotics

What is useful about such a grouping of drugs according to estimated magnitude of addictive potential? When all other factors related to addiction are equal (e.g., social context, doses, frequency of use, or genetic vulnerability), use of a drug with a higher potential for addiction is more likely to result in development of addiction than is use of a drug with a lower potential for addiction. Thus, if a person desires a lifetime relationship with a drug, that person should regularly use a drug with a higher addiction potential, such as nicotine, oxycodone, or methamphetamine. If a clinician recommends that the use of the potent analgesic oxycodone is in the best interests of a patient, then the patient should be strongly advised to use that drug in a prescribed manner that attempts to minimize the likelihood of addiction, and the patient's use should be monitored to ensure the patient is using the smallest effective doses as infrequently as possible. This advice is pertinent both to addictive drugs used as therapeutic tools and to addictive drugs used recreationally.

An assessment of the addictive potential of a psychoactive therapeutic drug, and of the vulnerability of the patient to addiction, should be taken into account when choosing the therapeutic drug and when determining a dosage regimen. The addictive drugs used as psychotropic medication fall into the "medium potential for addiction" and "lower potential for addiction" groups; one exception is oxycodone, as well as other clinically useful potent opioid analgesics having high addictive potential. Generally speaking, the addictive potential of psychotropic medications is not sufficient to curtail their therapeutic use, but it is sufficient to encourage vigilance.

Watchfulness regarding the use of an addictive therapeutic or recreational drug is important for two reasons. First, use of addictive drugs produces long-lasting neuroadaptations of the adult brain that can lead to compulsive drug use (Zahm, 2010). Second, use of addictive drugs by children or adolescents, whose brains are still developing, presents even greater risk of permanent changes in the brain and in behavior (Andersen & Navalta, 2004).

DRUGS CAN ALTER THE ORGANIZATION
OF A DEVELOPING BRAIN

Tony and Tyler are identical twins, and they were inseparable growing up. They played the same sports, they each succeeded academically, they enjoyed fishing and hunting together, and they even dated a few of the same girls! One difference—at the time not known to either of their parents—is the fact that Tony experimented with marijuana and alcohol while in high school, but Tyler did not. And only Tony is an alcoholic today. Tyler drinks socially, but he does not have a problem. Why only Tony? Is it a mere coincidence that he was the only one of the twins who exposed his brain at a fairly early age to recreational drugs? Or did that early exposure make the difference? Was Tony's high school experimentation with alcohol and marijuana an investment in his later becoming an alcoholic?

Some psychoactive drugs have the potential for reorganizing the functional neurochemistry of an adult brain. And some psychoactive drugs have the potential for altering the normal course of development of a brain that has not yet reached adult maturity. The developing brain is in the process of acquiring its fully mature adult functional neuroanatomy and neurochemistry. Pharma-cological interference with the normal course of development of the brain should cause alarm.

The cause for worry about this issue has increased in recent years with the increasing use of psychoactive drugs to treat psychopathology in children and adolescents (Andersen & Navalta, 2004; Olfson et al., 2002), including the increasing incidence of psychotropic polypharmacy in children and ado-lescents (Comer et al., 2010). Part of the rationale for treating children or adolescents with a drug that has been used successfully to treat adults is that, if the drug is demonstrated in clinical trials to show therapeutic benefit with acceptable risks in *adults*, then it is likely that the drug will have similar ben-efits and similar acceptable risks in *children and adolescents*. That is a bet—it is not a conclusion based on scientific evidence that supports the clinical use of that drug in children or adolescents.

It is possible to obtain evidence in clinical trials in children and adoles-cents to evaluate the effectiveness and relative safety of a drug, although clinical research in children obviously does present special ethical concerns, difficulties for constructing a scientifically sound clinical trial (Dubovsky & Dubovsky, 2007), and difficulties for measuring the effects of psychotropic drugs on the brain (Singh & Chang, 2012). But the degree of difficulty should not provide the excuse for not conducting the clinical studies necessary for acquiring information pertinent for *evidence-based* use of pharmacotherapy applied to the developing brains of children.

So what is known about the long-term effects of psychotropic drugs on the brains of children and adolescents? Not much (Singh & Chang, 2012), but there are some important facts worth keeping in mind when considering the use of psychotropic medications for children and adolescents:

- Most of the use of psychotropic medication in children and adoles-cents is off-label use (Bazzano, Mangione-Smith, Schonlau, Sut-torp, & Brook, 2009). This represents the use of a drug that has been approved by the FDA for one purpose (e.g., depression) or one population (e.g., adults) for a different purpose (e.g., anxiety) or in a different population (e.g., children), based largely upon the results of clinical trials in adults and upon clinical experience. At the point of approval for use in adults, there is little likelihood that anything would be known about the effects of such drugs on the brains of children or adolescents. The psychotropic drugs most fre-quently prescribed off-label to children and adolescents are stimu-lants and antidepressants (Andersen and Navalta, 2004; Olfson et al., 2002).

- The use of neuroimaging techniques to measure effects on the brains of children and adolescents receiving psychotropic medication for depression, anorexia nervosa, schizophrenia, autism, obsessive-compulsive disorder (OCD), ADHD, or bipolar disorder generally reveal *limited preliminary* findings consistent with the notion that pharmacotherapy can "normalize" some of the structural anomalies of the brain in children with these disorders (Singh & Chang, 2012). Further research is needed to determine the long-term effects of psychotropic medication on the brains of children and adolescents.

- Although there is very little information regarding the nature of long-lasting changes in the human brain for adolescents who engage in recreational use of alcohol (Spear, 2011), there is evidence consistent with the notion that use of alcohol during adolescence increases the likelihood of alcoholism in adulthood (Odgers et al., 2008). Moreover, ethanol and benzodiazepine drugs share the ability to enhance GABA neurotransmission, raising the possibility that benzodiazepines used therapeutically in children or adolescents have the potential to produce long-lasting changes in the brain that could contribute to behavioral or psychological abnormalities in adulthood.

Despite the scarcity of evidence that psychotropic drug use early in life produces long-term changes in the human brain, research findings in animals convincingly demonstrate long-term neuroadaptations elicited by psychotropic drugs, including these examples:

- Antipsychotic or stimulant drugs administered early in life to animals can have delayed effects on the maturation of structure and function of brain that are not apparent until adulthood (Andersen & Navalta, 2004).

- The SSRI fluoxetine administered chronically elicits opposite effects on serotonin neurotransmission (Bouet et al., 2012; Klomp et al., 2012) and behavior (Bouet et al., 2012) in adolescent versus adult rats. This kind of finding challenges the assumption that a psychotropic drug will affect the brain of a child in the same manner as it affects the brain of an adult.

- Methylphenidate administered chronically during adolescence has enduring effects on dopamine neurotransmission and behaviors that are evident in adult rats (Adriani, Zoratto, & Laviola, 2011; Marco et al., 2011).

- Nicotine administered chronically during adolescence (but not administration of nicotine during adulthood) increases expression of subunits of the acetylcholine receptor and increases the motivation for self-administration of nicotine in adult rats (Adriani et al., 2003). These findings demonstrate that early-life exposure of the brain to nicotine may alter maturation of brain neurochemistry in a manner that increases vulnerability to nicotine's addictive properties in adult animals, fueling speculation that something similar can happen in humans.
- Research in animals has not yet produced convincing evidence identifying the specific neuroadaptations to early-life exposure to various psychoactive drugs, or whether these drug-induced changes increase vulnerability to addiction (or to other psychiatric disorders) in adulthood. But the findings do indicate generally that adolescent animals are more sensitive than adults to the reward properties of psychoactive drugs, are less sensitive to withdrawal effects for addictive drugs, and experience structural and functional changes in areas of brain known to be involved in the rewarding characteristics of addictive drugs (Schramm-Sapyta et al., 2009).

The use of psychotropic medications in children and adolescents having diagnosed psychopathology is warranted currently as long as there is evidence that failure to treat children and adolescents would not be in their best interests. Ideally, treatments would involve the combined use of psychotherapy and pharmacotherapy that are *supported by the results of clinical trials in children and adolescents* (Wagner & Pliszka, 2009). This is not yet possible. Therefore, the current state of the art is to treat children and adolescents with approaches largely based on the results from clinical trials in adults, which leads to the off-label use of psychotropic medications in children and adolescents. Recognizing that mental health professionals have grown increasingly reliant upon the use of psychotropic medications despite these limitations, clinicians should proceed with caution and should urge that the necessary research be conducted, and parents should consider whether nondrug therapy might be in the better interests of their child.

SUMMARY AND PERSPECTIVE

Psychoactive drugs have short-term and long-term effects on brain neurochemistry. Drugs can enhance, inhibit, or prevent neurochemical transmission of information among neurons in the brain. The working assumption is that most psychoactive drugs produce their effects by altering the interaction of endogenous neurotransmitters and receptors in synapses. Some of the alterations of brain neurochemistry and synaptic neurotransmission are of short or long duration and are reversible, but other alterations may be enduring or permanent neuroadaptations, including some alterations in neurochemistry that accompany therapeutic success, and some neuroadaptations that accompany the development of addiction. These powerful effects of drugs on the human brain are evident in adults, and perhaps too frequently are present in children and adolescents who are increasingly exposed to therapeutic drugs and to recreational drugs during important periods of development of brain and nervous system.

THIS CHAPTER REDUCED TO A SENTENCE

A psychotropic medication will heighten or diminish the functional neurochemistry of the brain; use caution when it appears necessary to prescribe a drug for the developing brain of child or adolescent, and take precautions when prescribing a drug having addictive potential.

CHAPTER FOUR

Pharmacotherapy Should Be Evidence Based

Wally's therapist is disappointed, but not terribly surprised. The published clinical trials show that the drug can be effective in roughly two-thirds of subjects treated, and that the drug is more effective than placebo. It seems that Wally is among the one-third of patients who might be expected not to respond to the drug. So the psychiatrist will recommend an off-label prescription, based on anecdotal reports and his own clinical experience regarding a different drug's effectiveness for treating obsessive-compulsive disorder. If they are lucky, the off-label prescription will be effective. It probably will not matter to Wally that the therapist cannot tell him *why* the drug is effective, because the drug's mechanism of action is not known. If it works, it works—that will be enough to know. But she will do more than write the prescription. She will again attempt to convince Wally to consider that psychotherapy might be the better option for him. And she will need to prepare him for the possibility of further pharmacological disappointment.

A model therapeutic regimen might employ a drug as an adjunct to a method of psychotherapy. The medication and the psychotherapy together would be expected to improve symptoms, ultimately leading to full remission. The selection of the therapeutic drug, and the selection of the particular method of psychotherapy, would be based on published evidence from clinical trials demonstrating that each therapeutic option should be effective and relatively safe, and that combined drug and talk therapy should be more effective than either drug or talk alone. The patient would show a positive response to a small dose of the drug and would report that its side effects were tolerable. The patient-therapist relationship would be supportive and effective for enabling a shorter duration of drug therapy. The patient would be told the mechanism of action of the drug and would have full confidence that the drug was changing brain chemistry in a healthful manner. The behavioral strategies that the patient learned during psychotherapy would facilitate remaining free of symptoms for several years after discontinuing the drug therapy.

That scenario is a pleasant fantasy. A more realistic scenario is the following. A patient is prescribed a drug as an adjunct to a method of psychotherapy, both of which have been selected based on published results of clinical trials. The patient rejects the option of psychotherapy as being too time-consuming and too expensive. The drug regimen offers relief of symptoms, but one of the side effects is so troublesome that the patient becomes ambivalent about complying with the prescribed drug regimen and, after two months, demands a switch to some other drug. Although the first-line drug is somewhat effective, the drug's mechanism of action is unknown, making it impossible to select an alternative drug having a similar pharmacological profile. The therapist will make an educated guess when recommending an alternative drug, perhaps prescribing something off-label, and hope that a dose of good luck also would intervene. Annoyed by the therapist's apparent diminishing confidence, the patient also loses confidence and is now considering replacing the prescription drug with an herbal remedy that his mother swears by.

Each and every patient presents as a unique case, shaped by that individual's personal history, current circumstances, genetic and physiological characteristics, biases, attitudes, and expectations regarding the likelihood that a treatment program will be effective. Each and every psychotropic medication presents a unique chemical configuration and pharmacological profile, with a reputation based on common knowledge among prescribers along with more or less support from the results of clinical trials that encourage use without guarantee of success for any individual. But if each and every case is unique, and if each and every drug is an educated gamble, then how can a therapist expect to know what to recommend with confidence as therapy? How helpful is the published literature of clinical studies?

DRUGS CAN BE DEMONSTRATED TO BE ONLY RELATIVELY EFFECTIVE AND SAFE

Gert's mood is already so low owing to her depression that she does not need to hear the additional bad news that she is the rare patient who does not improve in response to fluoxetine. That is just another depressing piece of news coming on top of the fact that the drug does manage to make her mouth dry, does make her feel drowsy and anxious, but still does not lift her depressed mood. From her vantage point, the drug does have effects on her, but the only effects are negative. This whole business of pharmacotherapy appears to Gert to be a bit of a fraud, and she holds little hope for her own situation. She has read several of the published clinical trials evaluating the effectiveness of fluoxetine for treating major depression. The studies report the drug is effective, so what is the problem?

A carefully planned clinical trial is constructed to collect data useful for evaluating the effectiveness and relative safety of a drug for treatment of a particular disorder. Before a clinical trial is conducted in humans, information already has been collected regarding relative safety in preclinical experiments in animals and in humans. Thus, by the time a clinical trial is conducted in humans, there is some knowledge regarding the relative safety of the drug being studied. There is also likely to be preliminary information regarding the drug's effectiveness (a) in humans who have been given the medication as an experimental drug, and (b) in experiments using animal models for a particular human disorder. Therefore, the clinical trial is not a shot in the dark taking a chance that something good might come of it. It is an experiment constructed to ask a realistic specific question.

As any experiment, a clinical trial has its strengths and its limitations (Dubovsky & Dubovsky, 2007; McGrath, 2012; Shorter, 2011). The strengths of a clinical trial evaluating the effectiveness of a drug are those of a well-constructed and well-controlled experiment using humans as subjects:

- The independent variable of interest is selected or manipulated in a way that is precise; for example, a specific dosage of a specific drug is selected, and the clinical trial is limited to the use of that single dosage and drug.
- The effectiveness of a drug treatment is assessed by comparison with a control treatment; for example, one group of subjects receives the drug for some length of time, and a second group of subjects receives a placebo control treatment for the same length of time.
- The subjects used in the study are carefully selected for having the

disorder of interest; for example, the only people permitted in the study are determined to have the disorder based exclusively upon criteria in the *Diagnostic and Statistical Manual of Mental Disorders*. Ideally, subjects are randomly assigned to the various treatment conditions.

- The subjects used in the study diagnosed to have the targeted disorder usually have no other clinically defined psychopathology; people showing comorbidity usually are excluded from a study.
- The study will have a fairly short duration, rarely more than six months. Because the study is an experiment and not clinical treatment, ethical concerns arise if subjects with a disorder are not being helped by the experimental drug or placebo control treatment, especially if the study has a long duration.
- The dependent variables of interest are measured in a predetermined manner and typically include measures of the hallmark characteristics of the disorder of interest and an assessment of adverse effects.
- An objective assessment of the collected data is conducted using statistical analysis to determine whether or not the effects measured are of sufficient magnitude to be scientifically meaningful.

Thus, the strengths of the experimental clinical trial essentially are control of variables of interest, elimination of variables that would make interpretations difficult (e.g., comorbidity, use of other drugs), and quantitative assessment of outcomes. The control of variables serves to focus the experimental investigation so that it is a meaningful assessment of a *specific* question. It is this specificity of focus that lends the experimental clinical trial some inevitable shortcomings that are relevant to the eventual clinical utility of a drug:

- The limited selection of a single dosage does not allow generalization regarding the predicted effects of other dosages of the same drug.
- The limited duration of the study does not permit predictions concerning the ability of the drug to be effective in the long term or to be effective for maintenance therapy, and it usually precludes assessment of whether or not drug-induced improvement endures once drug therapy has ended.
- The elimination of subjects from the study who show comorbidity produces results that do not allow predictions regarding the drug's effectiveness in patients having comorbidities (which are likely to be fairly common).
- A demonstration that a drug has a statistically significant main

effect does not necessarily predict that the effect of the drug in a clinical setting will be *clinically* significant, that is, that the drug will meaningfully improve the quality of a patient's life. In addition, the demonstration of a statistically significant main effect of a drug for a group of subjects in a clinical trial does not mean that the drug is effective in 100% of the subjects in the trial; this fact predicts that the drug used in a clinical setting is not likely to be effective in *all* patients. Moreover, the results of a clinical trial cannot predict the magnitude of the drug's main effect in a clinical setting for an individual patient and cannot predict the identity and magnitude of side effects.

• The assessment of main effects in a clinical trial usually takes precedence over an assessment of side effects. Therefore, as difficult as it may be to predict whether or not an individual patient will improve in response to a drug therapy, it is even more difficult to predict with confidence the likelihood that an individual will experience specific side effects.

The clinical drug trial is perhaps the most important, necessary element in the collection of information to establish *evidence-based* use of psychotropic medications. Although the results of a clinical trial cannot predict effectiveness of the drug in any particular individual patient, the information gained from carefully conducted clinical trials serves as a guide for making a judicious choice of drug and dosage when formulating a therapeutic regimen.

Clinical trials are expensive to conduct. These expenses are largely carried by federal government grant support and by the pharmaceutical industry. The FDA requires that a drug manufacturer demonstrate through the use of clinical trials that a new drug is effective and relatively safe and that the drug's benefit outweighs the risks (Deyo, 2004). There is no requirement that a new drug be more effective than all older drugs to treat the same disorder. Thus, it is important for therapists and patients to keep in mind that newer drugs are not necessarily better drugs.

A THERAPEUTIC DRUG IS USED BECAUSE IT WORKS

Doris knows that her physician is disappointed that Doris has no interest in hearing the story of the unsolved mystery of lithium's therapeutic effect on the brain. She has experienced so much misery from her bipolar disorder and its history of remission and recurrence for these past 12 years that the details of why lithium might be helping her are of little interest. Lithium helps her. That is enough for Doris to know. "Show me the lithium!" Doris likes to say.

A patient mainly seeks help, and usually does not pursue detailed answers to questions about the oh-so-fascinating minutiae of psychopharmacology. The first priority for an effective psychotropic medication is that it be effective in relieving symptoms while producing side effects that are tolerable. Whether the drug is a selective agonist or an antagonist for a receptor subtype for a specific neurotransmitter, or whether the drug inhibits presynaptic transport for another neurotransmitter, is interesting but not essential information for patient or therapist. There are numerous examples of therapeutic options that are effective despite lack of sufficient understanding regarding the treatment's mechanism of action:

- Lithium carbonate, despite its potential for toxicity, has been used for decades to successfully treat mania and bipolar disorder. Lithium's mechanism of action remains unknown (Freeman, Wiegand, & Gelenberg, 2009).
- Bupropion has antidepressant properties and effects on multiple neurotransmitter systems, including inhibition of presynaptic transport for norepinephrine and dopamine and antagonism of nicotinic receptors for acetylcholine. But the precise mechanism by which buproprion relieves symptoms of depression is unclear (Clayton & Gillespie, 2009).
- Electroconvulsive shock therapy (ECT) remains a treatment of choice for major depression for patients who are resistant to drug and talk therapy. The mechanism of action for ECT's apparent antidepressant properties is unknown (McDonald, Meeks, McCall, & Zorumski, 2009).
- Psychotherapy can be effective for treatment of a variety of disorders, but the effects on brain produced by various methods of psychotherapy are only beginning to be studied.

Claiming to know the mechanism of action by which a drug relieves symptoms of a diagnosable disorder engenders a sense of intellectual security that can be misleading. To recognize this, consider the usual facts that lead to the claim of knowledge of a psychotropic medication's therapeutic mechanism of action. Begin with the fact that drug A relieves symptoms of a specific behavioral dysfunction in many of the patients treated with the drug. The second relevant fact is that drug A is measured to block receptors for neurotransmitter M in research conducted using animals as subjects. It is too easy to reach the seemingly logical conclusion that drug A relieves symptoms of that specific behavioral dysfunction by virtue of blocking receptors for neurotransmitter M. That conclusion is a speculation. It is a reasonable hypothesis—it is nice, simple, and neat. But the evidence supporting the hypothesis is weak. One reason it is weak is that the logic assumes that what the drug does in the animal brain predicts exactly and completely what the drug does to the neurochemistry of the human brain. This assumption does not always hold. A second reason that the supporting evidence for the hypothesis is weak is that it is possible that, although drug A does block receptors for neurotransmitter M, drug A also has other known and unknown effects on brain neurochemistry; it may be one or another of these effects, or some combination of these effects, that represents the mechanism of action for drug A's ability to improve symptoms of that specific disorder.

Despite the fact that many claims for a hypothetical mechanism of action are weak or imperfect, such a hypothesis does have its utility. For example, having a hypothetical mechanism of action permits the speculation that a behavioral dysfunction is caused by an abnormality in neurotransmitter M or in a receptor subtype for neurotransmitter M. This speculation is a comfortable one for many working within the Western medical model, in which one looks for specific organ dysfunction as a cause of symptoms. This speculation becomes an intellectual problem if one then assumes that the *only* thing wrong with a person exhibiting the specific behavioral dysfunction is a problem *only* with neurotransmitter M and a subtype of M's receptors. That conclusion is inconsistent with a biopsychosocial perspective. Reaching this imperfect conclusion can be useful, however, in encouraging a search for new, safer drugs that alter receptors for neurotransmitter M that might relieve symptoms of the behavioral dysfunction. This situation targets the development of new drugs for altering neurotransmitter M as an efficient way to discover new psychotropic medications.

In summary, it is not necessary, but it can be useful, to know the mechanism of action by which a therapeutic drug relieves symptoms. It can facilitate the development of new therapeutic drugs, and it can offer comfort to patients to be told that their disorder may have an identified underlying cause (however much a stretch of the imagination that requires).

DIETARY SUPPLEMENTS MAY OR MAY NOT BE EFFECTIVE AND SAFE

His cousin told Mike that when he becomes anxious or depressed he should just find the nearest health supplements store, walk the aisles, and be amazed that he will find on the shelves a cure for just about everything. The prices will be right, and no prescriptions will be needed. No need to see a physician or a psychologist. Just take a stroll and select an herbal remedy or a dietary supplement, and give it a try. Mike's intuition tells him that this sounds a bit too simple, too easy—things that come easily and inexpensively are often available and cheap because they are next to worthless.

As difficult as it is to predict for an individual patient whether or not an FDA-approved prescription drug will relieve symptoms with relatively little risk, it is even more difficult to predict whether or not a chemical marketed as a dietary supplement or herbal remedy will have positive or negative consequences. Drugs, some of which have psychoactive properties, are chemicals. Dietary supplements and herbal remedies, some of which have psychoactive properties, contain chemicals. The key distinction between chemicals sold as drugs and chemicals sold as supplements or herbals in the United States is that the FDA is responsible for regulating the availability of drugs but has no authority for regulating the dietary supplement industry.

This distinction contributes to several realities. The consumer can expect that a drug purchased by prescription, or over the counter, is a chemical that has been investigated in clinical trials to assess for its effectiveness and safety. Although such a drug may not be effective for each and every person who uses it, and may produce troublesome side effects in some users, that drug *has been examined* in experiments that produce data that address the issues of effectiveness and safety. In contrast, it is judicious to assume that no data from comparable scientific inquiry address the issues of effectiveness and safety for chemicals in a dietary supplement or herbal remedy. It would not be surprising, and it would not be illegal, if a dietary supplement sold for real money were found to be really ineffective. Moreover, it would not be surprising to find that a dietary supplement is labeled as having psychoactive properties when in fact its chemicals are without biological activity. This lack of assurance regarding the utility and safety of dietary supplements, or of herbal remedies, does not deter people from using them, and there are cultural differences regarding their perceived value and their use (Comas-Diaz, 2012). Clinicians should be vigilant regarding whether or not a patient is using a dietary supplement or an herbal remedy, because some supplements combined with prescription medications can produce serious adverse effects.

Perhaps the best advice to consider regarding the use of chemicals in dietary supplements, food additives, or herbal remedies is the following:

- A person who is troubled enough by symptoms of an emotional or cognitive disorder that they are considering self-medicating with a dietary supplement or herbal remedy should first consult with a physician or psychologist. Attempting to self-medicate using a dietary supplement that eventually proves to be of no help merely delays the initiation of perhaps more effective treatment with evidence-based pharmacotherapy or psychotherapy. Delaying effective treatment may be investing in a worsening condition that is more difficult to treat.
- A person who is using a dietary supplement should be prompted to be forthright when asked what other chemical treatments that person is using. It is important to indicate the use of a dietary supplement or herbal product in the event that its use has the potential to contribute to drug-drug interactions when that person begins using a prescription medication.
- A person using a dietary supplement, whether or not the supplement has been recommended by a therapist or physician, should be advised that there may be little or no scientific evidence supporting the supplement's effectiveness or safety.
- A person using a dietary supplement or an herbal remedy should be warned that there are few safeguards in place to assure the consumer that the supplement purchased does in fact have biological activity or psychoactive properties.

Despite these legitimate worries about the effectiveness and safety of chemicals sold as dietary supplements, there can be advantages for using a dietary supplement *if* the supplement is in fact effective and relatively safe: A dietary supplement is likely to be readily available without the need for a prescription, and without visits to a health professional. These facts can contribute to reduced cost of using dietary supplements and herbals compared with prescription medications. In addition to the advantage of reduced cost, some clients may find a dietary supplement or herbal remedy to be a more acceptable alternative than a prescription drug (although that perspective may not represent the reality of the situation). Viewing the use of a dietary supplement or herbal remedy as using a "more natural" treatment is a perspective that may support adherence to the recommended use of the substance. Finally, even a pharmacologically inert dietary supplement (i.e., one that has no biological activity) could conceivably have some therapeutic benefit owing to a placebo effect. If the person believes the supplement will improve symptoms, that belief may be sufficient to result in some benefit from taking the supplement.

PLACEBO CAN HAVE DRUG-LIKE EFFECTS

Tom feels certain that his symptoms of depression have improved, so he is a bit surprised to learn that he had been assigned to the "placebo group" in the clinical trial for a new antidepressant drug. One reason for his surprise is that Tom is dead certain that he was experiencing drug-induced side effects during the four months of the clinical trial. He wonders how a placebo could make him feel better and also have him believing that he was experiencing side effects.

A placebo has no pharmacological properties, but a *placebo does not do nothing* (Harris & Raz, 2012). Clinical trials evaluating the effectiveness of a drug compared with a placebo control treatment often produce results (a) demonstrating greater effectiveness of drug compared with placebo, and (b) also demonstrating that placebo improves symptoms (Finniss, Kaptchuk, Miller, & Benedetti, 2010). These placebo effects are sometimes of considerable magnitude. For example, in published double-blind, randomized, placebo-controlled clinical drug trials studying depression, the response rates for placebo treatment (often accompanied by supportive counseling during a trial) can range from 10% to 50% (Sonawalla & Rosenbaum, 2002; Walsh, Seidman, Sysko, & Gould, 2002), raising the prospect that placebo might have utility as an effective clinical tool (Koshi & Short, 2007).

The notion that placebo is doing nothing, because placebo is pharmacologically inert, is challenged by several facts. First, placebo is pharmacologically inert but not physiologically inert. For example, placebo can produce changes in brain processes, as measured by neuroimaging techniques employed in experiments and in clinical trials (Beauregard, 2009; Benedetti, Carlino, & Pollo, 2011; Benedetti, Mayberg, Wager, Stohler, & Zubieta, 2005; Mayberg et al., 2002; Pollo & Benedetti, 2009). Second, placebo can produce concurrent changes in brain neurophysiology and in symptoms of depression (Hunter, Leuchter, Morgan, & Cook, 2006; Leuchter, Cook, Witte, Morgan, & Abrams, 2002). Thus, there is accumulating evidence that placebo can be viewed as an *active* therapeutic intervention in some clinical contexts.

Despite the findings that placebo can change brain and improve symptoms, there certainly are ethical concerns regarding the use of placebo as clinical treatment (Brody, 1982). But perspective on the clinical utility of placebo has evolved (Ernst, 2007; Papakostas & Daras, 2001; Shorter, 2011), such that there is now a greater willingness to consider the use of placebo in a clinical psychiatric setting: There appears to be a trend toward increased use of placebo as treatment and also increased use of subtherapeutic dosages of drugs as treatment (Harris & Raz, 2012; Raz et al., 2011). While the debate regarding ethical dilemmas concerning the clinical use of placebo continues, there also are cautionary notes regarding cultural variations for the effects of placebo (Ernst, 2007; Moerman, 2000). And there are encouraging reports regarding the possibility that placebo treatment in the elderly (e.g., for antidepressant effects) might be effective for relieving symptoms and also provide a way to help diminish the prevalence of psychotropic polypharmacy (Cherniack, 2010).

An obvious ethical concern is that prescribing placebo requires deceiving the patient. Placebo as therapy need not require the use of deception (Kaptchuk et al., 2010)—that is, telling patients that they should improve despite that fact that the pill they are being prescribed is not a drug. Moreover, there is accumulating published evidence for beneficial clinical effects of placebo, and there are methods for constructing a client-patient therapeutic dialogue in a manner that recommends placebo without telling a lie (Finniss et al., 2010; Koshi & Short, 2007).

Prescribing a placebo essentially is asking patients to believe that the prescription will help—to believe that they will get better. This recognizes placebo as a reasonable and less expensive option than *some feature* of psychotherapy or the counseling associated with the dispensation of a medication, in which patients are told to think positively, adhere to the recommended drug regimen, and have confidence that their therapeutic outcome will be good. In fact, it is reasonable to view the dispensing of placebo as a simple form of talk therapy, in which the therapist simply is saying to the patient, "I'm going to prescribe something that may help you feel better." Believing those encouraging words, and adhering to the recommendation, can be sufficient to initiate a placebo effect.

PHARMACOTHERAPY IS BEST USED AS ONE AMONG SEVERAL TOOLS

This is Rose's fifth major confrontation with debilitating depression in her lifetime. The psychotherapy again has been helpful. It facilitates getting her to understand how the new sources of stress in her family life have been affecting her mood. And the advice she receives that provides ideas about how to adapt to those stresses, what changes to make in her daily routine, and who to call when things get really, really dark—all have been very useful. But none of that counseling was helping with the difficulty she was having sleeping. The insomnia was really wearing her out, until the fluoxetine regimen began. Rose is having more restful sleep now that she is using a drug. The talk and the drug each seem to have somewhat different, complementary roles in her recovery this time around.

There are numerous examples of evidence-based pharmacotherapeutic and psychotherapeutic interventions for the treatment of psychopathology (Nathan & Gorman, 2007). But the evidence that combined pharmacotherapy and psychotherapy can be more effective than pharmacotherapy alone or psychotherapy alone is relatively sparse. There are demonstrations and claims for combined drug and talk treatments being more effective than drug alone or talk alone for treating a variety of disorders (Beitman, Blinder, Thase, Riba, & Safer, 2003):

- *Depression* in adults (Peeters et al., 2012; Schramm et al., 2007; von Wolff, Holzel, Westphal, Harter, & Kriston, 2012), SSRI treatment-resistant adolescents (Lynch et al., 2011), and the elderly (Bottino, Barcelos-Ferreira, & Ribeiz, 2012)
- *Bipolar disorder* (Berk et al., 2010)
- *Schizophrenia* (Linden, Pyrkosch, & Hundemer, 2008)
- *Substance abuse* (Laniado-Laborin, 2010; Stitzer, 1999; Stitzer & Walsh, 1997; Zahm, 2010)
- *Bulimia nervosa* (Agras et al., 1992; Bowers & Anderson, 2007; Halmi, 2005; Walsh et al., 1997)
- *Obesity* (Vetter, Faulconbridge, Webb, & Wadden, 2010)
- *Anxiety* in children (Ginsburg et al., 2011; Strawn, Sakolsky, & Rynn, 2012; Walkup et al., 2008)

For these examples, the types of "talk" therapies considered to be useful are of a wide variety, including simply encouraging adherence to medication, advice for altering lifestyle, teaching coping skills, psychosocial intervention, cognitive behavioral therapy, and supportive psychotherapy.

Despite the lack of sufficient published evidence to assemble a manual (e.g., Sudak, 2011) detailing the best combinations of specific psychotropic medications and effective methods of psychotherapy to treat specific diagnoses of psychopathology, there is enough information to make it seem prudent at the very least to consider the use of drug and talk therapies in some combination.

One reason to encourage this approach is to compensate for the fact that, for better or for worse, the use of psychotropic medication seems increasingly to be preferred to psychotherapy for treating psychopathology: The use of psychotropic medication is increasing (Frank et al., 2005; Pincus et al., 1998) while the use of psychotherapy is declining (Chisolm, 2011; Mojtabai & Olfson, 2008). Are these trends favoring the use of psychotropic medication in the best interests of treatment for patients? Are these trends supported by clinical research findings, or are they simply responding to pressures that have little or nothing to do with choosing the most effective treatments based on the scientific evidence? For example, are these trends due to increased stigma associated with being treated with psychotherapy? Or are these trends due to increased costs or inconvenience associated with psychotherapy? Or are health management organizations and health insurers establishing policies that make it easier for a patient to acquire and pay for drug therapy and more difficult to justify psychotherapy? Are these trends due to the increased acceptance of the idea that psychopathology is caused principally by a problem in brain neurochemistry and that the most direct way to repair that problem is to use a psychotropic drug as therapy?

This notion that the use of psychotropic medication is the *only* way to rearrange neurochemistry of brain is difficult to maintain given recent findings. Take the case of major depression as an example:

- The SSRI paroxetine alters glucose metabolism in specific regions of the brain after a six-week drug treatment period during which symptoms of major depression improve (Kennedy et al., 2001).
- Cognitive behavior therapy alters glucose metabolism in specific regions of the brain after an average 26-week cognitive behavioral therapy (CBT) treatment program during which symptoms of major depression improve. Compared with paroxetine, CBT produces similar *and* distinct effects on changes in brain glucose metabolism (Goldapple et al., 2004).
- Venlafaxine, a serotonin and norepinephrine reuptake inhibitor (SNRI), alters glucose metabolism in specific regions of the brain after a 16-week drug treatment period during which symptoms of major depression improve. Compared with venlafaxine, CBT produces similar *and* distinct effects on changes in brain glucose metabolism (Kennedy et al., 2007).

Therefore, at least for the treatment of major depression using SSRI or SNRI medications or CBT, drug therapy and talk therapy can produce similar *and* different effects on brain processes that correlate with improvement in symptoms of depression. These findings demonstrate that CBT and SSRI or SNRI pharmacotherapy do some similar things, and some different things, when they alter brain processes during recovery from major depression. Thus, CBT and SSRI or SNRI not only share some aspects of therapeutic outcome but also share some aspects of changes induced in the brain during therapy. On the other hand, some effects on the brain are distinctly different for CBT compared with either drug therapy.

Taken together, these findings reveal, at least in terms of effects on brain, that (a) CBT may be a reasonable "substitute" for SSRI (or SNRI) drug therapy, but only to a limited extent, and that (b) CBT and SSRI (or SNRI) drug therapy do some things to the brain that are different, suggesting that the two therapeutic approaches may be somewhat complementary in their therapeutic effects. These kinds of findings encourage the consideration of the general idea that psychotherapy can complement and possibly *enhance* the effectiveness of pharmacotherapy (or the converse) by virtue of the similar and the different effects that the two therapeutic methods have upon the brain (Stahl, 2012). Moreover, it is reasonable to consider that pharmacotherapy may in fact offer some part of what psychotherapy can offer, considering that the full measured effect of a psychotropic medication is not due entirely to the pharmacological properties of a drug but is partially due to the drug's attendant "placebo effect" (Beitman et al., 2003).

SUMMARY AND PERSPECTIVE

Scientific evidence from well-controlled clinical trials demonstrates that pharmacotherapy can be effective and relatively safe, although such findings cannot ensure effectiveness and safety for any and every patient. Evidence from clinical trials also demonstrates that placebo can change behavior and brain processes, which supports the potential for use of placebo as active therapy in limited clinical situations. The effectiveness of pharmacotherapy or placebo therapy is not diminished by lack of knowledge about the neurochemical mechanism of action for a therapy. The effectiveness of either pharmacotherapy or placebo therapy may be enhanced by combining one or the other with some type of behavior therapy or psychotherapy. Pharmacotherapy, psychotherapy, placebo, and dietary supplement therapy should each be considered for their various advantages and disadvantages and for which combinations of therapeutic options might be in the best interests of an individual patient.

THIS CHAPTER REDUCED TO A SENTENCE

Know the particulars of the scientific evidence that supports the use of any psychotropic medication, and remember that the utility of a drug (or placebo) may be enhanced by psychotherapy or counseling.

CHAPTER FIVE

Availability of a Drug Depends Upon Many Factors

Bonnie's psychiatrist intends to prescribe lamotrigine to treat her bipolar disorder, which has not responded well to various drug therapies in the past. Bonnie is concerned about this idea for several reasons. She is surprised to not find lamotrigine listed among drugs approved and recommended for bipolar disorder and to learn that the drug is best known for treating epilepsy. Her physician assures her that the drug has a good reputation for its off-label use to treat bipolar disorder. She is also wary about using a relatively new drug. Her intuition tells her that less is known about the benefits and risks of something newer than something older. She is also worried about the cost. Wouldn't a newer drug be more expensive than an older drug? Will her health insurance cover the cost?

Various factors can increase or decrease the likelihood that a drug will be available to a patient. Some of these factors are related to the process of discovery and development of a new psychotropic medication, whereas other factors have to do with the variable policies and practices of regulatory agencies and other organizations and institutions.

SERENDIPITY CAN BRING NEW OPPORTUNITIES FOR PHARMACOTHERAPY

The role of good luck in the discovery of new psychotropic medications is surprisingly important. Perhaps the best-known example of this is found in the story of chlorpromazine: Appreciating the antihistamine-like sedative properties of chlorpromazine led to consideration of its utility for treating schizophrenic patients who show psychomotor agitation, resulting in the discovery of chlorpromazine's unanticipated antipsychotic properties (Jacobsen, 1986; Lehmann & Ban, 1997). Other examples of serendipitous discoveries from the 1940s and 1950s include (a) the evaluation of potential antipsychotic properties of imipramine, resulting in the discovery of imipramine's antidepressant effects, and (b) the search for new antibacterial drugs leading to the discovery of the anxiolytic properties of meprobamate and chlordiazepoxide (Ban, 2001).

The significance of such serendipitous discovery is best appreciated when it is considered against the rational planned development of new therapeutic drugs (Tollefson, 2009). For example, it is reasonable and convenient to think that a well-considered theory regarding the underlying neurochemical dysfunction in the schizophrenic brain would have led to the first discovery of drugs having antipsychotic properties. But in fact, the discovery of a clinically effective drug often precedes the development of a neurochemical theory for the cause of a disorder. A familiar sequence of events that ultimately leads to the development of newer and more effective psychotropic medications resembles the following:

- There is a serendipitous discovery that a drug has a particular unanticipated clinical effectiveness, despite not knowing how that drug is altering the neurochemistry of the brain.
- This drug, previously approved to treat a different disorder, quickly comes to be used off-label, taking advantage of the lucky discovery that it is also useful to treat another disorder.
- This same drug is then investigated in experiments in animals (usually rodents) to determine the effects of the drug on the neurochemistry of the brain.
- Knowledge of this drug's effects on animal brains, together with the results of experiments testing the effects of the drug in an animal behavioral model for a human disorder, reveal a putative mechanism of action for the drug's clinical effects and a theory for the underlying neurochemical basis of the disorder in humans.

This theory holds that the dysfunction of a single neurochemical in the brain is the principal cause of the disorder in humans.

- This overly simplistic neurochemical theory is useful for guiding the search for newer drugs that have the same mechanism of action, with the promise that some of the newer drugs will be at least equally effective with fewer side effects than the forerunner drug.

- The eventual discovery of newer, effective drugs reveals the involvement of other neurochemicals in the disorder, making clear how the original neurochemical theory was overly simplistic.

- The revised, now multifaceted neurochemical theory provokes the search for newer drugs having pharmacologically more selective or mixed effects on brain neurochemistry, which with more good luck will lead to the discovery and development of more effective pharmacotherapy.

Progress toward the discovery of new psychotropic medications is driven by opportunities for grants to be funded for academic research, revenue to be had by pharmaceutical companies, and demand from consumers for newer and better psychotropic medications.

CONSUMERS DEMAND NEW AND BETTER DRUGS

Roger saw the advertisement for the new antianxiety medication in this morning's newspaper and assumes that the drug must be the best because it is newer than the rest. As for the ad's detailed cautionary notes regarding potential adverse effects, Roger figures they do not apply to him, because he is young and robust. He clips the ad from the paper and will bring it to his next appointment with his physician and ask that he write a prescription. Roger's thinking is that it is better to be a step ahead of the doctor, if Roger intends to have some control over his own situation.

If each and every psychotropic medication has its benefits and its risks, it is not surprising that consumers would press for the discovery and development of newer and better drugs. The consumer-patient's active role in acquiring and using prescription medication has been facilitated by the FDA's 1997 guidelines on direct-to-consumer advertising (Donohue, Cevasco, & Rosenthal, 2007; Hilts, 2003; Rosenthal, Berndt, Donohue, Frank, & Epstein, 2002). The ensuing presence of advertisements for medications on television and in printed magazines and newspapers encourages consumers to contemplate whether they might have a particular psychopathology and to consider the use of psychotropic drugs (Dubovsky & Dubovsky, 2007). You don't need to be a scientist to read an advertisement in the *New York Times* or in a popular magazine, but you would require some college-level coursework to make some sense out of the primary published scientific literature on clinical effectiveness of psychotropic drugs. The advertisements in popular media and in professional journals draw the attention of patients and therapists to new drugs, and they provide for a patient some written documentation ostensibly supporting the use of particular medications.

Having a clipping or a written argument in hand to present to one's prescribing professional does have potential benefits for both client and clinician. First, it enables patients to take an active role in assembling their therapeutic regimen. Taking an active role encourages a patient to remain invested in the therapeutic process, as well as the outcome. That investment should encourage adherence to the therapeutic regimen that the patient *and* clinician agree upon. Second, the patient with written argument in hand (however biased an advertisement may be) may stimulate the prescribing professional to better prepare. Patients who are confident and assertive, believing they have useful knowledge and an important place in the conversation, are more likely to want a somewhat detailed and well-informed opinion from a physician or psychologist. Thus, the prescribing professional, when expecting professional opinion may be scrutinized or challenged, might be more likely to have done some pharmacology homework.

In addition to gently browbeating one's clinician, the consumer-patient can influence the availability of new drugs in other ways. Consumers can work with consumer advocacy groups toward the use of their tax dollars to support research aimed at solving the riddles of specific psychological disorders and at facilitating the development of new psychotropic medications. Consumers can also support lobbying for legislation that favors the ability of the pharmaceutical industry to invest in drug discovery and development. And consumers can ask their representatives in government to pressure the FDA to do a better job of bringing new therapeutic drugs to market.

The development of new psychotropic medications depends upon preclinical research using animals, principally rodents, as subjects in experiments. More important than merely testing for adverse or toxic effects of new drugs, experiments in animals are conducted to test for the potential clinical effectiveness of a new drug. This is done using animal models of human psychopathology, which is much easier said than done. After all, how can you tell when a rat is depressed? Would you recognize a schizophrenic rat if you chatted with one?

In recent decades the creation of animal models for human psychopathology often has begun with an assessment of the behavioral symptoms of disorders as they are classified in the *Diagnostic and Statistical Manual of Mental Disorders* (DSM). Beginning with that angle of approach for modeling, for an animal model to be *ideally* useful, an animal would show all of the symptoms of a specific disorder, have the relevant genetics and neurodevelopmental history for the disorder, be living among the appropriate environmental risk factors, and have the identical neurochemical pathology that produces the symptoms of the disorder in humans. If it met all of these conditions, an animal would present essentially complete construct validity for the human psychopathology—it would present a situation so close to the human condition that the animal model could be used to assess the effectiveness of a new drug in a way that should predict the effectiveness of that drug in humans. That kind of construct validity is virtually impossible to achieve, so we settle for less.

The less-than-ideal but still useful animal model is one in which there is partial validity or face validity. In other words, if an animal has or can be created to have some portion of the human psychopathology, then such a model might still be useful. For example, if an adult rat could be exposed to an environmental stressor in such a way that the stress induced a pathological neurochemical condition that caused one or two of the behavioral symptoms of a human psychopathology, that could be a useful animal model that may have predictive validity. It would have predictive validity if, for example, the stressed rat showed what appear to be measurable behavioral signs resembling those of depression, and those abnormal behaviors in the rat were improved by the administration of a proven clinically effective antidepressant drug. If a new drug also improved those symptoms in that rat model of depression, those results might well predict that the new drug has potential for diminishing analogous symptoms of depression in humans.

A drug's effectiveness in an experiment in laboratory rats might successfully predict the drug's effectiveness in a clinical setting in humans, or it might not. Encouraging results of experiments in animal models can bolster the justification for proceeding with the development of a drug, leading to testing of that drug in clinical trials in humans. Thus, preclinical research in animal models can be useful, is less expensive than clinical trials in humans, but it is not sufficient to demonstrate the ultimate clinical effectiveness of a new drug.

There are shortcomings regarding the recent use of animal models:

- The principal factor guiding how animal models are used often has been the pharmacological profile of existing clinically effective drugs. For example, the discoveries that chlorpromazine is an antagonist for D2 receptors for dopamine and that chlorpromazine can diminish behavioral abnormalities in rat models for schizophrenia and improve symptoms of schizophrenia in humans encourage the search for new drugs that can do the same as (or better than) chlorpromazine for antagonism of D2 receptors (Moore, 2010). That is an approach that encourages development of more of the same existing types of pharmacological tools, rather than novel therapeutics.

- The lack of sufficient understanding regarding the genetics, the neurodevelopmental history, and the environmental risk factors for a specific psychopathology limits the conceptualization of animal models essentially to simulation in adult animals of the behavioral symptoms of psychopathology in adult humans (Kaffman & Krystal, 2012).
- The lack of understanding regarding the neurochemical pathology causing specific symptoms of psychopathology also limits the creation of animal models (Edwards & Koob, 2012).
- The *DSM* establishes a limited frame of reference for conceptualizing animal models in relation to behavioral symptoms and not in relation to the underlying pathophysiology, or etiology, or genetics. Moreover, using the *DSM* as a guiding framework tends to constrain development of animal models to clusters of symptoms for the categories of diagnosable disorders in the *DSM*, which may not be the most productive way to conceptualize attempts to model human psychopathology. Alternative approaches have been proposed that incorporate genetic markers and neurochemical abnormalities, together with a reformulation of categories of behavioral dysfunction (Edwards & Koob, 2012; Fernando & Robbins, 2011; Kaffman & Krystal, 2012). Some one of these alternative frameworks eventually will improve upon the *DSM* as a frame of reference for the creation of animal models and as guidelines for diagnosis and treatment.

In summary, the recent history of the use of animal models to facilitate development of new psychotropic medications reveals models principally based on behavioral symptoms, and not upon underlying neurochemical substrates or neurodevelopmental antecedents to the adult psychopathology. Although this approach is now considered to be somewhat limiting (Cryan & Sweeney, 2011; Edwards & Koob, 2012; Fernando & Robbins, 2011; Fineberg et al., 2011; Hoffman, 2011; Kaffman & Krystal, 2012; Pratt, Winchester, Dawson, & Morris, 2012), and although the development of new drugs also has been limited by relying too heavily upon the preexisting pharmacology of useful psychotropic medications (Moore, 2010), the use of existing animal models and the development of new models remain important for facilitating the development of new psychotropic medications. But, a patient sitting in a clinician's office today cannot wait for the development of better animal models. The patient suffering symptoms relies upon the FDA to do its best to quickly bring new drugs to consumers.

THE FDA ATTEMPTS TO APPROVE NEW AND BETTER DRUGS

The responsibilities and the practices of the FDA have evolved over the past 80 years, as the FDA has responded to the changing needs of our society (Hilts, 2003; Howland, 2008a, 2008b; Lipsky & Sharp, 2001). The current responsibilities are broad, including oversight of the development and marketing of drugs, medical devices, and cosmetics for humans, as well as veterinary products, and foods. Given this long list of responsibilities, it is not surprising that limited staff and budgetary resources have often beset the FDA (Hilts, 2003).

The regulation of psychotropic medications is merely a piece of the FDA's work, yet the efforts toward bringing relatively effective and safe drugs to consumers require considerable time, money, and expertise. Psychotropic (and other) drugs in development work their way through preclinical and clinical phases of investigation—a sequence of drug development that can require 8–12 years (Howland, 2008c) and cost tens of millions of dollars. The costs of preclinical and clinical research for drug development are largely funded by the pharmaceutical industry and by government-supported research grants and, therefore, ultimately by consumers and taxpayers. Money and time remain prominent issues for the FDA and have led to concerns on the part of consumers, clinicians, and patients.

Concern about the pace with which the FDA allows new drugs and novel pharmaceuticals to come to market has been repeatedly expressed over the years and has been examined by research comparing the FDA's work in the United States with the work of comparable regulatory agencies in other countries. The FDA fares well in those comparisons: Generally speaking, the FDA is a leader in bringing novel pharmaceuticals—considered to be priority drugs or significant new medications—to market sooner and more frequently than happens in other countries (Downing et al., 2012; Kessler, Hass, Feiden, Lumpkin, & Temple, 1996).

Related to the issue of the speed with which a new drug comes to market is concern about the process by which new drugs are evaluated. For one example, in order to accelerate the review process, the FDA in the 1990s instituted so-called user fees paid to the FDA by the pharmaceutical company whose product is under review. A fee of tens of thousands of dollars or more supports costs related to expert panel review of the effectiveness and safety of a drug. User fees appear to have sped the approval process along (Deyo, 2004; Lipsky & Sharp, 2001), bringing new drugs to consumers months earlier than previously had been the case. The obvious concern about user fees is the potential for conflict of interest—the party that stands to profit from the approval of the drug is the party paying for the investigation of the product. This is a fine example of an ethical concern being trumped by the need for greater resources for the FDA to conduct its business in a timely manner.

Another way to shorten the length of time required to bring more new drugs to market is to lower the standards that must be met during the approval process. The idea that the FDA might be influenced to shift standards or shape decisions in response to pressure from citizens, politicians, and the executive branch of the federal government is credible. The commissioner of the FDA is a presidential appointee, and the biases of a political party can influence decisions regarding approval of drugs that are controversial (Hilts, 2003). One recent case in point regards the availability of contraceptive methods such as the so-called "morning-after" pill (Cleland, Peipert, Westhoff, Spear, & Trussell, 2012; Steinbrook, 2012; "Time for Plan B," 2013; Wood, Drazen, & Greene, 2005).

Shifting standards at the FDA might explain the controversy generated over the approval and subsequent rapid removal from the marketplace of the psychotropic weight loss medication "fen-phen"—the combination of fenfluramine and phentermine. This drug combination presented a potent appetite-suppressant effect that was unfortunately accompanied by a risk for damage to heart valves. This problem became apparent *after* fen-phen had been approved for sale—after several people using fen-phen had died. It is reasonable to surmise that this situation resulted from relatively lower standards in the FDA approval process, perhaps due to continuing intense market demand for new drugs effective for producing weight loss (Deyo, 2004).

Regardless of the standards and the pace of the review process, and whether or not the FDA faces an immense work load with a meager budget and insufficient staffing, the expectation is that the FDA will speedily approve new psychotropic medications. The problem of limited resources can be partially solved by outsourcing some of the responsibilities of the review process and research activities. One problem associated with subcontracting is the fact that many scientists outside the FDA, working in academia or in industry, may be asked to serve competing interests in their consulting responsibilities. For example, it would be no surprise to find that a first-rate academic pharmacologist might be conducting research funded by a pharmaceutical company and at the same time consulting for the FDA to consider the evidence submitted by that same pharmaceutical company requesting approval of a new drug that they have developed and hope to sell. This represents a less than ideal situation for obtaining a completely unbiased opinion on the efficacy and relative safety of a drug based strictly upon objective consideration of data submitted. (In fact, one of the articles cited in this book indicates that its author was a paid consultant for 31 pharmaceutical companies and was engaged in research funded by 11 of them!)

But even if one could do everything that reasonably can be done to ensure objectivity in the review process, the approval of effective and safe new drugs remains an imperfect business for several reasons:

- Clinical drug trials in humans are at the heart of the evaluation process, but even the best clinical trials are limited in scope. Some clinical trials have relatively small numbers of subjects. Even larger, multicenter clinical trials that have thousands of human subjects may use exclusion factors when selecting subjects, in the interest of establishing conditions of good experimental control. Exclusion factors—for example, excluding subjects with comorbidities—often diminish the generalizability of the results obtained from the sample of subjects in the study. Ultimately, clinical studies limited in scope will provide results that do not adequately predict effectiveness and safety for *all* individual patients.
- Many (if not most) clinical trials collect more and higher-quality data on main effects than on side effects. Thus, it is not surprising that only after a drug is approved and is being used more widely does it become known through postmarketing surveillance that it has side effects not fully anticipated based on the published results of clinical trials. There is irony in clinical drug trials being more effective for gathering data on main effects than on side effects: In the clinical setting, a decision regarding which psychotropic medication to prescribe, and the patient's willingness to comply with the prescribed medication regimen, is often determined more by the appearance and intensity of adverse effects than it is by the magnitude of the main effect.
- The understanding that no drug can have only one effect ensures that a drug that produces a main effect will also cause side effects; even those drugs approved for their impressive effectiveness in producing main effects in clinical trials will be accompanied by

some side effects. Thus, it simply is not possible to promise consumers that a drug will be *completely* safe, free of risk, and devoid of troublesome side effects. Expecting the FDA to approve for market only those drugs that are guaranteed to be effective and safe in all humans is too tall an order. A more realistic goal is to approve a drug for market that is effective in a substantial proportion of patients and is *relatively* safe or *relatively* free of risk or has tolerable side effects.

- Whereas the FDA requires, prior to approval, demonstrations in at least two clinical trials that a drug elicits *statistically significant* improvement in symptoms (compared with placebo), the FDA does not require that the data from a clinical trial be analyzed in such a manner as to demonstrate that the drug has *clinically meaningful* improvement. Therefore, the results of most clinical trials supporting the approval of a drug merely demonstrate that a patient might get better, but they do not demonstrate that this will represent a significant improvement in the quality of life for a majority of patients.

- Clinical trials in the United States generally present results collected from adult male Caucasians. Children, adolescents, elderly, people of color, and (until relatively recently) women often are poorly represented in samples of subjects in clinical trials, presenting problems for the generalizability of findings.

- The drug being investigated will be approved specifically for the purpose targeted in the clinical trials. The drug's effectiveness and relative safety will have been evaluated for that targeted purpose, but once approved by the FDA, the drug can be prescribed to treat disorders other than the one targeted in the clinical trials. This off-label use represents the use of the drug for a purpose for which there may be little or no scientific evidence ensuring the drug's effectiveness or safety.

OFF-LABEL USAGE HAS ITS ADVANTAGES AND DISADVANTAGES

Marcie was prescribed the "antipsychotic" drug chlorpromazine to treat her bipolar disorder. The chlorpromazine is helping her, the apparent side effects she is experiencing are tolerable, and that is all that really matters to Marcie.

A physician can prescribe for *any* purpose a drug that is approved by the FDA for a *specific* purpose. This off-label use of a drug has its advantages and disadvantages (Howland, 2012b). One advantage is that it gives the prescribing professional the flexibility to act in what might be considered to be the best interests of the patient; this may be especially important for treating the patient who has been refractory to other treatments. Off-label use also permits the prescribing professional the opportunity to use recent accumulating anecdotal evidence and clinical experience, despite limited or no published evidence, that a drug may be useful for a purpose other than the purpose for which it originally was approved. This opportunity mitigates unnecessary delay waiting for a formal approval process to be completed before a patient can be offered a potentially helpful medication.

Avoiding the need to await the completion of clinical trials that provide data necessary to work a new drug through a formal approval process also presents several problems. Perhaps the most worrisome problem is the fact that off-label use essentially represents use that is not supported by rigorous scientific evidence. To say this more harshly, off-label use is based on educated guesswork. This non-evidence-based use potentially exposes the patient to disappointment due to the lack of a drug's main effect, and also to unanticipated risk. Another disadvantage is that off-label use is often not supported by published guidelines recommending how to use the drug for an unapproved purpose.

Despite these obvious disadvantages for off-label prescribing, off-label use of psychotropic medications is increasingly common, although at times it appears to be imprudent:

- Off-label use of psychotropic medications, despite lack of published evidence to support it (Walton et al., 2008), is common for antidepressants, antipsychotics, and anxiolytics. In fact, off-label use of some antipsychotics (e.g., the atypical antipsychotic quetiapine) is sometimes more frequent than is the leading on-label use (Martin-Latry, Ricard, & Verdoux, 2007; Walton et al., 2008).

- Off-label prescribing of antidepressants, antipsychotics, and anxiolytics in *children* is common, despite limited knowledge of psychotropic drug pharmacokinetics in children (Novak & Allen, 2007). Off-label prescribing can occur in more than 50% of visits to pediatricians and general practitioners (Bazzano et al., 2009).

- Drugs used in pediatric medicine have a relatively small market share. Thus, there is little financial incentive for pharmaceutical companies to invest in clinical trials to evaluate effectiveness and safety for a drug to be used in children when that drug is already approved for use in adults. To address this problem, the FDA has attempted to provide incentives, for example, extending the period of the exclusive right to sell a drug (Novak & Allen, 2007).

The off-label prescribing of psychotropic medications has distinct advantages, but off-label prescribing has become so common in adults, children, and adolescents as to become worrisome. There is good reason to worry, because off-label prescribing is *not* evidence-based use of psychotropic drugs.

SUCCESSFUL USAGE ENCOURAGES INCREASED USAGE, FOR BETTER OR WORSE

Jane is demanding that her physician write a prescription for fluoxetine, despite his advice to consider cognitive behavioral therapy for treatment of her bulimia nervosa. Jane has read a few articles that praise fluoxetine's effectiveness for treating bulimia, and that is enough information for her to ask for the drug and not have to be bothered taking the time to deal with a psychotherapist.

A look at some of the facts regarding use of psychotropic medications provides support for the idea that the use of pharmacotherapy for treatment of psychopathology is in its heyday. There is a trend for increased use of therapeutic drugs (Frank et al., 2005; Pincus et al., 1998), which is accompanied by increased spending on therapeutic drugs (Horgan, Garnick, Merrick, & Hodgkin, 2009; Mark et al., 2012; Zuvekas, 2005) and decreased use of psychotherapy (Chisolm, 2011; Mojtabai & Olfson, 2008). The apparent increased availability of psychotropic medications has brought treatment for behavioral and psychological disorders to people who previously did not have access to treatment and has likely contributed to improving overall quality of care (Frank et al., 2005). On the other hand, increased use of psychotropic medications includes the use of *combinations* of drugs to treat psychopathology, heightening concern regarding the deleterious effects of psychotropic polypharmacy (Mojtabai & Olfson, 2010).

Taken together, these facts—the increased use of pharmacotherapy and psychotropic polypharmacy and the decreased use of psychotherapy—raise concern that the pendulum perhaps has swung too far toward the use of psychotropic medications. This trend may be driven principally by efficiencies in cost and time. However, it remains to be determined if this trend is serving the best interests of patients and improving their quality of treatment.

HEALTH INSURANCE PRACTICES CAN DETERMINE ACCESSIBILITY TO A DRUG

Randy has decided to use only a drug to treat his depression. Despite his physician's urging to also engage in psychotherapy, Randy sees this as unacceptable, but not because he is opposed to meeting with a therapist. His health plan will not cover enough of the cost associated with psychotherapy, whereas the plan is rather generous in its coverage of pharmaceuticals—especially for those drugs that have been around for some years, have proven their usefulness, and are available in generic formulations.

The patient and the prescribing clinician do not have complete control over the selection of the most appropriate therapeutic drug. There are multiple ways in which health insurance policies and practices can affect the availability of therapeutic options, including psychotropic medications.

Managed health care practices applied to mental health care have raised concerns regarding whether the best interests of the patient take precedence over cost efficiencies. For example, managed care practices can influence the likelihood of making a formal diagnosis (Danzinger & Welfel, 2001), can encourage a choice of pharmacotherapy over psychotherapy, can recommend ideal dosages (Robst, 2012), and can encourage the use of a presumably equally effective generic formulation instead of a more costly name-brand drug (Emanuele, 2011). In addition, mental health insurance coverage, which has traditionally been less generous than coverage for medical care, can impose limits upon the number of patient visits for mental health problems (McKusick, Mark, King, Coffey, & Genuardi, 2002), and in some situations the limits for mental health visits are more severe than the limits for medical care visits (Hodgkin, Horgan, Garnick, & Merrick, 2009).

The cost-sharing requirements of mental health insurance also can have an impact on accessibility to treatment, including psychotropic medications:

- The proportion of cost sharing can be higher for behavioral than for medical illness, and the range of mental health services selected can be differentially sensitive to the patient's cost-sharing burden. For example, the newer psychotropic medications can require greater cost sharing, and this can have an impact on the decision to switch from an older-generation drug that is ineffective for an individual patient to a newer-generation drug (Horgan et al., 2009).
- Cost sharing can decrease the rate of residential treatment for substance abuse (Stein & Zhang, 2003).
- Instituting a required copayment can decrease the likelihood of

utilizing mental health services; further increasing a copayment obligation can reduce the number of visits for mental health treatment (Simon, Grothaus, Durham, VonKorff, & Pabiniak, 1996). In addition, a small increase in copayment requirement can produce a disproportionate decrease in utilization of mental health treatment (Frank & McGuire, 1986).

- Imposing a limit on the dollars spent on psychotropic medications can decrease use of medications for the elderly and for schizophrenic patients (resulting in increased hospitalizations). Imposing a tiered copayment structure can increase the cost to patients for psychotropic medications for ADHD, resulting in decreased use of medication (Austvoll-Dahlgren et al., 2008).

Particular aspects of mental health treatment may be more or less sensitive to a patient's cost-sharing burden:

- Patients with more serious mental health problems are at higher risk for increased cost-sharing burden (McKusick et al., 2002). As the number of visits for mental health treatment increases, cost-sharing expenses to the patient can increase, while the cost-sharing expenses for psychotropic medication may not (Zuvekas & Meyerhoefer, 2006).
- Approximately 10% of substance abusers receive treatment; of these, half report cost constraints as an explanation for lack of care (Dave & Mukerjee, 2011).
- Different health insurance plans provide a wide range of access to the breadth of pharmacological options. For example, access to newer antidepressants and newer antipsychotics may require a greater cost-sharing requirement for some tiered formulary plans than for others (Horgan et al., 2009). In addition, publicly insured children and adolescents are more likely than privately insured children and adolescents to be prescribed antipsychotic medication (Aparasu & Bhatara, 2007; Olfson et al., 2006a).

There are differences across countries and cultures in the availability of resources for mental health (Saxena, Thornicroft, Knapp, & Whiteford, 2007), including psychotropic medications. A few examples specifically related to the use of pharmacotherapy for mental illness include the following:

- The lifetime prevalence rate for mental illness varies from approximately 10% to 50% globally, and access to treatments varies widely; the advent of psychotropic medications has increased access to treatment in those countries that can afford the cost of the drugs (Kohn, Saxena, Levav, & Saraceno, 2004).

- In some countries and cultures it is important to avoid the stigma associated with diagnosis and labeling (Patel, Chowdhary, Rahman, & Verdeli, 2011), diminishing the likelihood that psychotropic medication will be used.

- In some cultures the idea that mental illness results from a neurochemical problem in the brain is *not* the prevailing view, because it devalues the significant role of social stressors as a causative factor (Patel et al., 2011). The perception that the behavioral disorder is not a product of disturbed neurochemistry in the brain diminishes the likelihood that psychotropic medication will be valued.

- Although access to psychotherapy is severely limited in some countries, which likely would increase the reliance upon psychotropic medications (Patel et al., 2011), the prohibitive cost of newer and more expensive psychotropic medications limits their access.

In summary, there are a number of ways in which mental health insurance coverage, cultural biases, and economic factors can have an impact on selection of treatments and the use of psychotropic medications. The examples given here are not an exhaustive assessment of those topics. The changeable circumstances and policies of managed care programs and insurance underwriters make it difficult to offer enduring generalizations regarding how an individual patient's situation may be constrained by policies and practices of these organizations. Nevertheless, a clinician considering recommending a psychotropic medication should be aware of some of the economic factors outside of the patient-clinician relationship that can affect the selection of pharmacotherapy (or psychotherapy), the choice of drug, the duration of treatment, and the role of pharmacotherapy in the total treatment program. Awareness of these factors is important for keeping the best interests of the patient's mental health *the* priority when concerns about cost efficiencies threaten to become intrusive.

SUMMARY AND PERSPECTIVE

Patients and clinicians desire a broad range of useful therapeutic options, including new psychotropic medications that may be more effective and less troublesome than available older medications. The demand for newer drugs presses the FDA to provide streamlined processes for prompt review and approval of new medications. The efforts of the FDA are facilitated by a pharmaceutical industry eager for the profits that can be made from sale of newer medications, and sometimes are aided by anecdotal or serendipitous clinical findings. Preclinical studies in animal models can facilitate development of new drugs, and structured clinical trials evaluating effectiveness and relative safety of new drugs have their strengths and their limitations, but even the best clinical trials cannot predict the utility and safety of a drug for an individual patient. Once a new drug is approved for a particular purpose, that drug can be prescribed for virtually *any* purpose, which broadens the potential utility of the new drug, and also increases the likelihood of unexpected benefits and risks. This off-label use has contributed to the problem of increased pharmacotherapy for children, adolescents, and elderly without evidence from clinical trials to predict effectiveness and safety. Access to psychotropic medications is sometimes facilitated and sometimes hindered by practices of health management organizations, by mental health insurance coverage, and by cultural and economic factors.

Considering the ability to develop new psychotropic medications, the consumer demand for newer and better drugs, the demonstrable effectiveness of psychotropic medications, the flexibility afforded by off-label prescribing, the cost-effectiveness evident for pharmacotherapy versus psychotherapy, and the resultant extraordinary confidence in the clinical use of psychotropic medications, it is no wonder that the contemporary use of psychotropic medications may be reaching its zenith.

THIS CHAPTER REDUCED TO A SENTENCE

Scientific evidence supports the use of FDA-approved psychotropic medications, but not the off-label use of drugs, and FDA standards, mental health insurance practices, and cultural and economic factors influence the accessibility, cost, and ultimately the effectiveness of psychotropic medications.

CHAPTER SIX

A Patient Contributes to Effective Pharmacotherapy

Delaney is not going to use any more of that drug than he absolutely needs. Maybe he will take half of the recommended dosage, but he will not take all of it. His physician told him it is important to be committed to the drug regimen, but he did not offer information that convinced Delaney that it will be worth the bother. His physician also did not seem to be listening when Delaney told him how important it is that he not be troubled by a select few of the potential side effects. Delaney wishes to discuss whether or not there are some drug options, but his physician seems to be insisting that he begin with imipramine, advice that appears to be based on the physician's clinical experience. This whole situation annoys Delaney a great deal. Delaney is most concerned about his own experience, not his physician's biases based on professional experiences. He *does* want a drug to solve his problem, because there is no way he is going to make the time for any psychotherapy. At this point, he lacks confidence that things will get better, and he is beginning to dread the next appointment with his doctor.

The effectiveness of pharmacotherapy depends to some extent upon the quality of the relationship between the prescribing professional and the patient or, in the case of "split treatment," upon the quality of communication among the patient, the prescribing physician, and the psychotherapist (Tasman et al., 2000). The effort to establish trust and meaningful communication between patient and health care professionals ultimately represents an investment in the patient having realistic expectations for a drug's benefits, along with some degree of acceptance of a drug's side effects. The realistic anticipation of benefits and acceptable risks increases the likelihood of a patient's compliance with the recommended drug regimen. Establishing realistic expectations of treatment outcome begins with diagnosis.

DIAGNOSIS GUIDES CHOICE OF PHARMACOTHERAPY

Establishing a diagnosis for a behavioral and psychological problem is a task burdened with a degree of uncertainty and arbitrariness. The contemporary Western medical perspective on diagnosis of psychological problems has led to the creation of the *Diagnostic and Statistical Manual of Mental Disorders*, currently in its fifth edition (*DSM-5*). The approach to creating such a manual assumes that disorders can be identified as somewhat *distinct* entities, that *behavioral* symptoms currently provide sufficient data to assign people to specific categories of psychological illness, and that the specific categories that we enumerate *do in fact exist* in nature—that diagnostic categories are not merely fabrications of our professional imaginations turned loose to create convenient categories and labels.

Uncertainty regarding the integrity of diagnostic categories becomes apparent in several ways. First, some behavioral symptoms (i.e., diagnostic criteria) of one disorder can also be symptoms of another disorder—symptoms of depression and symptoms of anxiety being one case in point. Second, comorbidity is not unusual—it is common. What does it mean that someone may be diagnosed as having both a substance abuse disorder and bulimia nervosa? Is it possible that the comorbidity actually represents a distinct disorder—*not* concurrent substance abuse and bulimia, but some integration of the two that would be better understood and treated as being a separate category unto itself? Third, numerous drugs first identified to treat one diagnostic category of disorder, for example, depression, are not specifically and exclusively antidepressant in their effects. A so-called antidepressant drug can also be useful for treating some form of anxiety or bulimia nervosa. This breadth of a drug's effectiveness across diagnostic categories suggests that the different diagnostic categories have something in common, not only behaviorally but also perhaps at the level of neurochemistry of the brain, raising concern that the diagnostic categories are not so distinct after all.

The discomfort caused by the uncertainty regarding the distinctiveness of diagnostic categories can be alleviated somewhat by keeping in mind that a diagnosis is merely a working hypothesis regarding the patient's current condition. A *diagnosis is not a definitive determination*, and it certainly is not proof of a specific condition. It is not an end point but does provide a beginning to a process aimed at offering help.

However imperfect the process of categorization and diagnosis may be, making diagnosis is useful for a variety of reasons:

- Classification of categories and subcategories of psychopathology facilitates communication among professionals, patients, and families of patients. These categories of ailments also provide operational definitions of illness that are important for those doing clinical research. Scientists and clinicians can know what one another are speaking and writing about when using the operational definitions provided by the *DSM*.

- Naming a problem that a client is hypothesized to present offers some reassurance that the nature of the problem may be understood, ideally encouraging the patient to trust that help is on the way.

- Categories of illness ultimately become associated with treatments that have been successful (and dissociated from other treatments that have not been successful). This knowledge, emanating from clinical practice and published clinical trials, establishes a context guiding to specific therapeutic options, including psychotropic medications, that appear to best fit a specific category of illness for at least a sizable proportion of patients bearing that diagnosis.

Those advantages of categorization and diagnosis in most situations would appear to outweigh some of these disadvantages:

- Stigma can be associated with being labeled as psychologically ill. Fear of stigma may diminish the seeking of treatment and affect the patient's choice of treatment.

- Establishing a category with a label can facilitate an overly simplistic expectation that the disorder will have a specific unique solution, for example, the existence of a drug or class of drugs that will relieve symptoms in *all* patients having that specific diagnosis. This overly simplistic expectation can increase a patient's frustration when the recommended psychotropic medication is ineffective.

The imperfections in the boundaries of categories of psychopathology also are apparent when it is observed that many patients fail to respond to a specific drug therapy that is effective in other patients who bear the same diagnosis. This situation is common, and it demonstrates that the diagnostic categories are inadequate for distinguishing meaningful differences among people who are given the same diagnostic label. It also demonstrates that a clinician should expect that a drug known to have antidepressant properties will not inevitably relieve symptoms of depression in each and every patient diagnosed as having depression, and that the same drug with antidepressant properties may be useful for treating diagnosed disorders other than depression. These facts remind that perhaps it is better to regard a psychotropic medication as an intrusive chemical that can be deposited in the brain on an educated guess that it may improve symptoms, rather than a medication that has a specific calling to alter symptoms of one particular diagnosed psychopathology.

Perhaps the fundamental advantage of creating diagnostic categories for making diagnoses is that diagnostic categories eventually become associated with specific nondrug and pharmacological therapeutic options that are more likely to be successful for treating a sizable proportion of patients who fit a specific diagnosis (Nathan & Gorman, 2007). This knowledge, however imperfect, does provide a reference point for initiating the process of choosing among therapeutic options, including psychotropic medications. But the relative significance of the role of psychotropic medication for an individual patient, the details of *how* a drug can be most effectively used within a treatment program, can vary considerably among patients.

THE ROLE OF PHARMACOTHERAPY VARIES FOR DIFFERENT PEOPLE AND DIFFERENT DISORDERS

Frances is open to the idea of using a medication and seeing a psychotherapist, but she feels that she is much too agitated to benefit from conversation at the moment. She wonders whether a drug that reduces that agitation perhaps should be the first step in her attempt to get it together. Once she can feel less anxious, can concentrate better, can stay focused and think clearly, then she might benefit from some helpful conversation. Her psychiatrist agrees, and they make a plan to begin with a drug to even out her mood and then to follow in a few weeks with the start of psychotherapy.

It may be in the best interests of any patient to *at least consider* the possibility that the ideal path toward remission of symptoms is to employ a therapeutic program that includes some combination of drug and nondrug therapy—a therapeutic program that capitalizes on the advantages of psychotropic medication and of behavior therapy or psychotherapy (Beitman et al., 2003). There are several uncertainties to contemplate when attempting to design a therapeutic program that integrates drug and talk therapies:

- Is the patient willing to consider the utility of both drug and talk therapeutic options, and is the patient likely to fulfill the requirements of each? Will the patient take the drug as prescribed, and will the patient make the most of the opportunity to engage in psychotherapy? Does the patient, the patient's family, or the patient's culture harbor biases against the use of drug therapy or psychotherapy?

- Will the patient's mental health insurance coverage support a potentially more costly and more effective (e.g., Lynch et al., 2011) integrated psychotherapeutic and pharmacotherapeutic approach? Will the patient's obligation for cost sharing prohibit some aspects of an integrated approach? If the insurance coverage imposes some constraints, can the therapist work with the patient to construct a therapeutic program that serves the patient's best interests within a context of limited resources?

- What is the relative importance of the drug therapy and the talk therapy? Is drug therapy serving a more pressing need (e.g., making the patient sufficiently lucid to meaningfully participate in psychotherapy)? Is psychotherapy or counseling necessary to ensure compliance with the prescribed drug regimen? Is behavior therapy or psychotherapy necessary to address a longer-lasting solution (e.g., reorganization of perspective and changes in lifestyle)?

- Which drug and what dosage should be used in combination with which nondrug therapy? Can the use of a lower-cost generic psychotropic medication help to make a therapeutic program more affordable for the patient, and can a generic psychotropic drug substitute for a brand-name drug without diminishing effectiveness and without eliciting unexpected adverse effects (Emanuele, 2011; LaDue, 2011)?

- What should be the sequence and the duration of each treatment when employing multiple therapeutic methods?

- Can the patient be persuaded to take an active role partnering with the physician or therapist to construct a therapeutic program? Can the physician justify spending the extra time necessary to enable the patient to feel comfortable in an active collaborative role?

CLIENTS SHOULD BE ACTIVE PARTICIPANTS IN THEIR PHARMACOTHERAPY

Which drug? Generic or brand name drug? FDA-approved medication or off-label prescription? What dosage, and for how long? Which method of psychotherapy or behavior therapy, and for how long? Which therapist?

These questions are probably best answered in collaboration between patient and clinician to maximize the effectiveness of all treatment options. Decisions made in collaboration will be most useful when patients assume a comfortable collaborative role, confident that they have something to offer to the conversations and confident that their opinions are being heard (Levine & Foster, 2010). That confidence should encourage willingness to compromise and deference to the clinician when in doubt.

Patients' level of comfort in those conversations should increase as they acquire some relevant useful knowledge. When a patient lacks knowledge (e.g., regarding what a specific drug might be doing to the brain), the prescribing professional should take the time to educate the patient regarding some of the basics of the relevant pharmacology. The prescribing professional also should be able to recommend some relevant reading that is accessible to the patient. The prescribing professional should demonstrate a genuine interest in more than main effects and side effects; the patient should feel as if the drug dispenser is interested in the person as well as the drug's effects. The prescribing professional should lay out a plan of options in the event the drug does this or doesn't do that, discussing the likelihood of positive and negative outcomes. The patient's explicit hopes and expectations for treatment outcome should be a topic of conversation.

Most important, patients should be educated by their clinicians regarding a *realistic set of expectations* for the outcomes of drug therapy (or combined drug and talk therapies). A realistic set of expectations should include prioritization of which symptoms are the most meaningful to improve, the anticipated degree of improvement, and which side effects are the more likely, which must be avoided, and which would be tolerable (Ally, 2010). Having a realistic set of expectations will facilitate commitment to the therapeutic regimen and, as success is experienced, will reinforce a positive attitude important for facilitating continued improvement.

Attending to all of that will take time. That investment of time should in the long run increase the likelihood of successful treatment, because the investment should build trust and the patient's commitment to the therapeutic program. That investment should increase the likelihood of adhering to advice offered regarding the drug regimen and its place in the overall therapeutic program.

THERE ARE SOURCES OF USEFUL INFORMATION

Carl knows there is a world of information accessible through his laptop about absolutely everything he would ever want to know about psychotropic medications. Now if he just knew which sites and postings on the Internet can be trusted as being nonbiased and factual.

Patients will be more effective collaborators in constructing and fulfilling a therapeutic regimen the more they know about what they are being asked to do. They should benefit from being educated about their situation, and they can do some of the learning on their own. Other than advice from the professional health care workers involved with their case, there are numerous places where patients and family members can seek information relevant to their situation, in particular regarding the use of psychotropic medication.

Advertising in popular media.   Advertising is difficult for anyone to avoid; no one will need to search for it. The direct-to-consumer advertising in newspapers, magazines, and television do present opportunities for a client to get new information, which can have positive consequences:

- Direct-to-consumer advertising can increase a reader's awareness of symptoms, which can increase the likelihood of early treatment of a disorder. Advertising also can diminish the stigma associated with having a diagnosable disorder and can enhance interest in combining pharmacotherapy with psychotherapy (Donohue, Berndt, Rosenthal, Epstein, & Frank, 2004).
- Direct-to-consumer advertising, for better or worse, can increase the likelihood of psychotropic drug therapy (Donohue et al., 2004)—that is, after all, the principal goal of a pharmaceutical company spending money on advertising. This may be helpful when a patient is initially biased against the use of drugs.
- The advertisements provide information that can facilitate the initiation of a conversation between patient and therapist (Ally, 2010). This may be important for the patient who is likely to be intimidated by a physician's or a therapist's wealth of knowledge.

Reference books.   Just about any public library or university library will hold as a reference book the *Physicians' Desk Reference* (*PDR*). This large volume is useful for information regarding dosages, main effects and side effects, warnings, and drug interactions. There is an immense amount of useful information in the PDR, although the typical citizen may find a medical dictionary useful when consulting it. A common mistake that a patient can make when using the PDR is to believe that every single one of the side effects listed for a drug will be experienced by each user of that drug.

The original PDR is now complemented by more selectively useful volumes, including:

- The PDR for Nonprescription Drugs, Dietary Supplements, and Herbs
- PDR Health—a version intended for the lay reader
- The PDR Drug Guide for Mental Health Professionals

Academic books.   A variety of academic books may be useful reading for a patient, a patient's family, or a clinician:

- A patient or relative of a patient who is interested in the issues pertinent to structuring a treatment program that uses psychotropic medication should find the seventh edition of the Handbook of Clinical Psychopharmacology for Therapists (Preston, O'Neil, & Talaga, 2013) to be informative and helpful for facilitating conversation with a prescribing clinician or therapist. The treatment is thorough and does not require that a reader have an extensive background in medicine or psychology.
- An introduction to informed use of psychotropic medication that is thorough, objective, and accessible is The Medication Question: Weighing Your Mental Health Treatment Options (Diamond, 2011). Another book of this kind, written at a level more accessible to the clinician than to the patient, is Successful Psychopharmacology: Evidence-Based Treatment Solutions for Achieving Remission (Sobel, 2012).
- Detailed information regarding dosages, main effects, and side effects pertinent to psychotropic medications used to treat a broad range of psychopathology can be found in Clinical Guide to Psychotropic Medications (Dubovsky, 2005). This book would be useful for patients as well as clinicians.
- Wide-ranging advice for clinicians employing psychotropic medications can be found in Psychotherapist's Resource on Psychiatric Medications: Issues of Treatment and Referral (Buelow, Hebert, & Buelow, 2000). Patients might also find this book enlightening regarding the challenges facing the prescribing clinician.
- Someone who wants to have a broad understanding of psycho-

pharmacology should read a textbook that is challenging, yet readable, and covering a broad range of topics. My choice for the best such textbook available is the second edition of *Psychopharmacology: Drugs, the Brain, and Behavior* (Meyer & Quenzer, 2013). This is a college-level textbook.

- An introduction to the effects of psychotropic drugs on brain processes related to mental health is *The Unwell Brain* (Kraly, 2009).

- The clinical psychologist who is taking on the responsibility of prescriptive authority will find a wide variety of useful advice in *Pharmacotherapy for Psychologists: Prescribing and Collaborative Roles* (McGrath and Moore, 2010).

- A clinician who would like advice to facilitate establishing a working relationship with a patient should benefit from reading *The Doctor-Patient Relationship in Pharmacotherapy* (Tasman, Riba, & Silk, 2000).

- Advice for prescribing psychotropic medication to treat a range of disorders can be found in *Psychopharmacology for the Non-Medically Trained* (Dziegielewski, 2006).

- A clinician who treats patients from a cultural background different from one's own would learn useful things from *Multicultural Care: A Clinician's Guide to Cultural Competence* (Comas-Diaz, 2012).

Professional journal articles. Although published clinical trials evaluating effectiveness of psychotropic medication (and other treatments) are necessary reading for clinicians, such reading requires sufficient training to permit *critical* reading and interpretation of research findings. The typical patient does not have the background to critically read such professional publications. Advice for clinicians reading in the professional literature can be found in *Psychotropic Drug Prescriber's Survival Guide: Ethical Mental Health Treatment in the Age of Big Pharma* (Dubovsky and Dubovsky, 2007; see also McGrath, 2010).

Internet websites. A person's computer can provide access to numerous Internet websites that offer information and opinions about psychoactive drugs—drugs used therapeutically and recreationally. Some of these sites are trustworthy, offering balanced objective views. Other sites offer biased opinions, and some sites offer information that is flat-out erroneous. It is not a simple matter to know which sites can be trusted for accurate, unbiased information. Here is a list of some very useful sites on the Internet:

- Perhaps the best place to start when looking for objective information on psychotropic medications is the FDA website (http://www.fda.gov), which has such information as safety alerts, recalls, and news regarding approvals of new drugs. One of the more useful sections on the site is MedWatch (http://www.fda.gov/safety/medwatch/default.htm), which reports recent information gathered on adverse effects of medications.

- Another useful site for information about a broad range of issues in health is the National Institutes of Health's website (http://www.nih.gov). One can also visit the NIH's National Institute of Mental Health site (http://www.nimh.nih.gov/index.shtml) for information pertinent to a broad range of issues in mental health, including research and treatments for the range of psychological disorders.

- The website of the American Academy of Child and Adolescent Psychiatry has a page on "Psychiatric Medication" with useful advice for parents, families, and mental health professionals (http://www.aacap.org/AACAP/AACAP/Families_and_Youth/Resources/Psychiatric_Medication/Home.aspx).

- An excellent source of contemporary, thorough, evidence-based reviews of treatment approaches for a range of psychological disorders is Cochrane Reviews (http://www.cochrane.org/cochrane-reviews).

- *Monitor on Psychology*, a journal of the American Psychological Association, provides articles on its website pertinent to the judicious use of pharmacotherapy (http://www.apa.org/monitor/index.aspx).

- Websites of pharmaceutical companies can be useful, especially when seeking information for a specific product manufactured and sold by that company.

Patients should be encouraged to use some of these public resources to educate themselves. One reason to do so is simply to gain knowledge about the psychotropic medications that they are considering. Another reason is to facilitate meaningful conversations between patients and health professionals. Patients who have some familiarity with the professional language used by psychologists, psychiatrists, and physicians will be better able to converse using some of the terms of that language. Patients who have some familiarity will also be able to attend therapeutic sessions better prepared to take the best advantage of the limited time that they have with their physician or therapist.

SUMMARY AND PERSPECTIVE

The role of psychotropic medication in a therapeutic program is enriched when patients understand why that drug is being used to treat their specific diagnosis, and why a diagnosis is little more than a working hypothesis about their condition. Patients come to know more by having meaningful conversations in a collaborative relationship with prescribing professionals and other health care workers assigned to their case. Patients benefit the most from those conversations when they have taken the time to do some reading and to educate of themselves regarding their diagnosis and their treatment.

THIS CHAPTER REDUCED TO A SENTENCE

Remember that diagnostic categories of illness will not perfectly predict the best option for psychotropic medication for an individual patient; engage the patient as a valuable asset for successful pharmacotherapy, and get advice from trusted sources.

PART II

Principles and Recommendations Applied to Pharmacotherapy

Part II offers six chapters, each of which illustrates how research findings in humans (and sometimes animals) support the significance of the principles or recommendations presented in Part I. The topics chosen (obesity, schizophrenia, addiction, depression and bipolar disorder, attention deficit hyperactivity disorder, and anxiety) were selected for interest and importance, but also for their ability to readily illustrate some portion of the principles of pharmacology and recommendations introduced in Part I, as indicated under the headings within each of the following chapters. Each topic is considered in historical context regarding the use of psychotropic medications to treat symptoms of the behavioral disorder. Examples of how the use of psychotropic drugs to treat these disorders reveals the significance of principles of pharmacology are taken from published human clinical drug trials and from published research in animals. Each chapter includes a section of examples of the use of behavioral animal models relevant to issues in psychopharmacology. And there is a "Tidbits" section at the end of each chapter that offers brief topical examples to further illustrate each of the principles and recommendations presented in Part I.

Obesity

Quinn just loves to eat. For him, it is one of life's greatest plea-
sures. Sweet things, salty things, fatty things—they all are quite
exciting for Quinn. The very sight of a cannoli ends any dieting
that Quinn has attempted. But the weight gain does worry him
and his physician, who told Quinn that she could help him to lose
some weight with a prescription for phentermine. His physician
also told Quinn that he would have to commit to some changes in
his lifestyle. Quinn knows that swallowing the drug will be easy
enough, but denying himself unlimited oral access to all those
tasty foods is going to be a problem. Quinn wonders if he can just
stay on the drug forever, and if phentermine can be combined
with another drug to increase the drug therapy's potency—similar
to the way the combination of drugs called fen-phen had seemed
to be helpful to Quinn 15 years ago. Quinn thinks that he'd be
willing to tolerate a few additional side effects from a combination
of drugs. That would be a better approach for him rather than
have to give up the nightly beer and potato chips or, worse, those
thick, juicy cheeseburgers.

If there is an issue that is obviously a biopsychosocial problem, overeating
leading to being overweight is it (Lagerros & Rossner, 2012). Overeating and
subsequent weight gain certainly have their biological causes and consequences—for example, physiological signals for hunger and satiety, and dis-

posal of excess calories as body fat. Overeating leading to overweight also has its behavioral and psychological issues—for example, appetite and craving for foods, and eating tempting foods because they will taste so good. Overeating and weight gain also have social issues—for example, gatherings structured around sumptuous meals, and the advertisements depicting the lure of spectacular cheeseburgers and delicious pastries.

Given the biopsychosocial nature of overeating, overweight, and obesity, it seems clear that the most effective treatment would be a multifaceted approach that includes altering one or several physiological signals, counseling intended to change one's behavior, and restructuring one's local physical and social environment (Devlin, Yanovski, & Wilson, 2000; Ioannides-Demos, Proietto, & McNeil, 2005; Lagerros & Rossner, 2012). Given that perspective, what is the best way to employ psychotropic medication to treat what appears to be a three-component physiological, psychological, and social problem?

It seems quite reasonable to expect that a psychotropic medication can be developed that modifies neurochemical processes in the brain to inhibit appetite, thereby reducing food consumption and producing loss of body weight. On the other hand, it seems somewhat less likely that a drug can be developed that alters cognitive processes in a manner that results in a person making better decisions about which foods to eat and how much of them to consume. Moreover, it seems unrealistic to expect that a psychotropic medication can be developed that will change a person's local environment in a way that diminishes the ability of various external stimuli to encourage excessive eating. Considering the relative feasibility of these three approaches, the most effectual pharmacological approach to weight loss would employ a drug that directly reduces a person's appetite and eating. Such a psychotropic medication would best be employed as an adjunctive therapy in a multifaceted approach to reduce body weight that also includes (a) some method of counseling that encourages the client to change old behaviors or adopt new behaviors related to food (i.e., dieting), (b) a program of physical exercise, and (c) alteration of the client's local physical and social environment in such a way that decreases the likelihood of eating excessively.

This type of integrated approach for reducing eating and losing weight depends upon the availability of psychotropic medications that are effective and relatively safe to be used by people who bear the medical burdens that are secondary to being overweight or obese (recently defined as having a body mass index equal to or greater than 30 kg/m^2). If they are effective and safe, the drugs can be useful in two phases of treatment for obesity: the initial reduction of body weight and the longer-term maintenance of reduced body weight.

Such psychotropic medications are highly prized for several reasons: It is now common (Oliver, 2006) to consider obesity to be a disease of epidemic proportions (Campbell & Mathys, 2001; Chugh & Sharma, 2012; Devlin et al., 2000; Zhaoping et al., 2005) that is global in its prevalence (Heal, Gosden, & Smith, 2012; Lagerros & Rossner, 2012). This means that many adults, adolescents, and children are eligible to be treated for obesity—many potential consumers of diet books, counseling, exercise programs, and weight-loss medications. In addition, many consumers who do not meet the body mass index criterion for obesity still wish to use a drug to facilitate losing weight for what could be viewed as cosmetic reasons (Cerullo, 2006; Oliver, 2006). Given the size of that potential market, a pharmaceutical company that develops the psychotropic medication that becomes the treatment of choice for reducing appetite and producing weight loss stands to win big, especially considering that none of the current appetite-suppressing drugs measure up to expectations (Bray, 2011; Chugh & Sharma, 2012; Heal et al., 2012; Kennett & Clifton, 2010; Witkamp, 2011).

PROGRESS ON DEVELOPING DRUGS TO REDUCE APPETITE AND BODY WEIGHT

Obesity is a long story in my family, Doc. I know my grandmother lost weight using amphetamine by prescription maybe 50 years ago. And my mom had good success with one of those over-the-counter drugs that you can't buy anymore. And now you're telling me there are no drugs that are as effective? You can write me a prescription for something, but I'll still have to diet and work out to lose a great deal of weight? Are we not making progress here?

The history of the use of drugs to inhibit appetite and produce loss of weight is marked by three characteristics: (a) a search for a "magic bullet" drug that provides an easy, inexpensive way to lose weight and remain slim (Hirsch, 1998); (b) frequent renewed expectations for a novel effective weight-loss drug; and (c) an equal number of disappointments owing to the adverse effects of those new drugs. It has been very difficult to meet the goals enumerated for an anti-obesity drug to be considered successful (Kolanowski, 1999)—namely, that the drug produce a significant loss of body weight that is maintained throughout the period of treatment and beyond, and that the magnitude of reduction of body weight (and improvement in symptoms of cardiovascular and metabolic morbidity that are secondary to obesity) outweigh the adverse effects of the drug. The currently available anti-obesity drugs produce only modest reduction of body weight, *when* those drugs are combined with counseling that encourages behavioral changes such as new eating habits, lifestyle changes, and increased exercise (Devlin et al., 2000; Heal et al., 2012).

One problem that continues to hamper the search for effective appetite-suppressing drugs is the complexity of how the brain and nervous system control eating behavior. The physiological control of hunger (and satiety) is characterized by the integration of multiple neurochemical signals functioning at different sites in the brain, and numerous physiological and hormonal signals in the gastrointestinal tract and peripheral nervous system (Adan, 2013; Hirsch, 1998; Kaplan, 2005; Kraly, 2009; Morton, Cummings, Baskin, Barsh, & Schwartz, 2006). The complexity of such a system offers numerous potential targets for a drug that might inhibit appetite (or increase satiety), but at the same time, the complexity presents the possibility that the pharmacological alteration of a *single* neurochemical hunger signal may be ineffectual. In other words, if dozens of physiological signals provoke eating behavior, to what extent can eating be inhibited by pharmacologically blocking the activity of only one of those signals?

Drugs that have been used to produce loss of weight can be placed into essentially two groups—those having psychoactive properties that inhibit appetite and reduce eating, and those that diminish the ability of ingested calories to be stored in the body as fat. Drugs in this second group, for example, the intestinal lipase inhibitor orlistat, are not psychotropic medications. That is not to say that these drugs have no psychological consequences, but the effects of these drugs on behavior are likely secondary to the unpleasant gastrointestinal side effects they induce. In contrast, the psychoactive drugs that produce loss of weight are more likely to have as their principal effect the inhibition of appetite, leading to reduced caloric intake. It is this type of psychotropic medication that has a long history of use revealing limited success (Adan, 2013; Ioannides-Demos, Proietto, & McNeil, 2005). These medications can be assigned to one of three rather broad categories: drugs that enhance neurotransmission, drugs that have selective effects on neurotransmitter receptors, and drug combinations that have multiple effects.

Drugs that enhance dopamine, norepinephrine, or serotonin neurotransmission. Although several drugs were used prior to the 1950s (e.g., thyroid hormone) to produce weight loss, the first drug having psychoactive properties that was used to produce loss of weight is amphetamine (Table 7.1). Amphetamine was available beginning in the 1930s, and its use to suppress appetite peaked in the 1950s and 1960s. The FDA approved phentermine in 1959 to be used to produce weight loss, followed shortly by the availability of fenfluramine. The off-label combined use of fenfluramine and phentermine, known

TABLE 7.1

Evolution of use of drugs over the decades to produce weight loss.

DRUG	1930s	1940s	1950s	1960s	1970s	1980s	1990s	2000s	2010s
Amphetamine	x	x	x	x					
Phentermine				x	x	x	x	x	x
Phenylpropanolamine				x	x	x	x		
Fenfluramine					x	x	x		
Dexfenfluramine							x		
Fen-phen							x		
Sibutramine							x	x	
Orlistat								x	x
Lorcaserin									x
Phentermine + topiramate									x

Note: x indicates decade in which drug was prescribed. This table shows that the more recently introduced psychotropic medications generally have replaced the use of older medications, principally owing to improved side effect profiles of the newer drugs, not their greater effectiveness for producing loss of weight.

as fen-phen, began in 1992. The use of fen-phen ended in 1997 when the FDA removed fenfluramine and dexfenfluramine from the market over concerns about side effects, some of them potentially lethal (e.g., abnormalities in functioning of heart valves).

This lengthy period (1950s to 1997) was characterized by the use of drugs known to alter one or more of three neurochemical systems in the brain: norepinephrine, dopamine, and serotonin (Table 7.2). Amphetamine is known to have multiple effects that ultimately enhance the synaptic availability of dopamine, norepinephrine, and serotonin. Phentermine is known to enhance the availability of synaptic norepinephrine. Fenfluramine enhances the availability of synaptic serotonin, as does sibutramine, which was approved by the FDA in 1997 but subsequently withdrawn from the market in 2010 owing to adverse cardiovascular effects. Combining phentermine and fenfluramine enhances synaptic availability of norepinephrine and serotonin, thereby partially resembling the effects of amphetamine. These kinds of synaptic effects on one or several of three neurotransmitter systems, which are rather massive in their distribution in the brain, are not capable of directly and specifically targeting *individual* hunger or satiety mechanisms in the brain. These drugs were used principally because they were relatively effective, not because they selectively blocked one or several neurochemical signals for hunger.

Drugs that have selective effects on receptor subtypes.   It was apparent by the mid-1990s that the drug-induced enhancement of dopamine, norepinephrine, or serotonin neurotransmission could inhibit eating and produce loss of weight (Table 7.2), but at considerable cost in terms of adverse effects. This situation led to a period of drug development that focused on a search for drugs that might be more selective in their pharmacological properties— that could target specifically neurochemical processes important for appetite and, owing to this superior pharmacological selectivity, might present fewer troubling side effects. The newer drugs in this category that were approved or nearly approved by the FDA include lorcaserin, a selective agonist for a subtype of serotonin receptor, and rimonabant, a selective antagonist for a subtype of receptor for endogenous cannabinoids. This more recent approach for developing anti-obesity drugs has not yet been enormously successful. Lorcaserin's entry into the market in 2012 provides the first test case in the United States for clinical utility of a drug in this category.

Combinations of drugs producing multiple effects on neurotransmission. Recent drug development efforts have included the search for newer combinations of drugs that might simultaneously alter several neurochemical mech-

TABLE 7.2

Neurotransmitters and hormones altered by drugs that produce weight loss.

DRUG	DECADE INTRODUCED	NEUROTRANSMITTER OR HORMONE ALTERED								
		DA	NE	SER	CAN	OPIOID	ACH	LEPTIN	AMYLIN	?
Formerly or currently FDA approved										
Amphetamine	1930s	x	x	x						
Phentermine	1960s		x							
Phenylpropanolamine	1960s		x							
Fenfluramine	1970s			x						
Dexfenfluramine	1990s			x						
Fen-phen	1990s		x	x						
Sibutramine	1990s	x	x	x						
Lorcaserin	2010s			x						
Phentermine + topiramate	2010s		x							x
Failed FDA approval										
Rimonabant	2000s				x					
Combinations in development										
Naltrexone + buproprion	2010s	x	x			x	x			
Bupropion + zonisamide	2010s	x	x				x			x
Metreleptin + pramlintide	2010s							x	x	

Note: x indicates neurotransmitter or hormone that is known to be affected. DA, dopamine; NE, norepinephrine; SER, serotonin; CAN, cannabinoid; ACh, acetylcholine; ?, mechanism of action unknown. This table illustrates the relatively recent trend to explore the clinical utility of (a) drugs that alter neurotransmission of systems other than dopamine, norepinephrine, and serotonin, and (b) combinations of drugs.

anisms (Table 7.2). This approach is similar to that provided by the diverse pharmacological properties of amphetamine alone and the fen-phen combination. One such new combination is phentermine plus topiramate (a drug having anticonvulsant properties).

What is the current status of available medications for weight loss?

- In 2013 only four drugs have FDA approval in the United States for reduction of body weight: the psychoactive drugs phentermine, phentermine/topiramate combination, and lorcaserin and the lipase inhibitor orlistat (Adan, 2013).
- Medications for weight loss are recommended for use in the event that counseling for behavioral changes such as modifications in eating habits (dieting), changes in lifestyle, and exercise produce insufficient loss of weight (Chugh & Sharma, 2012).
- Approved medications, when combined with changes in eating habits, lifestyle, and exercise, can be expected to produce modest (5–10%) loss of body weight (Colman et al., 2012), but even this modest weight loss can diminish risk of cardiovascular disease and diabetes type II (Heal et al., 2009).
- The currently limited effectiveness of medications for producing weight loss allows dieting, exercise, changes in lifestyle, and bariatric surgery to be regarded as among the more effective treatments for obesity (Lagerros & Rossner, 2012).

The search for a potent and relatively safe drug to inhibit appetite and produce weight loss continues, propelled by advances in the study of neurochemical and neuroendocrine mechanisms that control eating and body weight, by consumers' general acceptance and appetite for psychoactive medications, and by the pharmaceutical industry's commitment to develop a product that will satisfy the consumer demand. Why, after approximately 60 years of searching for such a potent and safe drug, has so relatively little progress been made?

WHAT HAS BEEN THE PROBLEM WITH WEIGHT-LOSS DRUGS?

(No Drug Has Only One Effect.)

Anne has been handed a prescription for orlistat and has been instructed regarding its use. She is to take the medication prior to a meal, unless it is a meal that contains no fat. If the meal contains no fat, the orlistat will not be needed to block the absorption of fat. But if the meal contains fat, orlistat will prevent the absorption of that fat. She is smart enough to see that if she could manage to regularly eat meals having no fat, that she probably wouldn't be overweight and would not be holding a prescription for orlistat. She also can see that the warning of some unpleasant side effects (the oily stools, fecal urgency, and a few others), when orlistat is taken prior to eating that deep-fried haddock and French fries, will challenge her commitment to continue her use of orlistat.

The major reason for the halting progress in the development of psychoactive medications for obesity is the fact that all of the drugs approved (or very nearly approved) by the FDA have worrisome side effects.

Amphetamine. The principal difficulties with amphetamine are related to the fact that the appetite-reducing effects of amphetamine show tolerance. As tolerance develops, the daily dose of amphetamine necessary to suppress appetite increases to the point that it is sufficient to induce symptoms of psychosis and increase the likelihood of addiction (Berman et al., 2009). So marked are the symptoms of psychosis that users of large daily doses of amphetamine have been mistaken for having schizophrenia (Berman et al., 2009).

Despite the strong recommendations by the FDA and others to avoid prescribing amphetamine to treat obesity (Berman et al., 2009), amphetamine and other drugs having similar pharmacological properties (e.g., methylphenidate) continue to be available to those people wanting to use such drugs to lose weight. The principal legal avenue to gain access to amphetamine-like substances for the purpose of weight loss is through the off-label prescription use of these drugs, which are routinely prescribed for other FDA-approved purposes, most notably, the treatment of ADHD (Wigal, 2009). Such off-label use of amphetamine continues because the appetite-suppressant effects of the drug are potent and dose related (Silverstone & Kyriakides, 1982), despite side effects that can include symptoms of psychosis, addiction or substance abuse, insomnia, irritability, tremor, excessive perspiration, dry mouth, and gastrointestinal distress (Munro & Ford, 1982).

It is not surprising that amphetamine might have effects that are undesired. Amphetamine enhances the synaptic neurotransmission of dopamine, norepinephrine, and serotonin at synapses distributed throughout the brain—neurotransmitter systems known to be important for psychological processes such as cognition, emotion, pleasure, and movement. Thus, amphetamine—a potent psychomotor stimulant drug—essentially packs an extensive pharmacological wallop to the brain that is not limited to the desired main effect

of inhibition of appetite for food. Amphetamine simply is not a drug that selectively inhibits appetite for food. Amphetamine also enhances noradrenergic neurotransmission in the peripheral autonomic nervous system, which
would account for a variety of side effects related to cardiovascular and
gastrointestinal processes. Altogether, the mixture of amphetamine's adverse consequences, including unpleasant peripheral autonomic effects, drug-
induced psychosis, and potential for addiction, warn against prescribing amphetamine for its appetite-suppressing properties. Amphetamine's benefit/
risk profile for treatment of obesity is simply not favorable (Kolanowski,
1999).

Phentermine. The FDA in 1959 approved phentermine for treatment of
obesity. Compared with amphetamine, phentermine's effects on neurotransmission are relatively more limited, and phentermine's psychomotor stimulant properties are somewhat attenuated. Phentermine is identified principally
as a norepinephrine-enhancing agent (Table 7.2), having anorectic properties that are dose related (Silverstone & Kyriakides, 1982). Phentermine remains available for prescription as an appetite-suppressant treatment, despite
showing tolerance and many of the same side effects as does amphetamine
(Munro & Ford, 1982); rapid heart rate and transient hypertension can occur
and warn against using phentermine in people who have high blood pressure
(Ioannides-Demos, Proietto, & McNeil, 2005; Kaplan, 2005). Taken together, the benefits and risks of phentermine make it a drug best used for
short-term treatment in combination with diet and exercise (Zhaoping et al.,
2005).

Phenylpropanolamine. Phenylpropanolamine, perhaps best known for its
properties as a nasal decongestant, has been used alone and in combination
with caffeine for its relatively weak appetite-suppressant effects (Silverstone
& Kyriakides, 1982). Similar to phentermine, phenylpropanolamine principally enhances norepinephrine neurotransmission in the brain and in the
peripheral nervous system. For some years available as a nonprescription
medication, phenylpropanolamine in 2000 was limited to prescription status
in the United States, due to concern regarding its potential for causing cerebral hemorrhage (particularly in women). Phenylpropanolamine's benefit/
risk profile is not favorable for use as an appetite-suppressant drug (Campbell
& Mathys, 2001).

Fenfluramine and dexfenfluramine. Fenfluramine and its D-isomer dexfenfluramine were approved for use as appetite-suppressant drugs first in Europe (1963 and 1985, respectively) and then in the United States (1973 and

1996, respectively). Both drugs are known principally for their ability to enhance serotonin neurotransmission by inhibiting reuptake and increasing release of synaptic serotonin, and they have essentially no psychomotor stimulant properties. Although the results of clinical trials included few adverse effects, approval for the use of these drugs was removed in 1997 following reports of damage to heart valves and pulmonary hypertension (Kolanowski, 1999).

Fenfluramine was combined with phentermine for off-label use for suppression of appetite following demonstrations that this fen-phen combination was more effective than either drug alone, apparently without producing untoward side effects (Weintraub, 1992; Weintraub, Hasday, Mushlin, & Lockwood, 1984). That off-label clinical tryout, prompting approximately 18 million prescriptions for fen-phen (Hirsch, 1998), was short-lived once it became known that some people treated with the fen-phen cocktail developed serious cardiovascular abnormalities. Those serious side effects were ultimately attributed to the effects of fenfluramine (not phentermine), resulting in the removal of approved status for fenfluramine and dexfenfluramine (Campbell & Mathys, 2001). Despite the short clinical life and limited success of fen-phen, the fact that this particular drug combination was effective for producing weight loss did teach a potentially useful lesson that encouraged further exploration of drug combinations for the treatment of obesity.

Sibutramine. Sibutramine combines in one drug the ability to enhance both serotonin and norepinephrine (and dopamine) neurotransmission, similar to the effects achieved by combining fenfluramine and phentermine in fen-phen. Approved in 1998 by the FDA to be used in combination with dieting, sibutramine was effective for producing dose-related (Kolanowski, 1999), modest (5–10%) loss of weight when combined with nonpharmacological therapy for obesity (Kaplan, 2005), which could be maintained for up to two years in some clients (Ioannides-Demos, Proietto, & McNeil, 2005). Sibutramine's ability to increase heart rate and blood pressure somewhat limited its utility to those obese people without a history of cardiovascular abnormalities (Campbell & Mathys, 2001). Although other side effects of sibutramine are relatively tolerable (e.g., constipation, headache, dry mouth, insomnia), cumulative clinical experience with sibutramine revealed that the drug increases the risk of heart attack or stroke, ultimately leading to the FDA's 2010 decision to remove sibutramine from the market (Kang & Park, 2012).

Lorcaserin. Lorcaserin has been heralded as providing a novel approach for pharmacological inhibition of appetite, because its presumed mechanism of action is different from those of drugs that preceded it. Lorcaserin is a selective agonist of subtype 2C receptors for serotonin; thus, in contrast to drugs having indirect effects on *all* serotonin receptor subtypes by virtue of inhibiting serotonin reuptake or enhancing release of serotonin into synapses (e.g., fenfluramine, dexfenfluramine, sibutramine, tesofensine), lorcaserin's effect appears limited to enhancing activity at only one serotonin receptor subtype. Lorcaserin's greater selectivity for enhancement of serotonin neurotransmission might represent an opportunity to retain the serotonin-mediated anorectic effects of these other drugs while having fewer side effects. But remember, no drug has only one effect, so it is not surprising that lorcaserin can cause dizziness, headache, insomnia, fatigue, and dry mouth. These potential side effects, combined with the fact that the percentage of body weight loss induced by lorcaserin is modest (Fidler et al., 2011) and findings that rats treated with lorcaserin show signs of carcinogenicity, resulted in reluctance of the FDA to approve lorcaserin (Kang & Park, 2012). In other words, lorcaserin's perceived risks at first appeared to outweigh the modest benefit for reduction of appetite and loss of weight. Further study of the submitted data, however, resulted in FDA approval for lorcaserin in 2012 with recommendations delineating the appropriate conditions for use for treatment of obesity (Colman et al., 2012).

Topiramate plus phentermine. Topiramate plus phentermine combines two drugs having anorectic properties: topiramate, an agent having antiepileptic properties, combined with a lower dose of phentermine (a previously approved drug known to enhance norepinephrine neurotransmission). Topiramate's ability to reduce appetite was first apparent as a side effect of its use for reducing seizures (Adan, 2013), providing a fine example of how one user's side effect can be another user's main effect. Although topiramate can produce a variety of annoying side effects (dizziness, altered taste, fatigue, somnolence, and memory impairment, among others), and although there are concerns about its ability to increase heart rate and its teratogenicity (Kang & Park, 2012), the FDA in 2012 issued its approval of this drug combination with cautionary recommendations for proper use for treatment of obesity (Colman et al., 2012).

Orlistat. Although orlistat is not a psychotropic medication, it is effective for reducing body weight owing to its ability to inhibit the intestinal enzymatic process necessary to absorb ingested fat. Thus, you can eat your fat and not have it stored too, as long as you can tolerate the gastrointestinal side effects. Those side effects, including oily stools and spotting, fecal incontinence, abdominal bloating, flatulence, and dyspepsia, are common, but they tend to subside, especially when the patient learns to more effectively reduce ingestion of fats (Kang & Park, 2012). The irony here is that the side effects ultimately can become useful by providing negative reinforcement for ingestion of fats, thereby facilitating decreased ingestion of fats (Kaplan, 2005), that is, dieting! Orlistat has numerous other side effects (Campbell & Mathys, 2001), including malabsorption of fat-soluble vitamins (A, D, E, and K), which can be compensated by supplementation. Orlistat was approved by the FDA in 1999 and is still available in 2013. It is recommended for treatment of obesity when combined with exercise and dieting, and orlistat is to be taken prior to each meal (except when a meal includes no fat).

Rimonabant.   Rimonabant, a novel selective cannabinoid CB1 receptor antagonist, produces weight loss in a dose-related manner and improves markers of metabolic syndrome (Van Gaal et al., 2005), indicating reduced risk for cardiovascular disease and diabetes type II. Although it was briefly available as an anti-obesity medication in Europe, rimonabant failed in 2007 to gain FDA approval, owing to reports of depression and suicidal ideation in some patients treated with it (Christensen, Kristensen, Bartels, Bliddal, & Astrup, 2007). Despite the problems that beset rimonabant, it is probably too soon to give up hope that drugs that affect cannabinoid receptors can become candidates for treatment of obesity (Heal et al., 2012; Witkamp, 2011).

Herbal dietary supplements.   There is a relatively modest published literature that considers the utility of various herbal substances available as dietary supplements for the treatment of obesity (Hasani-Ranjbar, Nayebi, Larijani, & Abdollahi, 2009). Among these, the anorectic effects of ephedrine (which has amphetamine-like properties) combined with caffeine is perhaps the most impressive in terms of its effectiveness for producing loss of weight (Hasani-Ranjbar et al., 2009; Saper, Eisenberg, & Phillips, 2004), but the use of this combination can have worrisome effects on heart rate and blood pressure (Greenway & Bray, 2010; Ioannides-Demos, Proietto, & McNeil, 2005). Relatively little published evidence supports the use of herbal remedies or dietary supplements that can be considered to be effective and relatively safe for the treatment of obesity (Saper et al., 2004). Despite insufficient evidence to recommend use of these substances, nearly one-third of people who report a serious attempt to lose weight report having used a dietary supplement to facilitate their efforts, and the incidence of use varies with ethnicity (Pillitteri et al., 2008).

In summary, regardless of the presumed mechanism of action for the appetite-suppressant effects of the anti-obesity drugs that have been used over the past 60 years, in each and every instance no weight-loss drug has only that one effect—they all have side effects that can potentially compromise their clinical utility, whether or not the effects of a drug are pharmacologically broad or complex (e.g., amphetamine, sibutramine) or pharmacologically selective (e.g., lorcaserin, rimonabant). The side effects range from merely annoying to potentially lethal. The use of drugs to produce weight loss is a history of the need to assess the benefits and the risks for each drug, in order to determine whether the balance between the two can justify the use of the drug.

HOW MUCH WEIGHT LOSS IS ENOUGH TO TOLERATE ADVERSE EFFECTS?

(Compromise on Benefits and Risks is a Realistic Goal for Pharmacotherapy)

Brian stands 5 feet 8 inches and weighed 255 pounds when he started using lorcaserin every day. It has been six months now, and he has lost approximately 4% of his body weight—he now weighs 245 pounds. He has a headache virtually every single day, and he believes it is a side effect of the drug. In addition, the fatigue he feels makes it difficult to get off of the couch and into the gym. And his attempts at dieting have come to annoy him, because he keeps falling off that wagon. So, as far as Brian is concerned, he has struggled to maintain a diet, has a headache every day, and feels tired much of the time, with the end result of still appearing a bit like a human bowling ball after many months of trying. He wonders if it has been worth the aggravation.

A persistent challenge for pharmacological treatment of obesity is the need to find a reasonable point of compromise regarding the benefits and the risks of any potential drug therapy for obesity. To illustrate this point, let's consider the rationale supporting the evolution of drug therapy for obesity, beginning with amphetamine (Table 7.1). Amphetamine can elicit potent, dose-related inhibition of appetite and loss of body weight, but amphetamine is also potent for providing side effects, including some very serious ones, such as cardiovascular adverse events, risk of addiction and abuse, and amphetamine-induced psychosis. The question for amphetamine, then, becomes whether or not those serious risks outweigh the impressive anorectic effect of amphetamine; for example, an acute dose of amphetamine can inhibit eating by nearly 50% in humans (Silverstone & Kyriakides, 1982). The prevailing view has become that the risk outweighs the benefit, and now physicians, therapists, and patients are strongly advised not to use amphetamine to produce loss of weight.

Where does one go from there? One option is to search for a drug that is safer than amphetamine, recognizing that diminishing the side effect profile may or may not be accompanied by a diminished main effect. Phentermine then enters the arena in 1959 as a nonstimulant weight-loss drug, with side effects including increased heart rate and transient hypertension but, altogether, fewer risks than amphetamine and, fortunately, with relatively similar anorectic potency (Silverstone, 1972; Silverstone & Kyriakides, 1982).

Thus, phentermine improves upon amphetamine, but is less than ideal and is recommended for only short-term use. Continuing research brings fenfluramine in 1973, off-label use of the fen-phen combination in 1992, and dexfenfluramine in 1996. Fenfluramine can produce dose-related inhibition of eating of magnitude comparable to that induced by amphetamine (Silverstone & Kyriakides, 1982). And the fen-phen combination permits the use of lower doses of each drug (compared with their clinical use when given alone) to provide anorectic effects equal to that achieved using either drug alone and, at first glance, apparently fewer side effects (Weintraub et al., 1984). But jubilation is brief once it is discovered that fenfluramine and dexfenfluramine can increase risk of pulmonary hypertension (Abenhaim et al., 1996) and that fen-phen can cause heart valve abnormalities (Connolly et al., 1997). Fenfluramine, dexfenfluramine, and the fen-phen combination become banned in 1997 from being prescribed as pharmacotherapy for obesity, because the risks appear to outweigh the benefits. Now what?

Perhaps we can search for a better compromise regarding benefits and risks, by further lowering the expectations for anorectic potency in the hopes that the side effect profile also will be reduced. This adjustment in goals ultimately brings FDA approval for sibutramine, orlistat, lorcaserin, and the topiramate-phentermine combination. What attributes do these four pharmacological options share? They have these three characteristics in common: (a) the ability to produce only modest loss of body weight (between 5% and 10%), (b) side effect profiles that are mainly tolerable, and (c) the recommended use of these drugs as adjunctive therapy combined with dieting, increasing exercise, and changes in lifestyle (Colman et al., 2012; Derosa & Maffioli, 2012; Kang & Park, 2012). Let's take a closer look at the relationship among those three characteristics:

- The fact that the anorectic and weight loss main effects of these drugs are only modest raises the bar for expectations regarding side effects of these drugs. After all, if the benefit of the drug is merely modest, then what would be the point of tolerating significant side effects? Given this perspective, the more modest the desired effect of a drug, the relatively more salient the side effects in the overall consideration of the drug's clinical utility, making it less likely such a drug would smoothly sail through an approval process.

- The fact that the main effects of these drugs are modest, and the side effects are not insignificant, makes it difficult to justify the clinical use of *only* pharmacological therapy. Thus, the justification for approval of such a drug is aided by the qualifying recommendation that the drug be used as an adjunct to nonpharmacological treatment such as dieting, exercise, and changes in lifestyle.
- The fact that the drugs are recommended for use as adjuncts to behavioral therapy diminishes the perceived value of the drug as effective therapy, increases the perceived potential for effectiveness of nonpharmacological therapies, and reminds clinicians and patients that overeating, overweight, and obesity are biopsychosocial problems.

Thus, in 2013 the best psychotropic medications for treatment of obesity are not "magic bullet" pharmacological solutions for obesity. Each drug is merely one pharmacological clinical tool to be used along with other nonpharmacological clinical tools to treat the biopsychosocial problem of obesity.

Can we do better than this? Will the horizon reveal the possibility of drugs with greater effects on loss of body weight, fewer side effects, or both? As new drugs are developed that selectively target different neurochemical processes in the brain, as well as different neuroendocrine mechanisms in the gastrointestinal tract and peripheral nervous system, the holy grail treatment for obesity might be found (Chugh & Sharma, 2012; Heal et al., 2012; Kennett & Clifton, 2010; Lagerros & Rossner, 2012; Witkamp, 2011). Or it might not be found (Hirsch, 1998; Wilding, 2000), because it might not exist.

CAN A LARGER DOSAGE PRODUCE GREATER WEIGHT LOSS WITHOUT INCREASING ADVERSE EFFECTS?

(Desired Effects and Unwanted Effects Are Related to Dosage)

Melinda has used topiramate plus phentermine for six months now and has not lost an ounce of weight. So she is going to ask for a larger dose to be prescribed, despite the fact that her physician warns her that some people just don't lose weight when using the drugs. Well, Melinda does not want to be one of the people who are not helped by the medication, and she knows that larger doses are effective in some people.

Although it is easy enough to ask someone to have faith that the magnitude of each of the effects of a drug is related to the dosage of the drug, does that assertion play out in a clinically meaningful way for drugs used to treat obesity? Have sufficient data been collected on main effects and side effects of anti-obesity drugs to begin to answer that question? Let's address this issue by taking a look at such data for two drugs that have presented marginal cases to the FDA for their approval for clinical use: lorcaserin, which has succeeded in gaining approval, and rimonabant, which has failed.

Rimonabant.   There are published reports of the effects of rimonabant on main effects and side effects in large-scale, multicenter, randomized, double-blind, placebo-controlled studies in which two dosages of rimonabant were used in humans eating a reduced calorie diet (Pi-Sunyer et al., 2006; Van Gaal et al., 2005). These reports present sufficient data to consider whether main effects and side effects are related to dosage and whether main or side effects are differentially sensitive to dosage. There are numerous noteworthy findings regarding dosages and effects:

- Over 52 weeks, rimonabant significantly reduced body weight and waist circumference compared with placebo. The effect of rimonabant on weight loss was dose related: a significantly greater proportion of subjects receiving the 20 mg dose lost ≥5% of baseline body weight compared with subjects receiving the 5 mg dose. In addition, a greater proportion of people receiving the 20 mg dose lost ≥10% of body weight compared with placebo, whereas this was not true for subjects receiving the 5 mg dose. The effect of rimonabant on waist circumference was also dependent upon dose: 20 mg, but not 5 mg, significantly reduced waist circumference. Thus, the effects of rimonabant on loss of weight and on waist circumference were dose dependent (Van Gaal et al., 2005; see also Pi-Sunyer et al., 2006).
- Although 5 mg rimonabant produced significant loss of body weight, this dosage did not significantly change a variety of metabolic and cardiovascular risk factors (e.g., measures of cholesterol, triglycerides, fasting glucose, and insulin), whereas the 20 mg dose did improve a variety of these measures (Van Gaal et al., 2005). Thus, although 5 mg rimonabant can produce loss of body weight, it does not significantly improve indices of metabolic and cardiovascular risk, whereas 20 mg produces a magnitude of weight loss sufficient to improve numerous indices of risk.
- The total numbers of subjects reporting adverse events were similar for the 5 mg and 20 mg dose groups, and both groups reported

more adverse events than subjects receiving placebo. In addition, when considering a list of 15 "serious" adverse events (e.g., psychiatric, cardiac, gastrointestinal, renal), subjects receiving 20 mg reported only 8 of those 15 categories more frequently than did the group receiving 5 mg. On the other hand, when considering adverse events that led to discontinuation of the medication and dropping out of the study, subjects receiving 20 mg reported for 14 of the 17 categories more frequently than did the group receiving 5 mg. Thus, adverse events were reported with similar frequency for subjects receiving 5 mg or 20 mg rimonabant, but there was a tendency for adverse events caused by 20 mg to result more frequently in discontinuation. Moreover, although the absolute number of reports of adverse *psychiatric* events leading to discontinuation was relatively small for both the 5 mg and 20 mg groups, the proportional incidence of these reports was clearly greater for the 20 mg dose (Van Gaal et al., 2005; see also Pi-Sunyer et al., 2006).

Taken together, the results suggest that the 20 mg dose, which is more effective than 5 mg *both* for producing body weight loss and for reducing metabolic and cardiovascular risk factors, is the better choice for treatment of obesity, although the likelihood of discontinuing treatment may be greater for 20 mg than for 5 mg for some patients.

In summary, the effects of rimonabant in humans in multicenter clinical trials depend upon dosage. Taking into consideration the effects of rimonabant on main effects and side effects, the findings do not support the use of 5 mg rimonabant, because (a) 5 mg elicits reports of adverse events comparable to that of 20 mg, (b) 5 mg produces significantly less loss of weight than does 20 mg, and (c) 5 mg does not improve risk factors for metabolic and cardiovascular problems. These findings do appear to support the use of 20 mg of rimonabant, because 20 mg produces loss of weight accompanied by improvement in metabolic and cardiovascular risk factors, and although the reports of adverse events are greater than those after placebo treatment, the adverse events may be tolerable when weighed against the benefits. Or are they? Is rimonabant effective enough and relatively safe enough to be used?

Depressed mood was reported by approximately 2–4% of subjects taking 5 or 20 mg rimonabant (Pi-Sunyer et al. 2006; Van Gaal et al., 2005). Although those percentages are rather small, and not so different from subjects given placebo in those studies (approximately 1–3% incidence for placebo), reports of psychiatric adverse events and suicidal ideation during rimonabant treatment have caused great concern (Christensen et al., 2007; Johansson, Neovius, DeSantis, Rossner, & Neovius, 2009; Kang & Park, 2012; Padwal &

Majumdar, 2007; Rucker, Padwal, Li, Curioni, & Lau, 2007). This concern appears justified given that the clinical trials had excluded subjects with a history of depression or suicide attempt (Van Gaal et al., 2005), raising the possibility that the estimates of rimonabant's negative effects on mood were too conservative. Thus, this drug, which had some potential to induce depression and the possibility of suicide, and relatively modest benefit for producing weight loss, was removed from the market in Europe and did not receive FDA approval in the United States. On balance, considering the modest benefits and the potential for great risk for *some* users, rimonabant has been rejected as a weight-loss medication, but the search for an effective and relatively safe weight-loss drug that alters endogenous cannabinoid neurotransmission continues (Meye, Trezza, Vanderschuren, Ramakers, & Adan, 2012; Vemuri, Janero, & Makriyannis, 2008).

Lorcaserin. Lorcaserin presents a case with some similarities to that of rimonabant but with a different outcome following results obtained in clinical trials. Let's look at findings from a large-scale, multicenter, randomized, double-blind, placebo-controlled study in which the effects of two dosage regimens of lorcaserin (10 mg once daily or 10 mg twice daily) were studied in humans receiving diet and exercise counseling (Fidler et al., 2011):

- Over 52 weeks, 10 mg of lorcaserin once daily or twice daily produced statistically significant, modest, 5–10% loss of weight (compared with placebo treatment); 10 mg twice daily produced greater weight loss than 10 mg once daily. Thus, the effect of lorcaserin on weight loss was dose related (Fidler et al., 2011).
- Both dosage regimens produced decreases in waist circumference and in body mass index (compared with placebo), although the twice-daily regimen was more effective than the once-daily regimen for reducing body mass index (Fidler et al., 2011). Thus, the effect on body mass index, but not waist circumference, was dose dependent.
- The twice-daily 10 mg lorcaserin regimen significantly reduced total body fat and increased lean body mass (compared with placebo), but the once-daily 10 mg dosage did neither (Fidler et al., 2011). Thus, the effects of lorcaserin on total body fat and lean body mass were dose dependent.
- The twice-daily and once-daily 10 mg regimens had similar significant favorable effects on triglycerides and high-density lipoprotein cholesterol (Fidler et al., 2011). Thus, the effects of lorcaserin were not dose related for these risk factors.

- Both dosage regimens of lorcaserin produced greater reporting of adverse events than did placebo. The twice-daily 10 mg regimen produced greater reporting of every single category of adverse event than did the once-daily 10 mg regimen. Overall, the reporting of adverse events from either lorcaserin regimen did not indicate cause for concern (Fidler et al., 2011), but the adverse events of lorcaserin appeared to be dose related.

In summary, the effects of lorcaserin on loss of body weight, body mass index, total body fat, and lean body mass were dose related. In addition, the reporting of adverse events was dose related, but adverse events reported were not considered to be of major concern (headache being the most frequently reported, and depressed mood being the least frequently reported). Either dosage regimen of lorcaserin would appear to be useful (Fidler et al., 2011), with the once-daily 10 mg dosage producing marginal effects on weight loss with some complaints of adverse events. The twice-daily 10 mg dosage appears to produce greater, but still modest, effects on weight loss and is accompanied by more frequent complaints of adverse events. Compared with rimonabant, lorcaserin produces similar effects for modest loss of weight but appears to have a more favorable side effect profile. In addition, like rimonabant, lorcaserin is reported to improve risk factors for metabolic and cardiovascular disorders (Smith et al., 2010).

Lorcaserin has been approved by the FDA for use as an adjunct combined with dieting and exercise for treatment of obesity (Colman et al., 2012). On balance, with the modest effect of lorcaserin on weight loss, together with a side effect profile that does not yet appear to be worrisome and consumer demand for effective weight-loss medication, the FDA approved lorcaserin to enter the market amid continuing concerns about its effectiveness and safety (Bai & Wang, 2011; Bays, 2011). Postmarketing surveillance of lorcaserin will reveal whether lorcaserin's side effects become a concern (Colman et al., 2012).

Dose-response studies can reveal differences in magnitude of effects on main effects and side effects, as has been illustrated for rimonabant and lorcaserin. A thoughtful reading of the results of the clinical trials that used multiple dosages of rimonabant (Van Gaal et al., 2005; Pi-Sunyer et al., 2006) or lorcaserin (Fidler et al., 2011) reveals information that provides additional perspective:

- Conducting clinical trials demands extraordinary resources; they are time-consuming and expensive, even more so when multiple dosages of a drug are studied.

- With resources stretched thin, savings can be had by diminishing the assessment of adverse events. Most clinical trials provide more data and statistical analysis for main effects than for side effects.
- When the data regarding side effects are too few to be entirely convincing, the importance of postmarketing surveillance regarding adverse events is amplified.
- Regardless of the published findings for any dosage of any drug, the findings will not necessarily predict the main effect or side effect outcomes for that individual patient who walks into the physician's office.

Finally, if the results of a clinical trial reveal that a lower dose of a drug produces a relatively small loss of body weight, but also elicits fewer reports of side effects, might it be possible that the small dose could be even more useful when combined with a second drug? Are combinations of small doses of drugs that inhibit appetite a better target for the continuing search for novel pharmacological treatments for obesity?

WILL DRUG COMBINATIONS HAVE PREDICTABLE BENEFITS FOR WEIGHT REDUCTION?

(Drug Interactions Can Be Potent and Unpredictable.)

Although Anita discontinued her use of phentermine, because it seemed to cause dizziness, her physician wishes for her to try it again, but at a lower dose. Her doctor believes that using a lower dose might avoid the dizziness, and that the lower dose of phentermine, combined with a second drug (topiramate) that also can inhibit appetite, might help Anita to lose weight.

The idea that small doses of two prescription psychotropic medications combined for treatment of obesity could be more effective with fewer adverse effects was put to the test for the combination of fenfluramine and phentermine, with rather impressive initial results (Weintraub et al., 1984): The weight loss produced by the combination of fenfluramine plus phentermine was (a) more effective than placebo, (b) equivalent to weight loss produced by larger doses of either drug given alone, and (c) elicited fewer reports of adverse events than did larger doses of either drug given alone. This knowledge eventually led to the off-label clinical use of fenfluramine plus phentermine to treat obesity, which ended abruptly when reports of serious cardiovascular adverse events became known (Connolly et al., 1997). Although the clinical experience with fen-phen ultimately ended in failure, one useful lesson learned was that smaller doses of two drugs combined might be a successful approach for increasing the magnitude of the anorectic effects of psychotropic medications.

There are recent efforts evaluating the effectiveness of drug combinations to reduce appetite and produce weight loss (Greenway & Bray, 2010; Ioannides-Demos, Piccenna, & McNeil, 2011). Let's take a look at several of the more interesting ones.

Orlistat and sibutramine. The combination of orlistat, which inhibits the absorption of fat, and sibutramine, which decreases appetite presumably by its ability to enhance serotonin neurotransmission in the brain, has not been successful: The reduction of body weight produced by the drug combination was no greater than that produced by sibutramine alone (Sari, Balci, Cakir, Altunbas, & Karayalcin, 2004). One interpretation of this outcome is that when combining a drug that has effects outside the brain with a drug that has effects within the brain, the effect of the drug that alters brain neurochemistry is the determining factor, and the added peripheral manipulation is of little consequence (Greenway & Bray, 2010).

Topiramate and phentermine. This combines phentermine, approved by the FDA for treatment of obesity, with topiramate, used clinically for its antiepileptic properties but having the side effect of producing weight loss. One recent multicenter, randomized, double-blind, placebo-controlled clinical trial studied the effect of a combination of 7.5 mg phentermine plus 46 mg topiramate (and a second combination that doubled the doses) on weight loss, waist circumference, body mass index, metabolic measures, and adverse events (Gadde et al., 2011). The 7.5 mg dose of phentermine is below the typical dosage range (15–37.5 mg/day) recommended when used alone to treat obesity. A follow-up study measured the effects of these same drug combinations for 56 successive weeks (Garvey et al., 2012). The subjects in these studies were instructed to voluntarily reduce food intake by 500 kcal per day and to implement lifestyle changes. Highlights of the findings include the following:

- Both dose combinations of topiramate plus phentermine produced greater body weight loss than did placebo, but the larger dose combination did not produce significantly greater loss of body weight than the smaller one (Gadde et al, 2011; Garvey et al., 2012). Thus, the combination of topiramate and phentermine was effective for producing weight loss in sustained treatment, but the effects were not dose related in these two studies. An important exception to this conclusion was the fact that after 108 weeks of treatment, subjects with class III obesity ($\geq$40 kg/m^2 body mass index) had lost more weight when given the larger dose combination compared with the smaller dose combination (Garvey et al., 2012).

- A similar pattern of results was observed for changes in waist circumference, concentration of lipids, glycemia, and blood pressure (Gadde et al, 2011; Garvey et al., 2012).

- Adverse events generally were reported more frequently with both dose combinations than with placebo, and reporting of adverse events appeared to be dose related: The larger dose combination produced a greater frequency of adverse events for 17 of the 22 categories of adverse events (Gadde et al., 2011). Neither dose combination statistically significantly increased reporting of incidences of depression, but both dose combinations significantly increased reporting of disturbances in attention (Gadde et al., 2011). Psychiatric adverse events were minimal after 108 weeks of treatment (Garvey et al., 2012).

- Some obese subjects in the study were identified as being at risk for type II diabetes. For these people, by the end of the 108 weeks of the study, the lower dose combination had produced a 54% reduction in the progression to type II diabetes, and the higher dose combination had produced a 76% reduction (Garvey et al., 2012).

In summary, the two dose combinations of topiramate plus phentermine were effective for producing weight loss and for improving risk factors for metabolic and cardiovascular diseases, without apparent significant adverse effects. Thus, each of the two dose combinations seem to be effective, and the larger dose combination may be more effective for treating more severe levels of obesity. Moreover, each of the two dose combinations can reduce or delay progression to type II diabetes. Finally, the fact that subjects in the studies showed benefits without worrisome risks at the two-year mark following initiation of treatment suggests that the combination of topiramate and phentermine may be useful psychotropic medication for the initiation and the maintenance of weight loss when combined with diet and lifestyle changes. The FDA in 2012 approved this drug combination for clinical use. At present, no other psychotropic medication is approved by the FDA for long-term treatment of obesity.

Other combinations of drugs being considered for treatment of obesity (Chugh & Sharma, 2012; Heal et al., 2012; Kennett & Clifton, 2010; Witkamp, 2011) include the following (Table 7.2):

- *Naltrexone and bupropion.* Bupropion inhibits the reuptake of dopamine and norepinephrine and is an antagonist for nicotinic receptors for the neurotransmitter acetylcholine. It has been approved for clinical treatment of depression and addiction to nicotine. Its clinical use for treatment of smoking cessation revealed bupropion's anorectic effect (Hurt et al., 1997). Naltrexone is an antagonist for mu- and kappa-opioid receptor subtypes and has been approved for clinical treatment of alcoholism.
- *Bupropion and zonisamide.* Bupropion is here combined with zonisamide, which has been approved for clinical use for its anticonvulsant properties. Zonisamide, as well as the anticonvulsant topiramate, apparently has anorectic effects when given alone (Witkamp, 2011).
- *Pramlintide and metreleptin.* Pramlintide is an analogue of the peptide hormone amylin, which has anorectic effects. Metreleptin is recombinant human leptin, which also has anorectic properties. This novel approach showed promise in early clinical research but has more recently faced concerns about safety (Tam, Lecoultre, & Ravussin, 2011).

The most recent psychotropic medication approved by the FDA for treatment of obesity is the topiramate and phentermine combination. It is too soon to know if this drug combination will have greater clinical success than did fen-phen, but the drug combination approach is spurred on by the successful use of drug combinations to treat other medical conditions, such as hypertension and diabetes (Greenway & Bray, 2010). The effectiveness of the combination of topiramate and phentermine also has been examined in preclinical studies, which showed encouraging results in rats that become obese when they have free access to highly palatable foods.

CAN ANIMAL MODELS TEACH US ABOUT PHARMACOTHERAPY FOR OBESITY?

Ronnie the Rat is fat. But he has been told that if he lets Dr. Model put a fistula in his stomach (a hole!), Ronnie will be able to eat and eat forever and never get fatter. Better still, lapping up all that fatty food will drive the release of dopamine, stimulating dopamine receptors in the nucleus accumbens in his brain, making Ronnie feel mighty good as long as he keeps tasting the food that then drains out through the fistula in his stomach. What better proof than that for the idea that tasting food is pleasurable, satisfying, and rewarding in direct proportion to the release of dopamine in Ronnie's brain? Dr. Model also has promised Ronnie the Rat that eating with an open fistula in his stomach makes him a rat model for overeating, binge eating, or bulimia. Ronnie likes the idea of being a model. Being a model for big sizes seems like the perfect career for a big eater!

Overeating leading to overweight has been modeled in rodents in a variety of different ways for essentially two purposes: (a) conducting experiments intended to increase understanding of the physiological and neurochemical controls of eating behavior and (b) testing the ability of drugs to decrease appetite, inhibit food intake, and produce loss of body weight, trusting that the animal model has predictive value regarding a drug's potential clinical utility. Examples of useful animal models for obesity include:

- Destruction of the ventromedial area of the hypothalamus, which can produce a rat that overeats and becomes obese
- Surgical removal of the ovaries in female rats, which is followed by overeating and overweight
- Prenatal undernutrition, which can induce overeating and overweight
- Dietary-induced obesity produced by giving rats free access to high-fat or high-sucrose foods or to a wide range of tasty foods
- The *ob/ob* fatty mouse and the *fa/fa* Zucker fatty rat, both genetic models for obesity

These examples of animal models for overeating and obesity, only an handful of models of which have been used (Sclafani, 1984), illustrate methods for surgically altering brain or physiology to induce overeating, manipulating environment to facilitate voluntary overeating, or allowing genetics to produce the obesity. Any one of these models of overeating/obesity can be used to assess for the ability of a drug to inhibit eating and produce loss of body weight. The key to such an analysis is to be certain to determine whether the drug-induced inhibition of food intake (and weight loss) is due to the ability of the drug to reduce appetite and eating specifically—that the drug is not inhibiting ingestion (e.g., inhibiting eating and drinking) and is not inhibiting eating secondary to drug-induced or malaise or changes in other behaviors (e.g., hyperactivity). In fact, a drug that may be a prime candidate for being a clinically useful medication for overeating is one that specifically inhibits appetite for food and food intake and that also induces a behavioral sequence indicative of satiation, and not malaise (Vickers & Clifton, 2012).

There are many examples of the use of animals to assess for effectiveness

of drugs to inhibit eating. Here are a few examples, chosen because they evaluate the effectiveness of drug augmentation, drug combinations, or novel
drugs for inhibition of eating in a context in which rodents are overeating
because they have free or easy access to highly palatable foods.

Drug combinations or augmentation:
- In a model of dietary-induced overeating and obesity in rats, chronic daily administration of phentermine, topiramate, or the combination of phentermine and topiramate inhibits daily food intake and produces sustained loss of body weight (Vickers, Jackson, & Cheetham, 2011).
- In a model of dietary-induced overeating and obesity in rats, chronic daily administration of the intestinal hormone cholecystokinin alone fails to produce loss of weight. Augmentation of daily amylin administration with cholecystokinin enhances the ability of the pancreatic hormone amylin to produce weight loss, and augmentation of combined amylin and leptin administration with cholecystokinin enhances the ability of amylin plus the adipose-derived hormone leptin to produce weight loss (Trevaskis et al., 2010).
- Combining doses of rimonabant and sibutramine that alone are below the threshold for anorectic activity still fail to inhibit eating of a palatable mash food in rats (Tallett, Blundell, & Rodgers, 2010).
- In nondeprived, nonhungry mice eating sweet gelatinized milk "dessert," dexfenfluramine, phentermine, and the norepinephrine reuptake inhibitor thionisoxetine alone and in various combinations produce dose-related inhibition of eating (Rowland, Lo, & Robertson, 2001).

Novel anorectic drugs:
- In a model of dietary-induced overeating and obesity in mice, the experimental cannabinoid CB1 receptor agonist JD5037, whose activity is limited to the periphery (and does not directly affect the brain), is as effective for inhibiting eating as a CB1 agonist that does enter the brain (Tam et al., 2012).
- For rats pressing a lever to obtain palatable sucrose pellets, cannabinoid CB1 inverse agonists (e.g., rimonabant) inhibit eating, produce loss of weight, and induce anxiety-like symptoms in rats, whereas the CB1 neutral antagonist NESS0327 inhibits eating and produces weight loss without inducing anxiety-like symptoms (Meye et al., 2012).

The dietary-induced, or "cafeteria," overeating model and models that encourage rats or mice to overeat by offering select highly palatable foods have reasonable face validity for overeating and weight gain by humans. Rats, mice, and humans find fatty, sweet, and salty foods to be very palatable, and the overeating and gain in weight exhibited by animals having free access to these foods provides a reasonable paradigm in which to measure the effectiveness of a chronically administered drug for inhibiting overeating and for producing loss of body weight. The results of such experiments in animals may predict the effectiveness of a drug for inhibition of overeating and loss of body weight in humans.

TIDBITS ON PSYCHOPHARMACOLOGY LEARNED FROM THE TREATMENT OF OBESITY

The following are brief examples illustrating other principles of pharmacology or recommendations from Part I of this book, taken from the clinical treatment of obesity or from basic research on eating behavior and regulation of body weight:

- *Sensitivity to a drug varies from one individual to another.* This principle is illustrated by the fact that only 48% of people treated with the larger dose of topiramate plus phentermine (15 mg topiramate, 92 mg phentermine daily) experience greater than 10% loss of body weight, and only 5% of these people report any serious adverse events (Gadde et al., 2011). In other words, it works for some people and not for others, and it bothers some people but not others.
- *Sex, age, and genetics can determine the magnitude of effects of a drug.* The average weight loss produced by lorcaserin is greater for Caucasians than for African-American or Hispanic subjects (Fidler et al., 2011).
- *A person's drug history can affect a drug's effectiveness.* Tolerance develops to the appetite-suppressing effects of amphetamine.
- *Culture and community can affect the utility of pharmacotherapy.* Use of dietary supplements for weight loss is more common for African-Americans and Hispanics than for Caucasians (Pillitteri et al., 2008).
- *Drugs can mimic endogenous neurochemicals.* The drug CCK-8, a synthetic biologically active fragment of the intestinal hormone cholecystokinin, inhibits eating in obese men (Pi-Sunyer, Kissileff, Thornton, & Smith, 1982).

- *Drugs can block endogenous neurochemicals.* Blockade of subtype A receptors for the satiety signal endogenous cholecystokinin increases eating in humans (Beglinger, Degen, Matzinger, D'Amato, & Drewe, 2001).
- *Pharmacological effects on brain neurochemistry can be enduring.* Methamphetamine, a drug with anorectic properties that has been used to treat obesity, can produce downregulation of dopamine D2 receptors in the human brain (Volkow et al., 2001).
- *Drugs differ in their potential for addiction.* Following the strong recommendation that amphetamine no longer be used for treatment of obesity, all of the anti-obesity drugs subsequently approved by the FDA have little or no addictive potential.
- *Drugs can alter the organization of a developing brain.* The off-label use of anti-obesity drugs in children and adolescents occurs despite lack of knowledge of the effects of such drugs on the developing human brain (Sherafat-Kazemzadeh, Yanovski, & Yanovski, 2013).
- *Drugs can be demonstrated to be only relatively effective and safe.* All drugs that have ever been approved to treat obesity have side effects.
- *A therapeutic drug is used because it works.* The anticonvulsant drugs topiramate and zonisamide are used to treat obesity because they have anorectic properties, despite the fact that the mechanism(s) by which these drugs inhibit eating is unknown.
- *Dietary supplements may or may not be effective and safe.* Clinical trials have failed to identify dietary supplements for treatment of obesity that are effective and safe (Hasani-Ranjbar et al., 2009).
- *Placebo can have drug-like effects.* In a double-blind, placebo-controlled clinical trial of the effects of lorcaserin on weight loss, 75% of people in the placebo group reported adverse events (Fidler et al., 2011)!
- *Pharmacotherapy is best used as one among several tools, and the role of pharmacotherapy varies for different people and disorders.* Each of the current anti-obesity prescription medications is approved for use as an adjunct to dieting, exercise, and changes in lifestyle.
- *Serendipity can bring new opportunities for pharmacotherapy.* The anticonvulsant drugs topiramate and zonisamide have come to be used as appetite-suppressant drugs owing to the serendipitous discovery of their anorectic effects when being used to prevent seizures.
- *Consumers demand new and better drugs, and successful use encour-*

ages increased use, for better or worse. Millions of prescriptions for fen-phen were written despite lack of convincing evidence regarding the safety of the drug combination (Hirsch, 1998).

- *The FDA attempts to approve new and better drugs.* Lorcaserin and the combination of topiramate plus phentermine acquired FDA-approved status in 2012.
- *Off-label use has its advantages and disadvantages, and health insurance practices can determine accessibility to a drug.* The increased frequency of off-label prescribing of topiramate plus phentermine to treat obesity is likely one factor encouraging the ultimate FDA approval of the drug combination, because the cost of on-label use is more likely to be covered by insurance.
- *Diagnosis guides choice of pharmacotherapy.* People who meet the criterion for class III obesity (≥ 40 kg/m^2 body mass index) lose more weight when given the larger dose of the combination of topiramate plus phentermine than they do with the smaller dose (Garvey et al., 2012).
- *Clients should be active participants in their pharmacotherapy.* More than 60% of users of orlistat discontinue use after approximately one month (Hemo, Endevelt, Porath, Stampfer, & Shai, 2011); this rate of discontinuation is generally greater than that observed in clinical drug trials.

SUMMARY AND PERSPECTIVE

All drugs currently approved by the FDA for treatment of obesity have benefits and risks, and all are approved for use as adjuncts to dieting, exercise, and implementation of changes in lifestyle. Is this state-of-the-art situation good enough? The fact that all of the drugs currently approved are effective for producing only modest loss of weight, even when combined with simultaneous nonpharmacological treatments, is a characteristic that encourages the pharmaceutical industry to continue searching for more effective and safer medications. On the other hand, combining drugs with psychological and social modifications is effective for weight loss and improvement in risk factors for diabetes type II and cardiovascular disease, which can be viewed as the nearly ideal combination of treatments for a biopsychosocial problem such as obesity. From that perspective, having newer, better psychotropic medication options might improve the treatment of obesity, but searching for the "magic bullet" pharmacotherapy that would supplant the use of nonpharmacological interventions may be wrong-headed. This is especially so given that we have no evidence that there ever can be a psychotropic medication with no side effects—to treat obesity or any other disorder.

Instead of expecting that the development of the ideal drug for treating obesity is just around the corner, it may be more sensible to acknowledge that the current multifactor treatment of obesity represents a model paradigm for treating all behavioral and psychological disorders. If the heart of multifactor treatment of obesity is to be an assortment of nonpharmacological strategies supplemented by a psychotropic medication only when necessary (Lagerros & Rossner, 2012), then the search for the perfect anti-obesity drug is less important than is the development of newer, more effective nonpharmacological treatments.

CHAPTER EIGHT

Schizophrenia

Tim had listened to her voice for far too many years—constantly criticizing, humiliating, telling him he was wrong, foolish, and stupid. She would tell him when to eat, what to eat, when to go out, when to stay in, what to do, and she threatened to punish him severely if he did not obey. He also did some disturbing things under the control of her voice—things he could not tell people. Her voice seemed more distant when he stayed on his meds. The voice bothered him less—it was still there, but somehow was less intrusive. But the drug bothered him. It had side effects. He felt strange when using the drug—almost like he was awkward in the way he moved his arms and legs. So he stopped using the medication when he was feeling better mentally. And then inevitably her voice would return, more rancorous and more humiliating than ever. This recurrent cycle of misery repeated for some years. He is tired of it. He thinks he can end it by killing her voice, and he is now ready to do that. He will do that.

The advent of antipsychotic medication to treat schizophrenia represented a historic step forward in the evolution of the use of psychotropic medications, and of the study of the human brain and its relation to behavior. The serendipitous discovery of the clinical utility of a single drug, chlorpromazine, endowed with interest and excitement 50 years of research on the brain and the pharmacological treatment of psychological disorders.

Schizophrenia entered the 1950s as a familiar constellation of symptoms but with no known causes and no effective treatments. Discovering that chlorpromazine could ameliorate symptoms of psychosis induced two new hypotheses. First, if a chemical placed into the brain can diminish behavioral symptoms of a psychological disorder, then the symptoms very likely have some origin in the chemistry of the brain. This idea broke with the contemporary wisdom, which held that schizophrenia had no known organic cause and must therefore be considered a "functional psychosis." Second, if a chemical placed into the brain can alleviate symptoms, then knowing what that drug does to the brain will reveal something about the pathophysiology of the schizophrenic brain.

The 1952 introduction of chlorpromazine as a new clinical tool initiated the decline by 80% of hospitalized schizophrenic patients over the next 30 years (Nasrallah & Tandon, 2009). This stunning change of fate for those diagnosed with schizophrenia was accompanied by the implementation of new technologies to assist in the search for the neurochemical bases of schizophrenia in research in animals and humans, with the goal of improving the use of psychotropic medication for treatment of schizophrenia and other psychological disorders. The history of the pharmacological treatment of schizophrenia can be heralded as a prime example of the significance of basic research in medicine and neuroscience, but contemporary pharmacological therapy for schizophrenia is far from ideal.

PROGRESS ON DEVELOPING DRUGS TO TREAT SCHIZOPHRENIA

Billy has been in and briefly out of psychiatric wards for half of his adult life, until now. He has never really found remission using any of the drugs they prescribed for him. His psychotic symptoms remained despite trying a laundry list of drugs that did work for other schizophrenic patients. But Billy is no longer a "problem" schizophrenic patient, because the clozapine has healed Billy like a miracle. He has his life again. He is more lucid, so he now can attempt behavior therapy, and he can move toward getting himself back on a meaningful and productive track.

Which features of schizophrenia must an effective psychotropic medication target? What is known about the role of pharmacology as therapy, the role of behavior therapy, and how the two therapeutic approaches complement one another? How has the use of antipsychotic medications evolved?

It is possible to frame schizophrenia as a constellation of symptoms in three clusters (Tamminga, 2009): positive symptoms, negative symptoms, and cognitive impairment. Positive symptoms include delusions, disordered thinking, and hallucinations. Negative symptoms include flattened affect, lack of motivation, impoverished manner of speaking, and social withdrawal. Cognitive impairment includes deficits in attention, memory, and executive function. Individuals diagnosed with schizophrenia will show varying degrees of positive, negative, and cognitive symptom involvement, but all diagnosed schizophrenic patients will exhibit psychosis—believing the unreal is real, and lacking insight regarding their illness. Moreover, the three clusters of symptoms tend to respond somewhat differently to various psychotropic medications.

It is necessary for successful treatments of schizophrenia to be effective in one or more of three phases (Sobel, 2012): an acute phase in which psychosis is florid; a continuing treatment phase in which psychosis is diminishing, perhaps absent, but the patient still requires active treatment; a maintenance phase in which the principal goal is to prevent relapse. The utility of psychotropic medication is likely to vary across these three phases.

The use of medications to treat schizophrenia over the past 50 years has drawn from two categories of antipsychotic drugs: traditional (or first-generation) antipsychotics and atypical (or second-generation) antipsychotic drugs. There are similarities and differences in both the effectiveness and the side effects of these two categories of antipsychotic drugs. The differences between the categories are sufficient to recommend some guidelines for judicious use, based on what has been learned from clinical experience with various antipsychotic drugs.

First-generation, traditional antipsychotic drugs. Chlorpromazine was the first psychotropic medication to become available to treat schizophrenia. The good news about chlorpromazine was obvious in 1952: thousands of institutionalized schizophrenic patients improved and could be released. The bad news came in two parts: First, chlorpromazine has side effects, but that was to be expected; second, chlorpromazine does not help all schizophrenic patients—many did not respond to chlorpromazine, and it was not clear why. One way to adapt to the fact that not all patients showed improvement would be to develop a drug with pharmacological properties similar to those of chlorpromazine and hope that patients who did not respond favorably to chlorpromazine will respond to the new drug. That sounds simple enough today, but at the time chlorpromazine first displayed its antipsychotic efficacy, it was not known exactly what chlorpromazine was doing to the neurochemistry of the brain. Thus, the presumed mechanism of action that might explain how chlorpromazine improved symptoms of schizophrenia, and that would therefore offer a molecular target for efforts at drug development, was not known. It would be approximately 10 years before it became clear that chlorpromazine had effects on catecholamine neurotransmitters, dopamine in particular (Carlsson & Lindqvist, 1963). This knowledge facilitated a search for other first-generation antipsychotics, ultimately resulting in a list of approximately 50 drugs in eight classes (Nasrallah & Tandon, 2009), the two best known being the phenothiazines (e.g., chlorpromazine) and the butyrophenones (e.g., haloperidol).

It is possible to offer useful generalizations regarding the clinical utility of this large collection of traditional, first-generation antipsychotic drugs:

- The traditional antipsychotics do their best work by improving the positive symptoms of schizophrenia; these drugs do relatively little or nothing to improve negative symptoms or cognitive deficits (Tamminga, 2009).
- Approximately 25% of schizophrenic patients are refractory to treatment by any of these drugs (Nasrallah & Tandon, 2009).
- A pharmacological property shared by all traditional antipsychotics is their antagonism of the D2 subtype of receptors for dopamine. In fact, the measured clinical potency of these drugs correlates positively with their ability to block D2 receptors (Seeman, 2011).
- Each of the traditional antipsychotics does more than block D2 dopamine receptors. These drugs also have effects on other endogenous neurotransmitter systems, including acetylcholine, norepinephrine, and histamine, which explain some of their side effects (Nasrallah & Tandon, 2009).
- A common and particularly troublesome side effect of the traditional antipsychotics is extrapyramidal movement disorders, for example, tardive dyskinesia, which can be a major factor contributing to nonadherence to recommended medication regimen.
- It is not possible to predict which of the traditional antipsychotic drugs will be the best choice for an individual patient who is diagnosed for the first time as having schizophrenia.

Despite the fact that many of the traditional antipsychotic drugs have been in service for more than 50 years (Table 8.1), some of them still have their place in the contemporary treatment of schizophrenia, accounting for approximately 10% of prescriptions written (Nasrallah & Tandon, 2009). Haloperidol, developed in the 1950s, is at present the most frequently utilized drug in this category.

TABLE 8.1

Evolution of use of drugs over the decades to treat schizophrenia.

DRUG CLASS	1950s	1960s	1970s	1980s	1990s	2000s	2010s
First-generation antipsychotics	x	x	x	x	x	x	x
Second-generation antipsychotics				x	x	x	x

Note: x indicates the decade in which drug was prescribed. This table illustrates that the appearance of second-generation antipsychotic medications in the 1980s, and their continuing use, has not ended the utility of first-generation medications.

Second-generation, atypical antipsychotic drugs. Clozapine was the first atypical antipsychotic to make an appearance—first briefly in the 1960s, but then more assuredly in 1988 with evidence that clozapine could relieve symptoms in schizophrenic patients who were refractory to treatment with traditional antipsychotic drugs (Marder & Wirshing, 2009). It also became clear that treatment with clozapine presented less risk of extrapyramidal side effects, including tardive dyskinesia, than did the traditional antipsychotics (Kane, 2004; Keck, McElroy, Strakowski, & Soutullo, 2000). These facts together prompted a new look at molecular targets for development of antipsychotic medications, leading to the arrival of the second-generation drugs.

There are useful generalizations regarding the clinical utility of the second-generation, atypical antipsychotic drugs:

- This group of antipsychotic drugs, although now accounting for approximately 90% of prescriptions for antipsychotic medication, may or may not bring greater overall improvement in symptoms of schizophrenia compared with traditional antipsychotic medications (Leucht, Heres, Kissling, & Davis, 2012; Sharif, Bradford, Stroup, & Lieberman, 2007; Woo, Canuso, Wojcik, Brunette, & Green, 2009).
- Compared with traditional antipsychotics, second-generation antipsychotics generally are more likely to improve negative symptoms, and may also improve cognitive deficits (Leucht et al., 2012; Sobel, 2012).
- The second-generation antipsychotic drugs are generally less likely to induce extrapyramidal side effects, including tardive dyskinesia, than are traditional antipsychotics (Kane, 2004; Keck et al., 2000).

This fact is a major distinguishing characteristic of the atypical antipsychotic medications and represents a significant improvement over the traditional antipsychotic drugs, although not all atypical antipsychotic medications are equally benign regarding their potential for extrapyramidal side effects (Caroff, Hurford, Lybrand, & Campbell, 2011).

- Second-generation antipsychotics, in particular clozapine and olanzapine, can produce weight gain as a side effect, increasing the risk of type II diabetes (Woo et al., 2009).
- Although some second-generation antipsychotics have the ability to block D2 receptors for dopamine, dopamine receptor blockade is not their most prominent pharmacological property (Tamminga, 2009). The pharmacological properties of the second-generation drugs are mixed, but the distinguishing common feature may be that the drugs generally are more effective as antagonists for the 5-HT2A subtype of serotonin receptor than for the D2 dopamine receptor subtype (Iversen et al., 2009). Aripiprazole is an exception to this generalization—this drug combines mixed agonist and antagonist activity at D2 dopamine receptors, partial agonist activity at D3 dopamine receptors and 5-HT1A serotonin receptors, and antagonist activity at 5-HT2A serotonin receptors (Sharif & Lieberman, 2009).

Second-generation antipsychotic medications have largely replaced first-generation drugs as first-line pharmacological treatments for schizophrenia, despite lack of convincing published evidence that the newer drugs are always more effective and more safe (Caroff et al., 2011; Leucht et al., 2012). But an evidence-based case can be made for preferred use of second-generation drugs:

- Regarding the three clusters of symptoms (i.e., positive, negative, and cognitive deficits), the second-generation drugs are more likely than traditional antipsychotics to offer improvement of symptoms in all three clusters.
- Some second-generation drugs (most notably clozapine) are effective for the treatment-resistant schizophrenic patient—the patient who has not responded to one or several traditional antipsychotic drugs.
- Second-generation drugs generally are much less likely to produce extrapyramidal side effects than are the traditional antipsychotics.
- Generally speaking, the more favorable side effect profile of the

second-generation drugs may increase the likelihood of a patient adhering to the prescribed drug treatment regimen during the extended maintenance phase of treatment in particular, thereby decreasing the likelihood of relapse.

If approximately 25% of first-time diagnosed schizophrenic patients are likely to be refractory to treatment with a first-generation antipsychotic drug, then why not initiate treatment with a second-generation drug for each and every patient? Despite the advantages enumerated above, there are good reasons to exercise caution regarding the use of second-generation antipsychotic medications:

- Some second-generation drugs are more likely to produce weight gain than are first-generation antipsychotics.
- The longer history of clinical use of first-generation antipsychotics makes these older drugs less likely to offer unpleasant surprises than are the newer antipsychotics.
- Clozapine can produce potentially fatal agranulocytosis and can have other serious side effects, but clozapine is also identified as potentially having distinct advantages for treating schizophrenic patients who are treatment refractory, who show comorbidity for substance dependency or abuse, or who show high risk for suicide (Marder & Wirshing, 2009). These distinct advantages potentially increase the likelihood of taking the risks associated with prescribing clozapine.

In summary, the contemporary prescribing professional and the schizophrenic patient face choices regarding (a) which drug to choose from two categories of antipsychotic medications, all of which have somewhat unpredictable benefits and serious risks; and (b) how to use pharmacological therapy in a treatment program that integrates drug and nondrug approaches. The integration of drug and nondrug approaches is quite necessary for treating a disorder in which the hallmark characteristics include psychosis (including paranoia) and lack of insight into one's illness. For a patient who is believing the unbelievable, and also not appreciating the implications of that distorted worldview, it is unrealistic to expect that one merely needs to provide a prescription and give the patient instructions regarding how to use it.

Perhaps the ideal tack regarding how to integrate drug and nondrug therapies is to assume that each approach will facilitate the other (Marder, 2000; Woo et al., 2009): Patients initially presenting with florid psychosis will first need a drug that effectively brings them to a place where they can begin to accept and utilize therapy that depends on conversation with a therapist that they can trust. The drug that best accomplishes that initial step in an acute phase of treatment may well not be the same drug that is used in a latter phase of treatment. In addition, when the priority is to quickly diminish some of the positive symptoms, some risks regarding side effects might seem to be more acceptable for the short term. Continuing treatment past this acute phase, perhaps for one or two more years, will require behavior therapy that teaches coping skills and facilitates the likelihood of being compliant with instructions for using the medication. The drug therapy may increase the likelihood of talk therapy being efficacious, and the talk therapy may increase the likelihood the patient will stay committed to the drug therapy even as symptoms of psychosis abate during the continuing phase of treatment. The next phase of treatment, the maintenance phase, poses the challenge of obtaining a commitment from the patient to continue drug therapy for a period of perhaps four or five years with the purpose of preventing relapse (Robinson et al., 1999; Schooler, 2006). This extended commitment to pharmacotherapy will likely require a drug that poses few challenges in the way of side effects, *and* supporting psychosocial therapy that enhances the likelihood of maintaining that commitment. In addition, significant improvement in the patient's quality of life provides incentive to stay with the integrated therapeutic program. Switching from one medication to another from the acute to the continuing to the maintenance phase may be necessary to facilitate success. Unfortunately, there is no set of guidelines that will suit each patient regarding which drug to choose first and which to choose next. The particular needs of each patient will dictate the appropriate course of action (Sharif et al., 2007).

WHY DO SOME SCHIZOPHRENIC PATIENTS NOT BENEFIT FROM ANTIPSYCHOTIC MEDICATION?

(Sensitivity to a Drug Varies From One Individual to Another.)

Joseph has received little help from any of the antipsychotic medications that he has been prescribed over the years. A few of those drugs were combined with others—an antidepressant medication one time, an antianxiety medication another time, a second antipsychotic drug for several months another time. None of those combinations helped. In fact, they seemed to make things worse, leaving him to be a psychotic with drug-induced side effects. He even tried a newer medication—one that twice caused a seizure. After these many years of grief, he could tolerate a seizure or two if only the drug would also help with the psychosis. Joseph worries that he is doomed to a lifetime of psychosis, and no one has offered words that convince him to believe otherwise.

Drugs usually have effects that are dose related; the more drug you give, the greater effect you get, as a general rule. But the effects of antipsychotic drugs on symptoms of schizophrenia seem to be less abiding of that rule. One example is the fact that the main effects of most of the antipsychotic drugs do not appear to be dose related. An antipsychotic drug either improves symptoms of schizophrenia or it does not, and if a dosage of an antipsychotic has a relatively small main effect, increasing the dose for that patient is unlikely to increase the magnitude of that effect (Leucht et al., 2012). That situation is typically dealt with by switching to a different antipsychotic medication (rather than by further increasing the dose).

One possible explanation for this apparent lack of dosage-related effect is that a neurochemical threshold must be reached by an antipsychotic drug and that this threshold effect is close to the maximum neurochemical effect that can be achieved with that drug. This scenario essentially describes a pharmacological threshold that is near a pharmacological ceiling, leaving not much room to maneuver in between. To understand this in relation to antipsychotic drugs and their postulated mechanism of action, first remember that the clinical potency of antipsychotic drugs is robustly correlated with their ability to bind to and block D2 dopamine receptors, a correlation that holds for both first-generation and second-generation antipsychotic drugs (Seeman, 2011). Moreover, antipsychotic medications have a threshold range of values for D2 receptor antagonism that is necessary for a main effect of improvement in symptoms: a minimum of between 60% and 80% occupancy (blockade) of D2 receptors (Seeman, 2002). In addition, further increasing dose of these drugs to achieve more than 80% occupancy of D2 receptors is sufficient to produce extrapyramidal side effects (Seeman, 2002). With these facts in mind, the ideal clinical strategy would be to attempt to use a dosage of antipsychotic medication that produces close to but less than 80% occupancy of D2 receptors—this dosage would be just above the threshold for producing a main effect, and just below the threshold for inducing troubling extrapyramidal side effects.

That may sound like a nice and simple explanation for how antipsychotic drugs affect brain neurochemistry to improve symptoms of schizophrenia, but keep in mind that there remains a major conundrum: Many diagnosed schizophrenic patients fail to improve in response to any of the antipsychotic drugs, with approximately one-third of diagnosed schizophrenic patients showing limited or no response to antipsychotic medications (Lindenmayer, 2000).

Why are some schizophrenic patients refractory to drug treatment? Can we claim that the riddle of schizophrenia has been solved when as many as one-third of those diagnosed remain psychotic throughout pharmacotherapy? The fact that so many schizophrenic patients fail to respond to drug therapy is a significant failing given that medication is considered to be *essential* treatment for the acute psychosis that a schizophrenic patient initially presents, and for the prevention of relapse (Leucht et al., 2012; Preston et al., 2013; Sobel, 2012). Is there an explanation for the limited utility of antipsychotic medications for the treatment-resistant schizophrenic patient?

An explanation might be found in a study (Demjaha, Murray, McGuire, Kapur, & Howes, 2012) that used brain imaging to compare three groups of people: schizophrenic patients who responded successfully to antipsychotic medication, schizophrenic patients who were refractory to antipsychotic drug treatment, and healthy volunteers. Positron emission tomography measured the capacity for synthesis of endogenous dopamine in various regions of the brain. The treatment-refractory schizophrenic patients showed brain-region-specific reduced capacity for synthesis of dopamine compared with schizophrenic patients who showed a favorable behavioral response to antipsychotic medication. These findings suggest that antipsychotic medications that block receptors for dopamine may be less effective for relief of symptoms in those patients who have diminished capacity for synthesis of endogenous dopamine.

Regardless of the ultimate explanation for why so very many diagnosed schizophrenic patients are resistant to drug therapy, the contemporary utility of psychotropic medication for schizophrenia falls far short from being ideal for the following reasons:

- Between 10% and 60% of diagnosed schizophrenic patients show limited or no benefit from one or another psychotropic medication (Lindenmayer, 2000).
- First-generation antipsychotics are effective principally for relief only of positive symptoms, although second-generation antipsychotic drugs can be effective for improving positive and negative symptoms and, occasionally, cognitive deficits.
- Clinically effective dosages of antipsychotic drugs always have side effects, and in some situations the threshold clinically effective dosage is close to and sometimes even greater than the threshold dose for producing serious side effects (e.g., tardive dyskinesia and other extrapyramidal side effects, agranulocytosis, seizure, weight gain)—side effects so serious as to imperil adherence to reliable taking of medication.

- It is difficult to predict which individual patient will respond positively to which specific antipsychotic medication and which patient might be refractory to drug treatment.

The inadequacy of antipsychotic medication for providing predictable effects in individual patients, and the failure of these drugs to solve the problem of schizophrenia for all patients, emphasizes the importance of nondrug therapies for successful treatment of schizophrenia. Nonpharmacological approaches include skills training, family interventions, supported employment, cognitive behavioral therapy, behavior modification, token economy programs, and assertive community treatment (Kopelowicz, Liberman, & Zarate, 2007). The utility of these nondrug therapies is significant and can provide help even to those patients who are responding poorly to drug therapy. For example, cognitive therapy can improve symptoms of schizophrenia in patients who continue to show prominent negative symptoms while being medicated with second-generation antipsychotic medication (Grant, Huh, Perivoliotis, Stolar, & Beck, 2012).

In summary, it is very difficult to predict whether or not a schizophrenic patient will respond favorably to a first- or a second-generation antipsychotic medication, a fact that predicts the continuing utility of first-generation antipsychotic drugs for decades after second-generation medications became available (Table 8.1). Whether a response to medication is favorable will depend on what an individual patient is willing to accept as a compromise between the relief of symptoms and drug-induced side effects. The nature of an acceptable compromise will be determined in part by the sex, gender, and age of the patient.

DO WOMEN RESPOND MORE FAVORABLY THAN MEN TO ANTIPSYCHOTIC MEDICATION?

(Sex, Age, and Genetics Can Determine the Magnitude of Effects of a Drug.)

Zoe and her twin brother, Gordon, each have a history of schizophrenia. Gordon was diagnosed in his early twenties, and although he has found relief from his psychosis from time to time, he is all too familiar with relapse. The haloperidol has helped, but he has never been able to get life together long enough to hold a job and keep a meaningful relationship with the potential for marriage. Zoe watched much of this unfold for Gordon, and when her illness appeared in her forties, she feared the worst. But fortunately, she seems generally less troubled by her symptoms than does her brother, and she responds well to the haloperidol. She does not show the cognitive impairment that has so plagued her brother, and once her positive symptoms went into remission, she resumed her life as wife and mother.

Despite the emphasis on pharmacological treatment for neurochemical abnormality in schizophrenia, the disorder is surely a biopsychosocial problem that warrants treatment for its biological, psychological, and social parameters. This is apparent when examining the roles for sex and gender for the development of schizophrenia and its treatment. A variety of evidence demonstrates sex differences in schizophrenia (Abel, Drake, & Goldstein, 2010; Canuso & Pandina, 2007): There are sex differences in incidence of schizophrenia, with a ratio of approximately 1.4 to 1 for men versus women. Men generally exhibit earlier onset of schizophrenia than do women, and women more frequently than men are diagnosed later in life. Onset of psychosis is more insidious for men; onset for women occurs more abruptly. Men are generally more troubled by negative symptoms than are women, which leads to a poorer prognosis for recovery, greater likelihood of relapse, and less successful social functionality for men. Schizophrenic men are more likely than women to show comorbidity for substance dependence or abuse.

These differences between men and women may be a consequence of differences between males and females in development of brain processes (Goldstein et al., 2002b), and they also may be a consequence of the impact of the physical and social environments on the vulnerability for developing schizophrenia and for shaping the disease process (Abel et al., 2010). Considering the various ways in which schizophrenic men and women may differ, it might not be surprising to find that some of the differences have an impact on the effectiveness of various treatment approaches, including psychotropic medications:

- With schizophrenic men being relatively more burdened by negative symptoms, one might predict that more men than women would require a second-generation antipsychotic to capitalize on those drugs' greater ability to improve negative symptoms.
- With schizophrenic men being more burdened by negative symptoms and cognitive deficiencies—each of which can make adherence to drug therapy more difficult—one might predict that rates of relapse would be higher for men than for women.
- With more schizophrenic men showing comorbidity for substance dependence and abuse, one might predict greater difficulty successfully treating male schizophrenic patients, and greater polypharmacy being used to attempt to treat comorbidities.

These speculations or hypotheses seem reasonable, but it is difficult to collect data in clinical trials to evaluate such hypotheses, because it is difficult to construct the types of controlled experimental trials that would get at answers to such questions. Those clinical trials would need to control (i.e., hold constant) across groups of patients factors such as age, weight, ethnicity, premorbid symptomology, age of onset, magnitude of positive and negative symptoms, presence of cognitive deficits, drug, dosage, nondrug adjunctive treatment, duration of treatments, and more. Even the relatively simple question of whether or not men and women respond differently to various antipsychotic drugs does not find a clear answer. For example, some studies demonstrate no differences between men and women in response to first-generation antipsychotics (Pinals, Malhotra, Missar, Pickar, & Breier, 1996), whereas others do show differences; for example, first-episode schizophrenic women can show a better response to the first-generation antipsychotic haloperidol than do men (Szymanski et al., 1995), and first-episode and multiple-episode schizophrenic women can show a better response to the second-generation drug olanzapine than do men (Goldstein et al., 2002a).

Differences between men and women in the effectiveness—main or side effects—of an antipsychotic medication could be attributable to sex differences in pharmacokinetics or pharmacodynamics. There is evidence for sex differences in pharmacokinetics and pharmacodynamics for first-generation (Yonkers et al., 1992) and second-generation (Smith, 2010) antipsychotic medications; although there is some inconsistency in the details of those reported findings, generally women require lower doses than do men for equivalent main effect or side effects of antipsychotics.

Some of the differences between men and women depend on age. For example, the greater effectiveness of haloperidol for relief of symptoms in schizophrenic women versus men has been demonstrated for premenopausal women but not for postmenopausal women (Goldstein et al., 2002a). This finding and others (Canuso & Pandina, 2007; Kulkarni, Gavrilidis, Worsley, & Hayes, 2012) raise the possibility that the presence of endogenous estrogen in the premenopausal years combines with psychosocial factors to protect women from developing psychosis, which is consistent with the evidence for later onset of schizophrenia in women than in men (Abel et al., 2010). These findings also encourage the idea that estrogen adjunctive therapy may enhance the effectiveness of antipsychotic medications in both women and men (Kulkarni et al., 2012), which is supported by preliminary findings in treatment-resistant premenopausal women (Ghafari et al., 2013).

The age at which a person is diagnosed with schizophrenia is an important factor other than reproductive status for women. Generally speaking, the later the onset of schizophrenia, the better the prognosis for successful recovery, which is important to consider when a diagnosis of schizophrenia is determined for an adolescent. Early treatment for psychosis in adolescents is likely to begin with pharmacotherapy (Sharif et al., 2007), despite the lack of published evidence that the drugs approved for use in the treatment of adult psychosis will be effective and safe for off-label use in children or adolescents. It appears that second-generation antipsychotic medications are effective for treatment of adolescents diagnosed with early-onset schizophrenia spectrum disorders (Schimmelmann, Schmidt, Carbon, & Correll, 2013), although the data from clinical trials are not sufficient to support the use of one atypical antipsychotic drug over another. One exception is that clozapine appears to be the atypical antipsychotic drug of choice for treating adolescents who are refractory to other treatment (Schimmelmann et al., 2013). The relative lack of evidence to support the off-label use of any one specific antipsychotic medication, together with the fact that each of these drugs carries the risks of troublesome side effects, encourages choosing a drug principally on the basis of which side effect profile is likely to be most favorable to the individual patient (Schimmelmann et al., 2013).

Caution also should be exercised when considering the use of antipsychotic medication in diagnosed schizophrenic patients at the other end of the age continuum—the elderly. The elderly show approximately a five times higher rate of antipsychotic-induced tardive dyskinesia than do young adults, a fact that encourages the use of smaller doses and second-generation antipsychotics in this population (Jeste, 2004; Miller et al., 2005). Further supporting the use of a second-generation antipsychotic is the finding that olanzapine can be more effective than haloperidol for improving negative symptoms while running a lesser risk of extrapyramidal side effects in elderly schizophrenic patients (Barak et al., 2002). Despite the fact that the elderly appear to be better served by the use of second-generation rather than first-generation antipsychotic medications, the elderly remain more likely than young adults to experience a broad range of adverse events, including serious side effects, from any antipsychotic medication, in particular extrapyramidal motor disturbances and increased risk of cerebrovascular and cardiac abnormalities (Lindsey, 2009). This apparent greater sensitivity is likely attributable to age-related changes in pharmacokinetics and pharmacodynamics (Trifiro & Spina, 2011). The situation with the elderly schizophrenic patient is further complicated by the increased likelihood that an elderly patient will show comorbidity and age-related cognitive decline and be a candidate for polypharmacy (Le Couteur et al., 2004). Taken together, these findings encourage smaller doses of antipsychotic medications and the use of nondrug therapies, especially those intended to compensate for behavioral deficits related to aging.

HOW MIGHT DRUG USAGE ALTER THE EFFECTIVENESS OF ANTIPSYCHOTIC MEDICATION?

(A Person's Drug History Can Affect a Drug's Effectiveness.)

Helen is in a panic over the rumor that smoking will no longer be permitted on the premises of the hospital—not even in the rose garden! Several of the hospital staff are a bit panicky also, given their long history of using the smoking break and cigarette rewards to encourage the cooperation of psychotic patients and their compliance with the rules on the ward. Nearly every schizophrenic patient on the ward qualifies as a heavy smoker, and they smoke as if they really, really need it—as if the nicotine is medicine. No smoking anywhere at all on the premises of the hospital? Who the hell made that rule, and what were they thinking?

You don't much need a second prescription for a psychotropic medication to establish polypharmacy—the fact is that over 60% of schizophrenic patients are smokers (Sagud et al., 2009). Speculations regarding the explanation for such a high incidence of smoking include the ideas that the ingestion of nicotine is (a) a way to enhance release of dopamine to induce pleasure in a brain that is experiencing diminished dopamine neurotransmission as part of the disease of schizophrenia, (b) a means to enable nicotine-induced enhancement of cognitive processes, or (c) a method to reduce antipsychotic-induced extrapyramidal side effects. Regardless of the motivation for smoking and ingesting nicotine, the fact that such a sizable percentage of schizophrenic patients engage in such behavior begs for some understanding of the impact of nicotine ingestion on the effectiveness of antipsychotic medication.

Smoking and nicotine ingestion provide a pharmacokinetic interaction with a variety of first-generation (chlorpromazine, haloperidol) and second-generation (clozapine, olanzapine) antipsychotic medications (Kroon, 2007); as a consequence, the dose of antipsychotic drug may need to be increased in order to achieve the intended effectiveness for a schizophrenic smoker. This consequence of smoking is attributed principally to enhanced enzymatic degradation of many medications, including antipsychotic drugs. Thus, chronic smoking by the nicotine-addicted schizophrenic patient, owing to this enhanced enzymatic metabolism, will reduce the bioavailability of the antipsychotic medication, such that the smoking schizophrenic patient will on average require a larger dose of antipsychotic medication for the drug to have therapeutic value. Although this adjustment in dosage can be made (by an estimated increase of 1.5 times the antipsychotic medication dosage recommended for a nonsmoker; Haslemo, Eikeseth, Tanum, Molden, & Refsum, 2006; Kroon, 2007), a worrisome problem arises when the schizophrenic patient initiates abstinence from nicotine.

Abrupt cessation of smoking by the antipsychotic-medicated patient results in abrupt elevation of plasma levels of drug, which can cause overdose of medication, with potential consequences including seizure, unconsciousness, metabolic acidosis, or aspiration pneumonia (Bondolfi et al., 2005). To counter the consequences of abrupt cessation of smoking, a reduction of between approximately 35% and 50% of antipsychotic medication dose is needed to accommodate the abstinence-induced reduction in metabolism (Haslemo et al., 2006; Schaffer, Yoon, & Zadezensky, 2009).

In summary, smoking is a factor that must be monitored in order to ensure that the bioavailability of antipsychotic drug is sufficient to be effective. The use of nicotine products varies across ethnicity (Lariscy et al., 2013), as do attempts to abstain from smoking (Kahende, Malarcher, Teplinskaya, & Asman, 2011). These facts suggest that smoking, and its effect on the effectiveness of antipsychotic medications, may depend on factors related to ethnicity and culture.

HOW MIGHT ETHNICITY AFFECT THE UTILITY OF ANTIPSYCHOTIC MEDICATION?

(Culture and Community Can Affect the Utility of Pharmacotherapy.)

Stash is confused. He knows that his mother is disappointed and humiliated that her son has been labeled a schizophrenic and has been medicated for years. And his mother repeatedly has urged him to stop smoking, even going so far as to threaten to no longer make his favorite pierogi stuffed with sauerkraut filling. His mother talks about the cancer that will surely kill him if he keeps on with his "filthy habit," but his physician talks about the need to keep his nicotine intake stable so that his meds for psychosis will be effective. In fact, his doctor has warned Stanley that he can die if he quits smoking too abruptly while using haloperidol. Heck, 20 minutes after his most recent cigarette, Stanley always feels like he will die anyway if he does not get to smoke another one very soon.

The utility of an antipsychotic drug for relieving symptoms of schizophrenia is not simply a function of the extent to which the drug alters the neurochemistry of the brain—it also depends upon the drug's availability, and the ability of an individual patient to use it in a manner that maximizes its effectiveness. There is evidence that ethnicity plays a role in the utility of antipsychotic medications, and there are multiple ways in which ethnicity and cultural factors can have an impact on pharmacological treatment of schizophrenia (Lin, Smith, & Ortiz, 2001; Rey, 2006).

First of all, obviously a psychotropic medication stands a chance of being effective only if it has been prescribed, and antipsychotic medications may be prescribed more or less frequently, and in larger or smaller doses, depending upon race. For example, in the United States African-American schizophrenic patients are likely to be prescribed larger doses of antipsychotic medications, on average, than are Caucasian patients, attributed in part to the use of depot medications (Walkup et al., 2000), despite lack of evidence that there is a racial difference in effectiveness of those medications (Bakare, 2008). The reason for prescribing larger doses for African-Americans also may relate to subjective judgment regarding what is required of the pharmacotherapy; if African-Americans are perceived as being potentially more aggressive when the diagnosis of schizophrenia is made, prescribing a larger dose may follow from that perception (Bakare, 2008).

The choice of antipsychotic medication can also be affected by cost and cost-sharing obligations. The impact on choice and access determined by cost to the patient may vary across ethnic groups as socioeconomic status varies: Because newer psychotropic medications can require greater cost-sharing (e.g., with some tiered formularies), increased cost can influence the decision whether or not to switch from a first-generation drug that is ineffective for an individual patient to a more costly second-generation drug (Horgan et al., 2009).

The impact of cost on access to medications also varies widely globally. This is evident in the fact that access to the newer psychotropic medications is greater in those countries that can afford the cost of the drugs (Kohn et al., 2004). Another issue of international importance is the fact that the incidence of schizophrenia may be higher for people who have migrated. For example, increased incidence of schizophrenia is apparent in adolescents who have recently immigrated, perhaps due to the impact of the stress of being displaced from one's home country (Ampadu, 2011).

Aside from issues related to cost and access, schizophrenic patients of a particular ethnicity may require a larger (or smaller) dose owing to pharmacokinetic differences among races (Chen, 2006; Rey, 2006). For example, African-American schizophrenic patients metabolize the second-generation antipsychotic olanzapine approximately 25% faster than other races, thereby requiring a larger dose for equivalent therapeutic efficacy (Bigos et al., 2008).

Alternatively, differences in pharmacodynamics can require larger (or smaller) doses to achieve comparable therapeutic outcome across different races. One example of this is the report that Asian schizophrenic patients require lower doses of haloperidol than do Caucasian schizophrenic patients: Because there was no difference in bioavailability of haloperidol between the two ethnic groups, the fact that the Asian patients showed improvement in response to lower doses was interpreted as a difference in pharmacodynamics of haloperidol between Asian and Caucasian patients (Lin et al., 1989).

Finally, there may be ethnic differences in refractoriness to antipsychotic medication. For example, a Caucasian European is approximately twice as likely to be refractory to antipsychotic treatment as a non-Caucasian European (Teo, Borlido, Kennedy, & De Luca, 2013).

In summary, ethnicity can have an impact on the incidence of schizophrenia, choice of treatment, access to psychotropic medication, magnitude of antipsychotic effectiveness, and incidence of being refractory to treatment. Some of these differences may be attributed to racial or ethnic differences in pharmacokinetics, pharmacodynamics, stress, genetics, and social or cultural factors that are difficult to fully characterize.

CAN ANIMAL MODELS TEACH US ABOUT PHARMACOTHERAPY FOR SCHIZOPHRENIA?

Ronnie the Rat feels like he is spinning in circles. Well, he actually *is* spinning in circles—rotating toward his right side. Ronnie has become a rotating rat. A friend touches him on his right shoulder, and Ronnie rotates toward the right. A friend touches him on his left shoulder, and Ronnie again rotates toward the right. He is always moving toward the right, which is the wrong thing to do half of the time—even for a rat. This went on and on until one day Dr. Model gave Ronnie a prescription for chlorpromazine and explained the problem to Ronnie. It turns out that Ronnie has a lesion (or damage) to an area of the brain important for movement—the corpus striatum. And because the lesion is on the left side of Ronnie's brain, it results in that annoying tendency to turn to the right. So Ronnie has a lesion-induced behavioral dysfunction that causes the tendency to turn to the right. But chlorpromazine stops the rotating. Dr. Model explained this by offering that a large dose of chlorpromazine is able to so completely block so many D2 receptors for dopamine simultaneously on *both* sides of the brain, including Ronnie's damaged corpus striatum on the left, as well as the normal striatum on the right, that the drug balances the dopamine functioning across the two sides of the brain, making it temporarily normal again. As long as Ronnie the Rat takes his chlorpromazine, he stops rotating. If he goes off his meds, Ronnie relapses into rotating. Dr. Model has assured Ronnie that other drugs that block D2 receptors should also be good medication for Ronnie's problem. Dr. Model also asked Ronnie if he would like to be a subject in an experiment that is intended to evaluate the effectiveness of a new drug to treat schizophrenia. Ronnie nodded toward his right, affirming his interest.

The ability to speak is necessary to make evident that some of the symptoms of schizophrenia are present—that cognition is disturbed, delusions are present, voices are being heard and understood, emotions are disturbed. This fact makes it seem nearly impossible to create an animal model of schizophrenia that has impressive construct validity. But certain components of the positive, negative, or cognitive symptoms of schizophrenia might be effectively modeled, offering an animal model that could be useful for predicting the effectiveness of a new drug for treating schizophrenia. Examples of useful animal models for schizophrenia that have demonstrated some amount of predictive validity when testing the effects of potential antipsychotic medications include:

- Rearing of infant rodents in isolation, which can produce hyperactivity and deficits in cognition and social behavior as adults
- Amphetamine-induced changes in behavior indicative of the animal experiencing hallucinations
- Chronic NMDA receptor blockade by ketamine or phencyclidine, which can induce increases in locomotor activity and aberrant responding to nonreinforced cues, which in turn can contribute to apparent deficits in cognition (e.g., poor performance in a task demanding recognition of novelty or in an attentional set-shifting task)
- Lesions to the ventral hippocampus in neonatal rats that produce cognitive deficits
- Various genetically modified mouse models that demonstrate anhedonia, diminished motivation, cognitive deficits, and abnormalities in locomotion and social behavior (Chen, Lipska, & Weinberger, 2006; O'Connell, Lawrie, McIntosh, & Hall, 2011; Pratt et al., 2012)

These examples of animal models for schizophrenia, only a fraction of the models that have been used (Pratt et al., 2012), generally have limited construct validity and have not yet shown impressive predictive validity. Thus, the progress in development of novel medications for treating schizophrenia has been quite limited. Since the advent of the use of first-generation antipsychotic medications over 50 years ago, we now have second-generation antipsychotic medications and a handful of other drugs. This limited progress is partially attributable to the narrow approach of using animal models to measure the effectiveness of new drugs known to have the familiar pharmacological properties of the older clinically effective drugs (Moore, 2010). This approach has facilitated development of additional dopamine D2 receptor antagonists having pharmacological properties similar to chlorpromazine, and drugs with properties similar to clozapine that combine serotonin and D2 antagonism.

Here are three recent examples of the use of animal models for schizophrenia that assess the effectiveness of familiar antipsychotic medications or novel therapeutic drugs for treating behavioral deficits presumed to model some component of schizophrenia:

- In a model of rats reared in social isolation subsequent to weaning, the second-generation antipsychotic risperidone partially reverses their hyperactivity and their deficits in novel object recognition and conditioned emotional response learning (McIntosh, Ballard, Steward, Moran, & Fone, 2013).
- Chronic treatment of pubertal rats with the CB1 receptor agonist drug WIN55212-2 induces deficits in social recognition and interaction, which presumably model behavioral symptoms of schizophrenia; these deficits are reversed by acute administration of the second-generation antipsychotic quetiapine (Leweke & Schneider, 2011).
- Novel therapeutic D3 dopamine receptor antagonist drugs reduce locomotor hyperactivity and reverse the deficits in novel object recognition that are induced by rearing rats in social isolation (Watson, Marsden, Millan, & Fone, 2012).

The history of the successful use of animal models for schizophrenia leading to the development of novel medications is not impressive (Pratt et al., 2012). This is not surprising given that schizophrenia is a disorder that includes diverse clinical symptoms with a pathophysiology that remains poorly understood. Whether or not genetic mouse models of schizophrenia will be more productive for the development of new drug therapies remains to be seen (O'Connell et al., 2011).

TIDBITS ON PSYCHOPHARMACOLOGY LEARNED FROM THE TREATMENT OF SCHIZOPHRENIA

The following are brief examples illustrating other principles of pharmacology or recommendations from Part I of this book, taken from the clinical treatment of schizophrenia or from basic research on schizophrenia:

- *No drug has only one effect.* Each and every one of the traditional antipsychotic drugs are antagonists to the D2 subtype of receptor for dopamine, but each also (a) has effects on other neurotransmitter systems in the brain and (b) has undesired side effects (Seeman, 2011).
- *Compromise on benefits and risks is a realistic goal for pharmacotherapy.* Clozapine can improve symptoms of schizophrenia in patients who have been refractory to treatment using traditional antipsychotic drugs, but the patient using clozapine accepts increased risk for developing agranulocytosis and for experiencing seizures.
- *Desired effects and unwanted effects are related to dosage.* Neuroimaging of the human brain reveals that D2 dopamine receptor occupancy of 65–70% by a D2 antagonist drug is sufficient for maximal clinical antipsychotic effectiveness, whereas some side effects (e.g., extrapyramidal movements) will occur with occupancy greater than 72–78% (Nasrallah & Tandon, 2009).
- *Drug interactions can be potent and unpredictable.* Schizophrenic patients who show comorbidity with substance dependence or abuse are less likely to respond favorably to antipsychotic medication (Lubman, King, & Castle, 2010).
- *Drugs can mimic endogenous neurochemicals.* Adjunctive treatment using estrogen can enhance the effectiveness of antipsychotic medication (Ghafari et al., 2013).
- *Drugs can block endogenous neurochemicals.* The magnitude of antagonism of D2 receptors for dopamine robustly correlates with the clinical effectiveness of traditional antipsychotic medications (Seeman, 2011).
- *Pharmacological effects on brain neurochemistry can be enduring.* Chronic use of amphetamine can induce symptoms of psychosis that closely resemble schizophrenia.
- *Drugs differ in their potential for addiction.* Antipsychotic medications show no evidence of addictive potential.
- *Drugs can alter the organization of a developing brain.* The off-label use of antipsychotic drugs has increased for treatment of conduct disorder and ADHD in children and adolescents, despite lack of knowledge of the effects of such drugs on the developing human brain (Patten, Waheed, & Bresee, 2012).
- *Drugs can be demonstrated to be only relatively effective and safe.* All drugs that have ever been approved to treat schizophrenia have side effects.
- *A therapeutic drug is used because it works.* Chlorpromazine was

used clinically to treat schizophrenia for approximately 10 years before its mechanism of action was identified.

- *Dietary supplements may or may not be effective and safe.* No dietary supplements are known to be useful for treatment of schizophrenia.
- *Placebo can have drug-like effects.* It would very likely be considered unethical to use a placebo as treatment of patients showing symptoms of psychosis.
- *Pharmacotherapy is best used as one among several tools, and the role of pharmacotherapy varies for different people and disorders.* Goal-directed, individualized cognitive therapy (plus antipsychotic medication) once per week improves positive symptoms and overall functioning for low-functioning schizophrenic patients compared with antipsychotic medication alone (Grant et al., 2012).
- *Serendipity can bring new opportunities for pharmacotherapy.* The search for a drug with antihistaminergic sedative properties led to the discovery of the antipsychotic properties of chlorpromazine (Jacobsen, 1986; Lehmann & Ban, 1997).
- *Consumers demand new and better drugs, and successful use encourages increased use, for better or worse.* Off-label use of potent second-generation antipsychotic medications continues to increase for treatment of a long list of other disorders, including ADHD, anxiety, dementia, geriatric agitation, depression, eating disorders, insomnia, obsessive-compulsive disorder, personality disorder, post-traumatic stress disorder, substance use and dependence, and Tourette syndrome (Maher & Theodore, 2012). Phew!
- *The FDA attempts to approve new and better drugs.* There is no clear drug of choice for treatment of schizophrenia, so it is a good bet that quite a few people, institutions, and industries would like to find one.
- *Off-label use has its advantages and disadvantages, and health insurance practices can determine accessibility to a drug.* Frequent off-label prescribing of a variety of second-generation antipsychotics encouraged FDA approval of several of these drugs, which should make the cost of these medications more likely to be covered by insurance: aripiprazole for major depressive disorder and autism; olanzapine (combined with fluoxetine) for major depressive disorder and bipolar disorder; quetiapine for bipolar depression; risperidone for autism (Maher & Theodore, 2012).
- *Diagnosis guides choice of pharmacotherapy.* A schizophrenic patient presenting with comorbid substance dependence is more

likely to be treated with clozapine than some other antipsychotic drug, largely based on accumulating clinical experience rather than convincing published evidence demonstrating the superior effectiveness of clozapine (Marder & Wirshing, 2009; Woo et al., 2009).

- *Clients should be active participants in their pharmacotherapy.* Adherence to the antipsychotic medication regimen is the key to prevention of relapse of schizophrenia. There are many reasons that a schizophrenic patient, absent florid symptoms of psychosis, might fail to continue to comply with instructions to use antipsychotic medication: side effects, lack of insight regarding psychosis and the significance of medication, delusions regarding the use of medication, comorbid substance abuse, lack of a supporting environment. Psychosocial treatment that forges an alliance among the patient, therapist, and family (or supportive friends) is vital to facilitate the patient's adherence to the medication regimen (Marder, 2000).

SUMMARY AND PERSPECTIVE

Schizophrenia is a disorder with relatively low incidence but with devastating consequences for the individual diagnosed. Psychosis can be so severely debilitating to the patient that the significance of the role of psychotropic medication in treatment is magnified. This is surely the case for treatment of the acute phase of schizophrenia, in which early antipsychotic drug treatment can increase the likelihood of a more rapid and more complete remission (Loebel et al., 1992). Moreover, the steady management of schizophrenia using antipsychotic drug therapy continuously for five or more years also provides significant protection against relapse (Robinson et al., 1999). This central role of antipsychotic medication for treatment does not diminish the value of nondrug therapy for schizophrenia, especially considering the fact that a psychotic patient presents a rather high risk of discontinuing drug therapy absent consistent professional encouragement to stick with the drug regimen.

Antipsychotic medications provide a cornerstone of treatment despite their less than ideal effectiveness: Antipsychotic drugs do not relieve all symptoms, they all have the potential for serious adverse effects, and as many as one-third of diagnosed schizophrenic patients are refractory to drug therapy. No one antipsychotic drug is most effective, and no one antipsychotic drug is safest. Despite the disproportionate use of the newer, second-generation antipsychotics, one cannot make the case that an individual schizophrenic patient will be best treated with one of these newer drugs, because the side effect profile could very well lead to discontinuation of use of the drug. This situation emphasizes the importance of dealing with each individual schizophrenic patient as a unique case, in which the individual's sex, gender, diet, history of smoking, willingness to tolerate side effects, ethnicity, and treatment history are relevant and need to be considered when prescribing a medication as part of an integrated treatment program.

CHAPTER NINE

Addiction

Bill knew the likelihood of becoming addicted to marijuana was relatively small, and because his father is an alcoholic, he figured he'd best not drink alcohol. But he is now smoking weed much more frequently than he had planned. When he began, he used it because he enjoyed it in the evening. But now something is different. During the daytime he frequently thinks about using. He finds himself using it every day, and on some days he smokes before lunch. Bill is beginning to believe his behavior is starting to look like that of an addict.

Addiction is a chronic relapsing disease that is a biopsychosocial problem (Leshner, 1997; Levy, 2013). Becoming addicted requires behaving in a particular way to initiate the development of the disorder: Whether or not a person has a genetic vulnerability for developing addiction (Kreek, Nielsen, Butelman, & LaForge, 2005), an individual will develop an addiction only if ingestion of an addictive drug occurs, and occurs repeatedly. The likelihood of a person ingesting an addictive substance is very high in many countries, because social factors encourage consumption of legal and illegal addictive substances. And once the reinforcing neurochemical and psychological consequences of ingesting an addictive substance are experienced, drug ingestion tends to recur.

Psychoactive drugs that sustain addictive behavior are exogenous substances that powerfully activate one or another of the endogenous neurochemical systems in the brain that are normally activated by behaviors that bring pleasure or reward. Thus, psychoactive drugs used recreationally robustly tap into endogenous behavioral-brain mechanisms that function to keep humans well fed, hydrated, and happy (Volkow & Wise, 2005; Wise, 1998). The ability to activate those brain mechanisms gives psychoactive addictive drugs immense reward value. The euphoria induced by those drugs represents a resounding exogenous pharmacological whack to reward mechanisms normally activated by gentle endogenous neurochemical taps. It is no surprise, therefore, that humans are attracted to use drugs that can artificially, powerfully activate those brain mechanisms.

Ingestion of addictive drugs establishes the etiology of addiction—that much is certain. If you know what an addictive drug does to the brain and body, you know the drug-induced causes of addiction to that drug. A well-established but still evolving theory holds that all addictive drugs share the ability to directly or indirectly enhance dopamine neurotransmission in the brain (Kalivas & Volkow, 2005; Luscher & Malenka, 2011; Wise, 2013). These effects on dopamine neurotransmission are at the core of drug-induced neuroadaptations in dopamine and other neurochemical synapses that support the compulsive use of addictive drugs (Dietz, Dietz, Nestler, & Russo, 2009; Russo et al., 2010; Van den Oever, Spijker, & Smit, 2012).

Addictive drugs can be arranged into several categories based on their effects on neurochemicals in the brain:

- *Psychomotor stimulant drugs.* This category includes drugs that (a) enhance dopamine, norepinephrine, and serotonin neurotransmission (e.g., amphetamine, methamphetamine, and cocaine); (b) activate nicotinic receptors for acetylcholine (e.g., nicotine); or (c) block receptors for adenosine (e.g., caffeine, theophylline).
- *Sedative-hypnotic drugs.* This category includes drugs that are agonists for GABA-A subtype receptors for the neurotransmitter GABA (e.g., alcohol, barbiturates, and benzodiazepines).
- *Opioid agonist drugs.* These drugs bind to and activate one or more of the subtypes of receptors for endogenous opioids (e.g., heroin, oxycodone, hydrocodone, and morphine).
- *Cannabinoid agonist drugs.* The best-known drug in this category is marijuana, the principal psychoactive agent of which is delta-9-tetrahydrocannabinol; this chemical is an agonist for endogenous cannabinoid receptors.

Recreational users of these psychoactive drugs experience the acute pleasurable, reinforcing properties of the drugs. The chronic use of these addictive psychotropic drugs provokes the brain to adapt to the pharmacological assault that these drugs deliver (Nestler, 2009; Zahm, 2010): Repeated experience with these drugs teaches the user that ingestion can produce acute effects including intense pleasure or euphoria; motivation to get this intense pleasure can provoke frequent use; persistent use reorganizes brain neurochemistry to establish a neurochemical adaptation that supports a new psychological experience for the chronic user, namely, craving. Craving can establish compulsive use—use that temporarily diminishes an intense craving. Craving can also become conditioned to environmental cues, such as people, places, and objects associated with drug use. This conditioned craving phenomenon is a powerful mechanism by which environmental stimuli or experiences elicit drug use when a person was not intending to use a drug. Craving, conditioned craving, stress, and a single use of a drug can provoke relapse into addictive behavior.

Thus, the addict has repeatedly experienced the drug-induced euphoria, the craving, the fact that drug ingestion will temporarily diminish craving, and the conditioned craving leading to unexpected use. The addict also has achieved a level of familiarity and comfort with drug use, has developed a diminished perception of the risks associated with drug use, and likely has arranged a social context that facilitates obtaining and using addictive substances. All of those experiences provide the addict with a brain whose neurochemistry has been reorganized over an extended period of months or years by the behavioral features of drug addiction. It will require considerable work to attempt to reverse those changes in the brain and the impact that they have on the addict's behavior.

Not only does the ingestion of addictive psychoactive drugs initiate and maintain the development of changes in the brain and in behavior that support addiction, but also psychoactive drugs can be used to clinically treat the symptoms of addiction.

HOW HAVE DRUGS BEEN USED TO TREAT ADDICTION AND ABUSE?

They tell Marty that he needs to change his behavior and his social habits, avoid some of his friends, and take some medication. It seems as if they have prepared a program that is intended to get him to change his lifestyle. That seems like a pretty tall order for Marty—it is a lot for him to process and to commit to, but he thinks he can do it with the help of some medication. He has proven that he has the skill to take a drug, but he is not so confident he can manage all the rest of the changes that he needs to be making.

Given the contributions of an individual's brain, behavior, and living situation to the development of addiction, it seems reasonable that a treatment program should use methods and strategies intended to change all three—brain, behavior, and social context. Two aspects of recovery from addiction that must be addressed by a therapeutic program are detoxification and preventing or delaying relapse. Medication can assist counseling or behavior therapy toward both of these realistic goals. A medication can be used during the detoxification phase to prevent withdrawal symptoms as the addicted person is initiating abstinence. Medication also can be used to prevent relapse by diminishing the reinforcing value of the drug of addiction, abolishing the craving for the drug, or both.

Psychotropic medications for treating addiction would function best when used to accompany a nondrug therapeutic method(s) during both the detoxification phase and the prevention of relapse phase. Behavioral therapies might include cognitive behavioral therapy, community reinforcement, contingency management, 12-step treatment programs, and behavioral couples or family treatment (Carroll & Onken, 2005; Finney, Wilbourne, & Moos, 2007). What should the role of psychotropic medication be within that context? Aside from pharmacologically assisting the switch from active drug taking to abstinence, what might a medication do best? A medication could have pharmacological properties with the capacity to alter one or several of the addictive drug-induced neurochemical adaptations that support particular psychological and behavioral aspects of addiction, for example, the drug-induced euphoria or the onset of craving and its eliciting of compulsive drug ingestion.

Keeping in mind that there are a variety of neurochemical consequences of ingestion of the various drugs having addictive properties, what alternative pharmacological strategies might use psychotropic medications to treat addiction?

- Given that all addictive drugs appear to either directly or indirectly enhance dopamine neurotransmission, the therapeutic use of psychotropic medications might focus on strategies that alter dopamine neurotransmission. This approach is consistent with the perspective that addiction to one drug shares important neurochemistry with addiction to any other drug.
- Given that specific addictive drugs have selective effects on neurochemical processes, the therapeutic use of psychotropic medications might employ a variety of drugs that target an individual neurochemical process that is directly related to a *specific* drug of addiction.

- Craving is experienced for many drugs of addiction. If the psychological experience of craving has a neurochemical mechanism that is common to the experience of craving, regardless of the specific drug that is being craved, then a psychotropic medication that diminishes craving could be a useful tool for treating addiction to any drug for which craving can occur. On the other hand, if, for example, craving for cocaine is a different neurochemical-psychological phenomenon than craving for alcohol, then different medications might be necessary to treat cravings for these different drugs.

Of these various strategies for pharmacologically obstructing or reversing some of the neurochemical mechanisms of addiction, the general approach most frequently taken is one that attempts to treat addiction for the specific drug that the patient is compulsively using. Within that context, the use of psychotropic medications falls into three tactics for pharmacological intervention; a single medication could serve one or more of these tactics:

- *Blockade of the euphoria* induced by the specific addictive drug to diminish the motivation to seek and experience the drug-induced pleasure
- Substitution of a medicinal drug for the addictive drug to *forestall the onset of withdrawal* following the initiation of abstinence
- *Inhibition of craving* for a specific drug to prevent drug seeking and relapse

A variety of options for pharmacotherapy can diminish use or inhibit craving for addictive drugs (Table 9.1). Some of these medications appear to have the ability to affect use for more than one addictive drug. And for some addictive drugs, there are multiple options to consider for treating addiction, in the event that the first choice of medication is not effective for an individual patient. None of the medications is expected to provide successful monotherapy for treatment of addiction; combinations of these drugs are occasionally used clinically, and all of these therapeutic drugs have side effects (van den Brink, 2012). Let's take a look at psychotropic medications used to treat addiction to drugs that have different pharmacological properties: nicotine, alcohol, opioids, cocaine, and marijuana.

Nicotine. Nicotine is a nicotinic receptor agonist for the neurotransmitter acetylcholine. Nicotine can indirectly enhance the release of dopamine in synapses in the nucleus accumbens served by dopamine neurons originating in the ventral tegmental area in the brain.

TABLE 9.1

Psychoactive medications and their presumed synaptic mechanism of action for treatment of addiction to various addictive drugs.

MEDICATION	PRESUMED SYNAPTIC MECHANISM	ADDICTIVE DRUG				
		NICOTINE	ALCOHOL	HEROIN	COCAINE	MARIJUANA
Nicotine	ACh	x				
Varenicline	ACh	x				
Mecamylamine	ACh	x				
Naltrexone	Opioid	x	x	x		
Rimonabant	Cannabinoid	x	x		x	
Topiramate	GABA	x	x		x	
Baclofen	GABA		x		x	
Bupropion	DA, NE, SER	x				
Nalmefene	Opioid		x			
Methadone	Opioid			x		
Buprenorphine	Opioid			x		
Acamprosate	Glutamate, GABA		x	x		
Propranolol	NE				x	
Ondansetron	SER		x			
Modafinil	DA				x	

Note: x indicates the drug has clinical utility for treating addiction. ACh, acetylcholine; GABA, gamma-aminobutyric acid; DA, dopamine; NE, norepinephrine; SER, serotonin. This table illustrates a lack of selectivity of some medications for treatment of addiction to various drugs. For example, the opioid receptor antagonist naltrexone has been used to treat addiction to nicotine (an acetylcholine agonist), alcohol (a GABA agonist), and heroin (an opioid agonist). Despite the rather long list of medications useful for treating addiction, none of them—including the cannabinoid antagonist rimonabant—have demonstrated utility for the treatment of chronic use of marijuana.

- *Nicotine* itself has been used for nicotine replacement therapy (as nicotine patch, gum, inhaler, nasal spray, or lozenges) to aid in stopping the use of tobacco to ingest nicotine.
- *Varenicline*, a partial agonist for nicotinic receptors for acetylcholine, has been used to delay relapse of addiction to nicotine.
- *Mecamylamine*, a nicotinic receptor antagonist for the neurotransmitter acetylcholine, has been used (sometimes in combination with nicotine replacement therapy) to attempt to reduce nicotine ingestion in smokers.
- *Naltrexone*, a receptor antagonist for multiple receptor subtypes for endogenous opioids, has been used to attempt reduction of nicotine ingestion in smokers.
- *Rimonabant*, a cannabinoid receptor antagonist, has been used to attempt to prevent relapse of smoking in patients abstaining from nicotine use, but there are worries over rimonabant's psychiatric side effects.
- *Topiramate*, a drug with anticonvulsant properties that enhances GABA neurotransmission, has been used to prevent relapse of addiction to nicotine.
- *Bupropion*, a drug with antidepressant properties that can inhibit reuptake of dopamine and norepinephrine, and also acts as an antagonist at acetylcholine receptors, has been used to inhibit craving and delay relapse in smokers who are abstaining.

Alcohol. Alcohol enhances GABA neurotransmission by binding to the GABA-A receptor subtype. Alcohol also has effects on other neurotransmitter processes, and it indirectly enhances dopamine neurotransmission.

- *Disulfiram* inhibits aldehyde dehydrogenase, thereby diminishing the catabolism of alcohol, resulting in the accumulation of acetaldehyde, which causes intense illness. This pharmacological manipulation gives the ingestion of alcohol severe negative consequences. This result is easy enough to avoid by failing to take one's disulfiram medication—a fact that has compromised the utility of disulfiram therapy for addiction to alcohol, except when conducted with intensive supervision.
- *Naltrexone* has been used to diminish the euphoria induced by ingestion of alcohol and the craving experienced by an alcoholic during abstinence.
- *Nalmefene*, an opioid receptor antagonist with a longer duration of action and fewer side effects than naltrexone, has been used to

attempt to reduce consumption of alcohol or to prevent relapse in patients abstaining from alcohol.

- *Topiramate* also has been used to prevent relapse of addiction to alcohol.
- *Baclofen*, an agonist for the GABA-B receptor subtype, can indirectly inhibit release of dopamine in the nucleus accumbens; baclofen has been used to forestall symptoms of withdrawal from alcohol and to delay or prevent relapse for addiction to alcohol.
- *Acamprosate* has antagonistic effects on NMDA receptors for glutamate, and effects on GABA neurotransmission. Acamprosate has been used to diminish craving to prevent relapse during abstinence for patients addicted to alcohol.
- *Rimonabant*, the cannabinoid receptor antagonist, has potential for delaying relapse of addiction to alcohol.
- *Ondansetron*, an antagonist for the serotonin 5-HT3 receptor subtype, has potential for delaying relapse of addiction to alcohol.

Heroin, oxycodone, and hydrocodone.   Heroin and other opioids (such as oxycodone and hydrocodone) activate mu-opioid receptors to indirectly increase dopamine neurotransmission.

- *Naltrexone*, a receptor antagonist for multiple receptor subtypes for endogenous opioids, once was heralded as a potential solution for addiction to heroin (Pert, Pasternak, & Snyder, 1973). The idea was that heroin's ability to induce a rush would be blocked by naltrexone, discouraging the heroin user from self-administering heroin. This approach is effective for the addict who is highly motivated to remain abstinent (Goldstein, 1976) but has proved to be less effective than the use of methadone or buprenorphine (Bart, 2012).
- *Methadone and buprenorphine*, partial agonists for endogenous opioid receptors, have been used as substitution treatment to prevent relapse of addiction to opioid drugs. Both drugs have longer duration of action than heroin. Buprenorphine runs a lesser risk of overdose by respiratory suppression than does methadone.
- *Acamprosate*, an antagonist for NMDA receptors for the neurotransmitter glutamate, has been used to delay relapse of heroin addiction.

Cocaine.   The ability of cocaine to inhibit reuptake of dopamine is the principal means by which cocaine is reinforcing and has addictive potential.

Various drugs in such classes as anticonvulsants, antidepressants, antipsychotics, and dopamine agonists have been considered in the treatment of addiction to cocaine, with the conclusion that no drug has been identified as particularly useful for this purpose. Several drugs have been used clinically with limited effectiveness.

- *Topiramate* has been used to prevent relapse of addiction to cocaine.
- *Disulfiram* has been used to prevent relapse of addiction to cocaine.
- *Modafinil*, which may inhibit synaptic reuptake of dopamine, has been used to inhibit craving, thereby preventing relapse of addiction to cocaine.
- *Propranolol*, an antagonist for beta-adrenergic receptors, has been used to prevent relapse of addiction to cocaine.
- *Baclofen*, an agonist to the GABA-B receptor subtype, has been used to delay relapse for addiction to cocaine.
- *Rimonabant*, the cannabinoid receptor antagonist, has potential for delaying relapse of addiction to cocaine.

Marijuana.   Marijuana, the most heavily used illegal psychoactive substance in the world, has as its principal psychoactive component delta-9-tetrahydrocannabinol—an agonist for CB-1 cannabinoid receptors.

- *Rimonabant*, a cannabinoid CB-1 receptor antagonist, has not demonstrated utility for the treatment of chronic use of marijuana.

In summary, numerous psychotropic medications have proved to be useful or have potential for treating addiction (Table 9.1). No one medication has evidence-based support for being the best choice for diminishing the reinforcing value of addictive drugs, and no one medication has evidence-based support for being the best choice for inhibiting craving, thereby delaying or preventing relapse. These facts reinforce the perspective that medications for treating drug addiction perhaps are best used as adjuncts for nondrug behavior therapies that encourage the addict to make changes in lifestyle and social environment, assisted by psychotropic medication. One pertinent example of the utility of a multimodal therapeutic program is provided by attempts to quit smoking: Abstinence alone can produce a 3–5% success rate after one year, behavioral interventions alone can produce a 7–16% success rate, and pharmacological plus behavioral treatment can produce a 24% success rate (Laniado-Laborin, 2010).

The toolbox of psychotropic medications for treating addiction contains drugs that alter one or several of a group of neurochemicals, including endogenous opioids, dopamine, serotonin, norepinephrine, GABA, glutamate, acetylcholine, and cannabinoids (Table 9.1). This fact provides perspective on the state-of-the-art understanding of addiction. First, it reminds us that, although the behavioral features of addiction (e.g., compulsive use) appear similar for addictions to a wide variety of recreational drugs, the processes that underlie addiction engage multiple neurochemical processes and sites in the human brain. Addiction is not *only* about dopamine synapses in the nucleus accumbens of the brain. In other words, psychological processes such as reward, pleasure, reinforcement, craving, conditioned craving, and compulsive use engage multiple neurochemicals and numerous sites in the brain. Second, the variety of useful drugs in the toolbox for treating addiction reminds us that addictions to different drugs may engage neurochemicals and sites in the brain in different ways. For example, the manner in which the brain organizes craving for cocaine may be somewhat different from the way the brain supports craving for alcohol; this is consistent with the fact that naltrexone pharmacotherapy may be useful for diminishing craving for alcohol but not craving for cocaine.

Thus, the ultimate goal for understanding in what way the brain is disordered during addiction is to understand how each individual drug with addictive properties is causing neuroadaptations in the brain, such that the brain becomes addicted specifically to the drug the addict is using. The key to understanding the addicted brain is not in knowing that all addictions to all drugs have something to do with dopamine neurotransmission and dopamine neuroadaptations. Rather, the key is found in knowing how nondopamine neuroadaptations are interacting with dopamine neuroadaptations to support behavioral features of addiction for a specific addictive drug. Acquiring that knowledge is aided by clinical experience in using psychotropic medications to treat addition. For example, discovering in a clinical setting that the opioid antagonist naltrexone can delay relapse for a patient addicted to the acetylcholine agonist nicotine ultimately enriches the neurobiological theories of addiction and guides the search for new options for pharmacological therapy.

IS OVEREATING AN EXAMPLE
OF ADDICTIVE BEHAVIOR?

Larry and his spouse appear to have somewhat similar problems. Six months ago he was addicted to cocaine, and Teri was obese. One similarity was the professional advice they both received to approach solving their maladies. Both of them were told that they first needed to use less of the substance being overused, and that they also needed to change some related behaviors: Larry needed to quit using cocaine, and needed to abstain completely. Teri needed to eat less food, and needed to quit eating so many fried, fatty foods. They are now in the midst of their second phase in their recoveries, and again there are similarities: Larry needs to maintain his abstinence in the face of multiple environmental cues that bring on his craving for cocaine. He needs to avoid relapse. And Teri needs to maintain her dietary restrictions in the face of multiple environmental cues that tempt her to eat more than she needs. She must avoid returning to her unhealthy habits with food, if she is to maintain her loss of weight. Is Larry a recovering drug addict and Teri a recovering food addict? Have they both been "substance" abusers?

Recovery from addiction is essentially a two-stage process, and so also is reduction of eating to lose body weight. There are similarities in the behavioral aspects of recovery: The addict must stop using the drug and must remain abstinent to avoid relapse. The overweight or obese person must alter choices about food and reduce eating and must maintain reduced food intake to maintain loss of weight.

There also are similarities in the manner that the brain organizes eating behaviors and addictive drug-taking behaviors: There is an evidence-based argument for the idea that the neurochemical processes in the brain that control ingestion of food overlap to a considerable extent with the neurochemical processes in the brain that control ingestion of drugs (Wise, 1997; Volkow & Wise, 2005). At the heart of that argument is the fact that eating palatable foods, or the ingestion of addictive drugs, immediately elicits the release of endogenous dopamine in the nucleus accumbens of the brain (Volkow, Wang, Tomasi, & Baler, 2013a; Wise, 2013). Thus, the neuronal circuitry of brain that utilizes dopamine to produce the experience of pleasure is important for enabling eating behavior or drug-taking behavior to become the compulsive behaviors of addiction (Volkow, Wang, Tomasi, & Baler, 2013b). Finally, both overeating and drug addiction are biopsychosocial problems that are affected by many factors—genetic, neurochemical, psychological (e.g., craving), environmental (e.g., conditioned cues), and social (Liu, von Deneen, Kobeissy, & Gold, 2010; Volkow et al., 2013b).

Although these are interesting and important ideas for those who study the relation between brain processes and ingestive behaviors, the notion that overeating to obesity is a form of addiction has facilitated only to a limited extent the development of drugs that can serve as pharmacotherapy *both* for overeating and for addiction. For example, the drugs currently being used or being considered as medications to treat some component of overeating *and also* drug addiction are these few: naltrexone, topiramate, bupropion, and rimonabant. Despite this short list, there is a rather long list of at least 20 endogenous peptide hormones and neurotransmitters known to be involved in the reinforcing properties of food and of addictive drugs (Volkow et al., 2013b); these identified hormones and neurochemicals may provide the opportunity for the development of novel medications that are potentially useful for the treatment of addiction to food and addiction to drugs.

HOW DO ADDICTIVE DRUGS ALTER NEUROCHEMICAL PROCESSES IN THE BRAIN?

(Drugs Can Mimic Endogenous Neurochemicals.)

Art was and still is drug dependent. He was having an intimate relationship with an illicit substance. He craved it every day, he used it every day, and it was quite inconvenient but necessary to acquire it frequently enough to maintain his habit. His need for the illicit drug was dominating his life. Now he is receiving help for his addiction. He is taking a medication daily, although it is a bit of a pain to have to fulfill his prescription weekly at a pharmacy that is an hour drive from his home. But he needs the medication every day, or else he is likely to relapse into taking his illicit drug. Taking his medication precisely as prescribed, and structuring his days to avoid certain places and people, have become of central importance for keeping his life together. Art is still drug dependent, but now he's medication dependent—without his medication, it all falls apart.

Addiction is a process that can be bracketed by psychoactive drugs—recreational psychoactive drugs that create addiction by reorganizing brain neurochemistry and behavior, and medicinal psychoactive drugs that help to remedy the neurochemistry and behaviors of addiction. Some of these recreational drugs and medicinal drugs mimic or partially reproduce the effects of endogenous neurochemicals.

It is no surprise that an ingested exogenous drug that induces pleasure may be mimicking the effect of an endogenous neurochemical that plays a role in the normal neurochemistry of pleasure, particularly dopamine or endogenous opioids (Volkow & Wise, 2005; Wise, 1998). Some of these recreational pleasure-inducing substances are receptor agonist drugs that bind to and activate one or another subtype of receptor for a neurotransmitter: Nicotine is a receptor agonist for acetylcholine; alcohol is a receptor agonist for the GABA-A receptor subtype; heroin, oxycodone, and hydrocodone are agonists for opioid receptors; delta-9-tetrahydrocannabinol, the principal psychoactive chemical in marijuana, is an agonist for receptors for endogenous cannabinol; LSD is a partial agonist for 5-HT2A serotonin receptors.

Other recreational drugs are not receptor agonist drugs but enhance synaptic neurotransmission for one or several neurotransmitters. For example, inhibition of presynaptic transport (i.e., reuptake) of a neurotransmitter results in increased or prolonged access of a neurotransmitter for synaptic receptors: cocaine, amphetamine, and methamphetamine enhance release and inhibit reuptake of dopamine, serotonin, and norepinephrine.

Some drugs with therapeutic value for treatment of addiction act as agonists for receptors for endogenous neurotransmitters (Table 9.2). Varenicline is a partial agonist for nicotinic receptors for acetylcholine and thus mimics some but not all of the effects of nicotine at those receptors. Baclofen is an agonist for the GABA-B receptor subtype. Methadone is a full agonist, and buprenorphine is a partial agonist, for mu-opioid receptors;

TABLE 9.2

The presumed synaptic mechanism of action for receptor agonist and antagonist medications used to treat addiction.

MEDICATION	RECEPTOR TYPE	ADDICTIVE DRUG			
		NICOTINE	ALCOHOL	HEROIN	COCAINE
Agonist					
Nicotine	Acetylcholine	x			
Varenicline	Acetylcholine	x			
Methadone	Opioid			x	
Buprenorphine	Opioid			x	
Baclofen	GABA		x		x
Antagonist					
Mecamylamine	Acetylcholine	x			
Naltrexone	Opioid	x	x	x	
Nalmefene	Opioid		x		
Rimonabant	Cannabinoid	x	x		x
Acamprosate	Glutamate		x	x	
Propranolol	Norepinephrine				x
Ondansetron	Serotonin		x		

Note: x indicates the drug has clinical utility for treating addiction. GABA, gamma-aminobutyric acid. This table illustrates that agonist drugs that activate receptors and antagonist drugs that block receptors can both serve as medications for addiction to various drugs.

buprenorphine mimics some but not all of the effects of heroin at the mu-opioid receptor.

In summary, direct pharmacological activation of receptors, or indirect enhancement of synaptic neurotransmission, can artificially and powerfully enhance neurotransmission in neurochemical systems (e.g., endogenous dopamine and opioids) that normally serve the psychological process of reward or pleasure. In addition, pharmacological activation of receptors can provide a strategy for treating addiction. Both of these facts make clear that targeting synaptic receptors for pharmacological manipulation is a powerful tactic for altering behavior.

Let's take a closer look at three cases in which both the drug of addiction and the therapeutic drug are agonists for the same endogenous neurochemical.

Nicotine. If you would like to have a lifetime relationship with a legal drug, choose to use nicotine. The addictive potential of nicotine is immense, perhaps most evident in failure to quit rates between 90% and 100%. The global use of tobacco products is also immense and increasing, and smoking tobacco is predicted to kill more than one billion people in this century (Laniado-Laborin, 2010). Why is it so very difficult to quit smoking, and what are the options for treating addiction to nicotine?

Nicotine is an agonist for nicotinic acetylcholine receptors. The nicotinic receptor is a receptor complex composed of five subunits. One of these subunits, the beta-2 subunit, is of primary importance for the reinforcing effects of nicotine, which depends upon the ability of nicotine to release dopamine in various regions of the brain, including the nucleus accumbens, prefrontal cortex, and corpus striatum (Benowitz, 2008). Nicotine also can indirectly alter neurotransmission for norepinephrine, acetylcholine, serotonin, GABA, glutamate, and endorphins, but it is nicotine's ability to enhance release of dopamine in synapses of the nucleus accumbens, and enhance release of opioids (Berrendero, Robledo, Trigo, Martin-Garcia, & Maldonado, 2010), that is central to its addictive potential. Ultimately, nicotine's effect on release of dopamine in the nucleus accumbens depends upon the interaction of nicotine's direct effects on nicotinic acetylcholine receptors and its indirect effects on glutamate and GABA neurotransmission (Benowitz, 2008). Thus, it is a multiplicity of direct and indirect neurochemical effects of ingested nicotine that establishes the drug's compelling capacity for addiction.

Chronic use of nicotine provokes neuroadaptations in the brain, including the upregulation of nicotinic receptors. Initiating abstinence from nicotine quickly causes a decline in synaptic release of dopamine and other neurotransmitters, which may provide an explanation for the general malaise that accompanies abstinence. Smoking a cigarette can quickly relieve this malaise, providing powerful incentive to resume smoking during abstinence.

Thus, smokers use nicotine for a variety of reasons: Nicotine's acute effects include pleasure; heightened arousal, vigilance, and performance; relief of anxiety or depression; and the relief from symptoms of withdrawal that appear during abstinence. Given all that, it is a lot to ask for a therapeutic drug to reduce the motivation to use tobacco to get nicotine. Let's take a look at two receptor agonist drugs that have been used to treat addiction to nicotine: nicotine and varenicline.

The use of nicotine as medication for addiction to nicotine—nicotine replacement therapy—is basically an approach that allows the addict to have the nicotine but not have to smoke or use tobacco to get it. There are advantages and disadvantages to this strategy. One principal advantage is the simple fact that the nicotine-addicted smoker can avoid withdrawal symptoms during abstinence from smoking by taking nicotine by a different route. The avoidance of withdrawal symptoms does not abolish desire or craving for the pleasurable acute effects of nicotine, but the desire may be blunted by nicotine replacement therapy. The obvious shortcoming to this approach is that allowing the addict to continue to use the drug of addiction surely is not itself a remedy for addiction. On the other hand, it is a step toward a remedy in the following way: The reinforcing or rewarding characteristics of rituals associated with smoking behavior may be eliminated or extinguished in the person no longer smoking to get the drug. Those smoking rituals (e.g., tamping down tobacco, lighting up, assuming a fashionable posture, blowing smoke) may be replaced by behaviors associated with taking the nicotine in gum, in a lozenge, in a nasal spray, by inhaler, or through a patch, but those new self-administration behaviors may not themselves acquire secondary reinforcing value, because they do not mimic the rapid transit to the brain for a dose of nicotine obtained by smoking (except perhaps for nasal spray or inhaler). Thus, nicotine delivered by chewing gum and other means provides relatively less pleasure than does smoking. This diminished reward value of nonsmoked nicotine, together with diminishing the withdrawal symptoms that normally follow cessation of smoking, provides two steps toward being able to stop smoking and nicotine use. Getting to that sustained abstinence end point, however, will require more than nicotine replacement therapy. It will also require some type of supportive counseling and changes to lifestyle.

An alternative receptor agonist drug with potential to treat addiction to nicotine is varenicline. Varenicline has high affinity for the beta-2 subunit of the nicotinic acetylcholine receptor. When this subunit of the nicotinic receptor is activated by nicotine, nicotine has its full impact on the release of dopamine in the nucleus accumbens associated with nicotine-induced pleasure. When acting as only a partial agonist and binding to this same receptor subunit, however, varenicline has only partial effect (approximately one-half that of nicotine) on release of dopamine. In addition, a sufficiently large dose of varenicline will bind to and *occupy* nicotinic receptors, thereby preventing nicotine from binding to and activating those receptors. Taken together, the ability of varenicline to bind to nicotinic receptors, and only partially activate them while fully occupying them, enables varenicline to (a) provide only some fraction of the pleasure normally associated with nicotine use, (b) diminish craving while further preventing the usual magnitude of pleasure associated with smoking, and (c) diminish withdrawal symptoms (Benowitz, 2008; Laniado-Laborin, 2010).

Thus, the advantage that varenicline has over nicotine for pharmacological therapy for nicotine addiction is due to varenicline's more *selective* pharmacological effects as a *partial* agonist for nicotinic receptors. This selectivity makes varenicline a different tactical tool compared with nicotine replacement therapy. The results of clinical trials assessing varenicline's effectiveness show promise, but there are concerns about varenicline having adverse psychiatric effects in some users (Laniado-Laborin, 2010).

Alcohol.   Although alcohol may have relatively less potential for addiction than nicotine, the global use of alcohol is enormous, with approximately 140 million people meeting criteria for alcohol dependence or abuse (van den Brink, 2012). Alcohol has a variety of effects on receptors for GABA, glutamine, acetylcholine, dopamine, adenosine, and glycine, but its ability to act as an agonist for the GABA-A receptor subtype has long been considered to be significant for understanding the reinforcing effects of alcohol on behavior, which also depends upon release of dopamine and endogenous opioids (Koob et al., 1998).

Alcohol's ability to enhance GABA-A receptor-mediated neurotransmission has encouraged consideration of manipulation of receptors for GABA as a tactic for treating addiction to alcohol. Baclofen is a GABA-B receptor agonist that shows promise for its ability to maintain abstinence from alcohol ingestion, thereby preventing relapse (van den Brink, 2012). Evidence from clinical trials supports the idea that baclofen can diminish craving for alcohol, decrease alcohol intake, and prevent relapse (Addolorato et al., 2002).

Heroin, oxycodone, and hydrocodone.   Heroin had been for some time the opioid of choice for addicts, but the abuse of prescription analgesics such as oxycodone and hydrocodone has increased so dramatically in the United States that some consider the problem to have reached epidemic proportion (DuPont, 2010; Hernandez & Nelson, 2010). Heroin, oxycodone, and hydrocodone are agonists for mu-opioid receptors. Pharmacological activation of mu-opioid receptors in the brain is followed by inhibition of GABAergic neurotransmission, thereby causing increased release of dopamine in the nucleus accumbens (van den Brink, 2012).

Among pharmacological tactics to treat addiction to heroin, oxycodone, and hydrocodone is the use of either methadone or buprenorphine. This approach is somewhat analogous to using varenicline to treat addiction to nicotine, in that methadone and buprenorphine are both agonists for mu-opioid receptors, and therefore can essentially substitute for the drug of addiction. There are pharmacological differences between methadone and buprenorphine: Methadone is a full agonist for mu-opioid receptors, but buprenorphine has complex effects as a partial agonist for mu-opioid receptors, partial or full agonist for delta-opioid receptors, and antagonist for kappa-opioid receptors. Either drug can be used clinically to substitute for the drug that the patient is dependent on. Substitution can forestall the symptoms of withdrawal during abstinence, diminish the reinforcing effects of the drug of addiction, and inhibit craving for the addicted drug.

Methadone and buprenorphine have established utility for treatment of addiction to heroin (Pierce, O'Brien, Kenny, & Vanderschuren, 2012; van den Brink, 2012), but their use for treating addiction to oxycodone or hydrocodone has not yet been convincingly demonstrated (Holmes, 2012). In addition, as with nicotine replacement therapy, substitution maintenance therapy does not represent a complete remedy for opiate addiction, because persons maintained on daily doses of methadone or buprenorphine are still drug dependent, although their situation has improved to some degree.

In summary, the use of a receptor agonist drug as medication for an addiction to a receptor agonist drug permits the patient to switch from being addicted to one drug to being dependent on a different drug. There are advantages to this switch (e.g., cost, legality, access, social acceptability), but the addict remains drug dependent until nondrug therapeutic methods can initiate and maintain sustained abstinence from both the drug of abuse and the medication.

CAN BLOCKADE OF THE EFFECTS OF AN ADDICTIVE DRUG TERMINATE ADDICTIVE BEHAVIOR?

(Drugs Can Block Endogenous Neurochemicals.)

Janey completely understands the explanation that naltrexone will prevent the heroin from producing its rush, as long as she takes the naltrexone as instructed and does not take a larger than usual dose of heroin. But Janey also knows dollars and cents, and she knows that when she needs a rush, she'd be stupid to waste the heroin on which she had spent good money. So, she is smart enough to not take her naltrexone on a day when she intends for heroin to be her medication of choice.

A drug that prevents an endogenous neurochemical from activating a receptor is a useful tool in research aimed at studying the functions of neurochemicals in the brain. It is assumed that such a receptor antagonist drug can be used in a manner that reveals the functional role of the endogenous neurochemical that is being pharmacologically blocked by the antagonist drug. The same assumption can be made about a receptor antagonist drug when it is used as a therapeutic device. For example, if a receptor antagonist drug inhibits the euphoria induced by a recreational drug, that fact reveals that the blocked receptor type and the endogenous neurochemical that normally activates that receptor type are at least partially responsible for the euphoria induced by the recreational drug.

A look at the clinical utility of the receptor antagonist drugs used to treat addiction to various recreational drugs supports the following conclusions:

- Mecamylamine's clinical utility reveals a role for nicotinic receptors and endogenous acetylcholine in the reinforcing effect of nicotine.
- Naltrexone's clinical utility reveals a role for mu- or kappa-opioid receptors and endogenous opioids in the reinforcing effects and craving for nicotine, alcohol, and heroin.
- Rimonabant's potential clinical utility reveals a role for the CB-1 cannabinoid receptor for endogenous cannabinol in the craving for nicotine, alcohol, and cocaine.
- Nalmefene's clinical utility reveals a role for mu-opioid receptors and endogenous opioids in the reinforcing effect and craving for alcohol.
- Acamprosate's clinical utility reveals roles for NMDA receptors for glutamate in the craving for alcohol and heroin.
- Propranolol's clinical utility reveals a role for beta-adrenergic receptors and norepinephrine in the craving for cocaine.
- Ondansetron's clinical utility reveals a role for 5-HT3 receptors for serotonin in the craving for alcohol.

When considering the demonstrated clinical utility of these seven receptor antagonist drugs (Table 9.2), it is apparent that three different receptor antagonist drugs are useful for the treatment of addiction to nicotine, five are useful for the treatment of addiction to alcohol, two for the treatment of addiction to heroin, and two for the treatment of addiction to cocaine. Of these antagonist drugs, naltrexone has the longest and perhaps the most interesting track record of clinical utility and thus is worthy of a closer look.

Naltrexone was originally heralded for its potential utility for treating addiction to heroin (Pert et al., 1973), but in just several years time it became clear that naltrexone pharmacotherapy would be effective only in heroin addicts who were highly motivated to abstain (Goldstein, 1976). The logic for using naltrexone to block the reinforcing properties of heroin made sense in pharmacological terms: The mu-opioid receptor antagonist in sufficient doses should be able to prevent the reinforcing properties of the mu-opioid receptor agonist heroin. But addiction is not only a pharmacological phenomenon—it is also a biopsychosocial phenomenon, and as such, an addict's behavior, cognitions, emotions, and social issues are powerful factors that determine choices made. In the case of naloxone medication for addiction to heroin, it is too easy for an addict to choose to not adhere to the recommendation for proper daily use of naltrexone. Addicts with heroin that desire its euphoria can simply skip their naltrexone that day. In the end, the utility of naltrexone for treatment of addiction to heroin is limited (Goldstein, 2001; O'Brien & Dackis, 2009; Bart, 2012).

Naltrexone has found a role for treatment of addiction to alcohol. This opportunity originated in research in animals that demonstrated a role for endogenous opioids in the reinforcing properties of alcohol (Trigo, Martin-Garcia, Berrendero, Robledo, & Maldonado, 2010). Several findings suggested the potential clinical utility of naltrexone:

- Ingestion of alcohol by rats increases the release of dopamine in the nucleus accumbens; naltrexone can block this alcohol-induced release of dopamine and can inhibit the self-administration of alcohol (Gonzales & Weiss, 1998). These findings suggest that the reinforcing properties of alcohol can be diminished by naltrexone, which predicts that naltrexone might inhibit alcohol ingestion in humans.
- Mice who lack the mu-opioid receptor subtype fail to self-administer alcohol (Roberts et al., 2000). This finding suggests that activation of the mu-opioid receptor is necessary for the reinforcing properties of alcohol, predicting that naltrexone-induced blockade of the mu-opioid receptor might inhibit alcohol ingestion in humans.
- The ability of conditioned cues to provoke relapse of alcohol in-

gestion is blocked by naltrexone in rats (Liu & Weiss, 2002). This finding suggests that naltrexone might diminish conditioned craving for alcohol in humans.

Findings such as these were enough to provoke attempts to use naltrexone in clinical settings to treat alcoholism. Naltrexone can inhibit alcohol intake and craving for alcohol in humans (O'Malley, Krishnan-Sarin, Farren, Sinha, & Kreek, 2002), but its effectiveness varies considerably (O'Brien & Dackis, 2009). Some of the variability may be attributable to genetic factors, because there is some evidence that a family history of alcoholism can moderate the effectiveness of naltrexone on alcohol intake (Capone, Kahler, Swift, & O'Malley, 2011; Ray & Hutchison, 2007; Rohsenow, Miranda, McGeary, & Monti, 2007). Moreover, there is evidence that, among people with a family history of alcoholism, men are more likely than women to benefit from naltrexone pharmacotherapy (Krishnan-Sarin, Krystal, Shi, Pittman, & O'Malley, 2007).

Naltrexone may also prove to be useful for treating addiction to nicotine. Nicotine's reinforcing properties depend upon its ability to enhance release of both synaptic dopamine and endogenous opioids (Berrendero et al., 2010; Trigo et al., 2010). The evidence supporting naltrexone's clinical effectiveness for treating addiction to nicotine is relatively slight (van den Brink, 2012) but holds promise while showing sex-related differences in effectiveness. For example, naltrexone augmentation of nicotine replacement therapy increases the success rate for cessation of smoking (O'Malley et al., 2006), and naltrexone produces higher rates for cessation of smoking for women than for men compared with placebo (King et al., 2006). In addition, naltrexone is more effective in women than in men for prevention of weight gain during extended abstinence from nicotine (King et al., 2012). Moreover, naltrexone has greater benefit for reducing alcohol consumption for alcoholic smokers than for alcoholic nonsmokers (Fucito et al., 2012).

In summary, naltrexone selectively blocks opioid receptors and can be useful for the treatment of addiction to heroin, alcohol, and nicotine, despite the facts that heroin is an agonist for mu-opioid receptors, alcohol is an agonist for GABA-A receptors, and nicotine is an agonist for nicotinic acetylcholine receptors (Table 9.2). These findings demonstrate that the reinforcing properties or the craving for heroin, alcohol, and nicotine share an endogenous opioid mechanism in humans.

A wide variety of receptor agonist and antagonist drugs for an extensive list of endogenous neurochemicals have clinical utility for treating various aspects of addiction to numerous drugs (Tables 9.1 and 9.2). This situation exemplifies the complexity of neurochemical processes involved in addiction to drugs.

HOW DOES A DRUG CHANGE BRAIN NEUROCHEMISTRY TO CREATE CRAVING?

(Pharmacological Effects on Brain Neurochemistry Can Be Enduring.)

Will has used crack cocaine for a very long time. The binges are frequent and have occurred over a period of five or six consecutive years. He craves cocaine between binges, and he continues to experience craving even now, despite not having used cocaine for more than 8 months. It seems to Will as if the crack has changed his brain forever.

Chronic ingestion of addictive psychoactive drugs produces a variety of changes in synapses (Van den Oever et al., 2012) and in postsynaptic intracellular processes (Luscher & Malenka, 2011; Russo et al., 2010). These changes are considered to be neuroadaptations to drug-induced assaults upon neurochemistry of the brain.

Among these neuroadaptations, psychomotor stimulant drugs (e.g., cocaine, methamphetamine) can produce enduring changes in dopamine neurotransmission. For example, abusers of methamphetamine have lower dopamine D2 receptor availability in the caudate nucleus and the putamen and abnormal glucose metabolism in the orbitofrontal cortex (Volkow et al., 2001). These abnormalities in D2 receptors and orbitofrontal cortex are significantly correlated and can be interpreted as a drug-induced dysfunction that ultimately contributes to symptoms of addiction—one idea is that chronic ingestion of methamphetamine drives down D2 receptor density in synapses, which in turn causes an abnormally functioning orbitofrontal cortex, resulting in compulsive drug use (Volkow et al., 2001).

Consistent with this idea are findings from the study of dopamine and its relation to conditioned craving for cocaine. Using a neuroimaging strategy that employed the D2 receptor antagonist drug raclopride to provide an indirect measure of the availability of synaptic dopamine, cocaine-related visual cues increased availability of dopamine in the striatum, and the magnitude of dopamine availability correlated with the reported intensity of craving (Volkow et al., 2006b). The speculation is that the conditioned dopamine-related increase in craving reveals an enduring change in the brain induced by chronic use of cocaine (Fowler & Volkow, 2009). Whether or not such drug-induced changes in the brain are relatively permanent or are neuroadaptations that can subside during abstinence or be reversed by pharmacotherapy remains to be determined.

WHY IS METHAMPHETAMINE MORE ADDICTIVE THAN MARIJUANA?
(Drugs Differ in Their Potential for Addiction.)

John regularly uses several drugs—alcohol, nicotine, methamphetamine, and marijuana, but mostly meth and weed. He is a polysubstance abuser and probably addicted to several of them. He is driven, sometimes absolutely obsessed with using the methamphetamine. He enjoys the marijuana and uses it daily but never really craves it. He can live without the other drugs, but he absolutely needs the methamphetamine and will do just about anything to get it.

Chronic use of addictive psychoactive drugs induces measurable acute and long-lasting changes in the human brain (Fowler & Volkow, 2009; Urban & Martinez, 2012). The enduring changes include neuroadaptations that are to some extent reversible, and others that may be permanent, resulting from the neurotoxicity of an addictive substance. In addition, some drugs present a greater or lesser risk of addiction and produce greater or lesser lasting impact on brain processes. A consideration of these issues by contrasting the effects of methamphetamine and cannabis on brain and on behavior reveals clues regarding how some drugs differ in their potential for addiction.

Methamphetamine is a highly addictive psychomotor stimulant drug. In fact, it is a scourge owing to its ugly effects on physiology and behavior. Chronic use of methamphetamine also has measurable, enduring effects on the brain. One of its principal effects is on dopamine neurotransmission, which may designate the core of methamphetamine's addictive potential. Some of methamphetamine's effects on brain neurochemistry are due to the drug's neurotoxicity at dosages chronically self-administered by humans. For example, methamphetamine appears to produce permanent damage to presynaptic dopamine transport processes (i.e., the synaptic reuptake process): Impairment of reuptake of released synaptic dopamine causes persistent overabundance of dopamine in synapses, which can decrease the availability (i.e., downregulate) of D2 dopamine receptors, which can in turn produce dysregulation of glucose metabolism in the orbitofrontal cortex. It is this collection of neuroadaptations that is presumed to sustain the craving and compulsive use of methamphetamine (Fowler & Volkow, 2009).

Many of the neurochemical, psychological, and behavioral abnormalities induced by chronic use of methamphetamine persist after abstinence from drug use, including loss of presynaptic transport processes for dopamine, downregulation of dopamine receptors, hypometabolism in specific sites in the brain, memory loss, depressive symptoms, anxiety, and craving (Fowler & Volkow, 2009). A lengthy period of abstinence from methamphetamine use can result in at least partial recovery of some of these functions, but some neurochemical and behavioral abnormalities can persist for as long as a year after initiation of abstinence (Fowler & Volkow, 2009). Some of the persistent abnormalities are site specific (e.g., the striatum, including the nucleus accumbens) and are consistent with the documented neurotoxicity of methamphetamine on dopamine and serotonin neurons (Urban & Martinez, 2012; Wang et al., 2004).

In summary, methamphetamine not only is powerfully addictive but also can have persistent and perhaps permanent effects on specific regions and specific neurochemical processes in the human brain. How similar is this to what is observed in chronic users of cannabis?

Despite the fact that marijuana is the most frequently used illegal drug in the world (Cooper & Haney, 2008), relatively little is known about its effects on the human brain, perhaps because it generally has been assumed that cannabis has little or no addictive potential, and because cannabis is known to be a CB1 receptor agonist and therefore presumably not a potent agent for altering dopamine neurotransmission. But cannabis does indirectly alter dopamine neurotransmission (Oleson & Cheer, 2012), although there are differences compared with the effects of methamphetamine, amphetamine, or cocaine (Urban & Martinez, 2012).

The ability of cannabis to enhance release of dopamine in the nucleus accumbens of rats appears to depend upon its ability to inhibit GABA-mediated inhibition of dopamine release (Oleson & Cheer, 2012), which distinguishes it from methamphetamine, which directly enhances dopamine release (Iversen et al., 2009). Moreover, neuroimaging studies of the brains of chronic users of cannabis reveal no abnormalities in dopamine release or availability of D2 receptors for dopamine (Stokes, Mehta, Curran, Breen, & Grasby, 2009, Stokes et al., 2012; Urban et al., 2012). Thus, the effects of cannabis on dopamine neurotransmission are indirect and are not as potent as the effects produced by psychomotor stimulant drugs such as methamphetamine (Volkow et al., 2001). In addition, chronic use of cannabis appears not to produce enduring effects on dopamine neurotransmission in humans (Urban & Martinez, 2012), although other abnormalities in brain structure have been identified in heavy users of marijuana (Yucel et al., 2008).

The effects of cannabis on CB1 cannabinoid receptors are substantial: Chronic administration of delta-9-tetrahydrocannabinol in animals causes downregulation of CB1 receptors (Chang & Chronicle, 2007; Sim-Selley, 2003), but these changes appear to be reversible (Sim-Selley et al., 2006). Cannabis-induced downregulation of CB1 receptors also has been measured in humans who chronically use marijuana, but these effects are reversible following as little as four weeks of abstinence (Hirvonen et al., 2012).

In summary, methamphetamine has much greater addictive potential than does cannabis. Methamphetamine also has more direct and much more profound effects on enhancement of dopamine neurotransmission than does cannabis. Some of methamphetamine's effects on brain neurochemistry may be permanent owing to the drug's neurotoxicity, or, if not permanent, some of methamphetamine's effects may be only partially reversible during abstinence. In contrast, it appears that the effects of cannabis on brain neurochemistry may be reversible during abstinence. The differences in the magnitude of the effects of methamphetamine and cannabis on brain neurochemistry are consistent with the differences in potential for addiction of these two psychoactive drugs.

DOES DRUG USAGE DURING ADOLESCENCE INCREASE THE RISK OF ADDICTION IN ADULTHOOD?

(Drugs Can Alter the Organization of a Developing Brain.)

Barb has heard that there is no research demonstrating that use of marijuana causes addiction or has permanent effects of any kind. Barb's mother has begged her to not use the drug—or any drug, for that matter. Barb has decided to not use any "hard" drugs but that she can safely use marijuana. Nearly everyone at the high school is using it now and then. She believes that using it will be no problem.

The acute effects of a drug on adult humans do not necessarily predict the effects of the drug on adolescents. Moreover, the effects of a drug on a still developing adolescent brain may be more deleterious in the long term than are the effects of the same drug on a mature adult brain (Andersen, 2003; Andersen & Navalta, 2004). This situation has implications for the impact of use of addictive psychoactive drugs during adolescence on the vulnerability to addiction for adolescents and for adults. For example, those who initiate use of cannabis during adolescence are two to four times more likely to exhibit symptoms of drug dependence within the two years after initiating use compared with people who initiate use of cannabis as adults (Chen, Storr, & Anthony, 2009b). This kind of finding provokes asking whether a drug with addictive properties produces neuroadaptations in the developing brain that are enduring or irreversible, and whether those neuroadaptations increase the vulnerability to addiction. Those are important and timely questions to consider, because the use of marijuana has increased for adolescents and adults, and increasing numbers of people support the legalization of marijuana use (Gonzalez & Swanson, 2012).

Although relatively little is known about the effects of cannabis on the developing brain of human adolescents, what is known suggests that adolescents may be more vulnerable than adults to the deleterious effects of marijuana. Adolescent chronic users of marijuana do show neurobehavioral abnormalities: During a three-week abstinence period, adolescent chronic users of marijuana exhibit impaired verbal learning and memory, suggestive of cortical and subcortical abnormalities in the brain (Hanson et al., 2010). It is not yet clear whether these and other neurobehavioral abnormalities reported for adolescent users of marijuana persist after prolonged periods of abstinence (Schweinsburg, Brown, & Tapert, 2008).

Long-term use of marijuana during adolescence can produce an enduring decline in cognitive processes (Meier et al., 2012): Adolescents who initiate chronic use of marijuana, and persist using chronically over a 20-year period, show a decline in IQ, whereas those who initiate chronic use during adulthood show only a slight increase in IQ. Moreover, cessation of use of marijuana for one year or more is not sufficient to reverse the measured functional decline.

Experiments using animals as subjects provide better opportunities for measuring developmental changes in brain neurochemistry (Ellgren et al., 2008) and whether exposure to drugs during adolescence produces enduring changes in brain neurochemistry and increases vulnerability to addiction. There are convincing demonstrations that early exposure to cannabis has profound effects on adult brain and behavior. For example, rats administered delta-9-tetrahydrocannabinol every third day during adolescence, compared with adolescent rats administered a placebo, (a) self-administer more heroin at lower doses as adults, indicative of increased appetite or increased sensitivity to the heroin, and (b) show elevated availability of a marker for mu-opioid receptors in the nucleus accumbens, which is correlated with their increased self-administration of heroin (Ellgren, Spano, & Hurd, 2007). These findings in animals demonstrate that early exposure of a developing brain to cannabis can induce enduring changes in neurochemistry that can sustain increased self-administration of heroin, revealing changes in the brain and in behavior that may represent an increase in vulnerability for developing addiction as an adult.

These kinds of findings in humans and animals are important for understanding how adolescent behavior can have effects on brain and behavior that linger into adulthood. These findings urge caution regarding the use during adolescence of addictive drugs, including marijuana—a drug that has increasingly come to be perceived as being relatively harmless.

CAN ANIMAL MODELS TEACH US ABOUT PHARMACOTHERAPY FOR ADDICTION?

Ronnie the Rat has never had it so good. Just several days ago, a quite mysterious lever showed up on a wall in his cage. Then one day, encouraged by his new friend Morony Mouse, Ronnie pressed on that lever and wow—his brain seemed to get a jolt of pleasure! So he proceeded to press that lever vigorously, and he pressed it frequently, getting a similar reward each and every time. He seems to need to press it more and more frequently as the days go by, in order to feel as satisfied as he had on that first day. If he gets distracted and fails to press the lever for some hours, he'll get a little jittery and anxious, but those feelings subside as soon as he resumes pressing the lever. And just today, Dr. Model showed up and suggested that he inject a little naltrexone or maybe a new experimental drug into Ronnie to see if either drug will reduce Ronnie's attraction to the lever.

Knowing that it is the ingestion of addictive psychotropic drugs that produces measurable neuroadaptations in the brain of a human who becomes a compulsive drug user has facilitated the design of animal models for addiction and provides advantages for the development of medications to treat addiction. Animal models provide some degree of construct validity or face validity for three components of behaviors indicative of various stages of chronic drug use: (a) the repeated use of a drug to obtain the drug's rewarding properties—the pleasure, (b) the behaviors and emotions resulting from abstinence or withdrawal from an addictive drug that has been chronically used, and (c) the craving that can lead to the resumption of drug use following a period of abstinence—the relapse. In addition, models for drug-induced neuroadaptations in young animals show increased likelihood of compulsive drug self-administration as adults. Examples of useful animal models for addiction include the following.

Models of drug ingestion to experience pleasure:
- Lever pressing by animals to deliver electrical stimulation to sites in the brain that organize feelings of pleasure or reward
- Self-administration of drugs

- Conditioning of preference for a place in which a drug that induces pleasure is obtained—that is, conditioned place preference

Models of behaviors during abstinence or withdrawal:
- Measures of changes in the reward threshold values for electrical stimulation of sites in the brain that organize feelings of pleasure or reward
- Conditioning of aversion for a place in which withdrawal symptoms are experienced—that is, conditioned place aversion
- Increased attempts to self-administer drugs during abstinence or withdrawal
- Withdrawal-induced increase in behaviors indicative of anxiety

Models of resumption of drug use at relapse and models of craving:
- Relapse induced by drug ingestion
- Relapse induced by stress
- Relapse induced by conditioned cues—that is, conditioned craving

Models of drug-induced vulnerability for addiction in young animals:
- Chronic drug administration to adolescent rodents

Animal models for addiction (Gardner & Wise, 2009; Koob, Lloyd, & Mason, 2009) generally have served two purposes: (a) examine behavioral, physiological, and neurochemical processes that occur during development and various stages of addiction and (b) evaluate the potential clinical effectiveness of medications to treat addiction.

Here are examples of the use of a variety of animal models for addiction, chosen from a lush published literature; many of these include an assessment of the effects of a drug used clinically to treat some aspect of addiction:

- Pressing a lever to self-administer a sweet alcohol solution for drinking elicits the release of dopamine in the nucleus accumbens in the brain, as measured through a chronic microdialysis probe in the rat. Administration of naltrexone inhibits this self-administration of alcohol and prevents the alcohol-ingestion-induced release of dopamine (Gonzales & Weiss, 1998).
- Rats that are dependent on alcohol, trained to press a lever to self-administer alcohol for drinking, demonstrate hypersensitivity to the effects of the beta-adrenergic agonist propranolol, which suppresses the self-administration of alcohol more effectively in

alcohol-dependent rats than in nondependent rats (Gilpin & Koob, 2010).

- Rhesus monkeys press a lever to self-administer intravenous methamphetamine; bupropion decreases this self-administration of methamphetamine, but methylphenidate does not (Schindler, Gilman, Panlilio, McCann, & Goldberg, 2011).

- Rats show a conditioned preference for the place in which they have received injections of nicotine. Administration of the cannabinoid CB1 receptor antagonist rimonabant diminishes the preference they had previously acquired. In addition, rimonabant diminishes the ability of the administration of nicotine to reinstate a previously established conditioned place preference (Fang et al., 2011); that is, rimonabant appears to deter drug-induced relapse.

- Mice bearing the genetic defect of having no mu-opioid receptors (i.e., mu-opioid knockout mice) fail to self-administer alcohol and exhibit an aversion to alcohol (Roberts et al., 2000).

- A rat addicted to nicotine that can press a lever to deliver electrical stimulation to its brain exhibits an increase in the threshold values for electrical stimulation (i.e., stimulation appears to be less rewarding), concurrent with somatic behavioral symptoms of withdrawal, when abstinence from nicotine is initiated. These effects can also be induced by administration of an antagonist for nicotinic receptors, suggesting that nicotine replacement therapy may prevent these behavioral symptoms of withdrawal (Epping-Jordan, Watkins, Koob, & Markou, 1998).

- A rat dependent on alcohol will press a lever to self-administer alcohol for drinking. During enforced abstinence from alcohol, environmental stress or presentation of a conditioned cue signaling availability of alcohol will reinstate the extinguished lever pressing for alcohol. Stress and the conditioned cue are additive in their ability to reinstate lever pressing to obtain alcohol. Administration of naltrexone can prevent the conditioned cue from reinstating self-administration of alcohol, and administration of a drug that is an antagonist for corticotropin-releasing factor can prevent stress from reinstating self-administration of alcohol (Liu & Weiss, 2002).

- Rats administered repeated frequent injections of delta-9-tetrahydrocannabinol throughout adolescence exhibit as adults heightened sensitivity to the effects of self-administered intravenous heroin, evident in greater lever pressing to obtain heroin and increased consumption of heroin (Ellgren, Spano, & Hurd, 2007).

- Rats administered daily injections of nicotine throughout adolescence exhibit as adults heightened sensitivity to the effects of self-administered intravenous nicotine, evident in greater lever pressing to obtain nicotine and increased consumption of nicotine (Adriani et al., 2003).

In summary, there is an impressive history of the successful use of animal models for addiction leading to (a) increased understanding of the development of addiction, (b) identification of the underlying neurochemical processes of addictive behaviors, and (c) the development of novel medications for treatment of addiction (Edwards & Koob, 2012; Koob et al., 2009).

TIDBITS ON PSYCHOPHARMACOLOGY LEARNED FROM THE TREATMENT OF ADDICTION

The following are brief examples illustrating other principles of pharmacology or recommendations from Part I of this book, taken from the clinical treatment of addiction or from basic research on addiction:

- *No drug has only one effect.* Although the addictive properties of cocaine are primarily attributable to cocaine's ability to inhibit presynaptic transport of dopamine, cocaine also has profound effects that enhance neurotransmission of norepinephrine and serotonin, including effects in the peripheral autonomic nervous system (Iversen et al., 2009).
- *Compromise on benefits and risks is a realistic goal for pharmacotherapy.* Buprenorphine, a partial agonist for mu-opioid receptors, provides a risk of abuse when being used to treat addiction to heroin, oxycodone, or hydrocodone, because buprenorphine can induce euphoria. This risk can be diminished by combining buprenorphine with the opioid antagonist naloxone in a formulation (Suboxone) that diminishes part of buprenorphine's effects (van den Brink, 2012).
- *Desired effects and unwanted effects are related to dosage.* The mu-opioid receptor antagonist naltrexone can abolish the euphoria induced by the mu-opioid agonist heroin. Increasing the dose of heroin can overcome this antagonistic effect of naltrexone. Unfortunately, this maneuver, which allows heroin to successfully compete with naltrexone for mu-opioid receptors, can increase the likelihood that heroin produces a fatal suppression of respiration.

- *Drug interactions can be potent and unpredictable.* Naltrexone treatment differentially affects alcoholic smokers compared with alcoholic nonsmokers (Fucito et al., 2012): Smokers are more likely to withdraw prematurely from naltrexone treatment and are more likely to drink alcohol less often during the course of treatment.

- *Sensitivity to a drug varies from one individual to another.* Naltrexone is more effective for inhibiting alcohol consumption in heavy-drinking alcoholic subjects who show higher antisocial traits, compared with heavy-drinking alcoholics who show lower antisocial traits (Rohsenow et al., 2007).

- *Sex, age, and genetics can determine the magnitude of effects of a drug.* Under certain treatment conditions, naltrexone can produce greater reductions in smoking for men than for women, and greater prevention of weight gain for women than for men abstaining from smoking (King et al., 2012). An individual with a family history of alcoholism, who has increased availability of D2 dopamine receptors in caudate and ventral striatum, appears protected from development of alcoholism (Volkow et al., 2006a).

- *A person's drug history can affect a drug's effectiveness.* Baclofen reduces alcohol consumption and use of cocaine for alcohol-dependent, cocaine-using patients, and baclofen is most effective in patients with the highest levels of cocaine use at the initiation of therapy (Shoptaw et al., 2003).

- *Culture and community can affect the utility of pharmacotherapy.* Use of traditional medicines (e.g., St. John's wort) to treat alcoholism is considered an important therapeutic option in China (Liu et al., 2011).

- *Drugs can be demonstrated to be only relatively effective and safe.* All drugs that have ever been approved to treat addiction have side effects.

- *A therapeutic drug is used because it works.* The mechanism by which bupropion diminishes craving for nicotine is not known (O'Brien & Dackis, 2009).

- *Dietary supplements may or may not be effective and safe.* St. John's wort produces no benefit compared with placebo for attenuation of symptoms of nicotine withdrawal or for sustaining abstinence from smoking in mostly Caucasian-American subjects (Sood et al., 2010).

- *Placebo can have drug-like effects.* Ingestion of a placebo appears to increase the benefit of meeting with a medical professional for patients attempting to recover from addiction to alcohol (Weiss et al., 2008).

- *Pharmacotherapy is best used as one among several tools.* Any pharmacotherapy for addiction should be used as an adjunct to non-drug therapy (O'Brien & Dackis, 2009; O'Brien & McKay, 2007).
- *The role of pharmacotherapy varies for different people and disorders.* For a thorough review of evidence-based drug therapies for addiction that speaks to this issue, see van den Brink (2012).
- *Serendipity can bring new opportunities for pharmacotherapy.* Methadone, the drug with the longest history of successful treatment of heroin addiction, was initially developed as an analgesic (Pierce et al., 2012).
- *Consumers demand new and better drugs.* The FDA approved in 2002 the combination of buprenorphine and naloxone, which has become a preferred treatment for heroin addiction because the combination has a lower risk of death than does methadone (Pierce et al., 2012).
- *Successful use encourages increased use, for better or worse.* Despite the risk of death due to respiratory depression or cardiac arrhythmias, methadone has been used to treat addiction to heroin for over 50 years (Pierce et al, 2012).
- *The FDA attempts to approve new and better drugs.* There is no clear drug of choice for treatment of addiction to cocaine, but that fact has advanced the exploration of the potential for developing a vaccine to prevent addiction to cocaine (Shen, Orson, & Kosten, 2012).
- *Off-label use has its advantages and disadvantages.* Despite lack of effective FDA-approved pharmacotherapy for addiction to cocaine, methamphetamine, or marijuana, there also are no recommended off-label drug treatments for these addictions.
- *Health insurance practices can determine accessibility to a drug.* Treatment of addiction has not yet achieved full parity with treatment of other medical conditions. Full parity will be realized when there is (a) equal access to services for addiction compared with services for other medical and surgical services, (b) equal opportunities for education for professionals wishing to specialize in treatment of addiction, (c) equal compensation for services provided for treatment of addiction compared with treatment for other medical disorders, and (d) equality in professional recognition and status for those specializing in treatment of addiction (Roy & Miller, 2010).

- *Diagnosis guides choice of pharmacotherapy.* The use of the terms *addiction* and *dependence* was part of the deliberations for revising the most recent edition of the *Diagnostic and Statistical Manual of Mental Disorders, DSM-5.* The term *addiction* is considered to be too negative or pejorative, whereas the term *dependence* is considered to encourage less appropriate treatment (O'Brien, Volkow, & Li, 2006).
- *Clients should be active participants in their pharmacotherapy.* The major problem with the use of naltrexone as treatment for addiction to heroin is noncompliance with its prescribed use (Goldstein, 1976).

SUMMARY AND PERSPECTIVE

The psychopharmacology of addiction encompasses the use of psychotropic drugs for etiology and for therapy. Drugs of either sort—addictive or medicinal—can be agonist drugs that mimic or enhance one or more neurochemical processes in the brain, or antagonist drugs that block neurochemical processes. Most drugs having addictive potential are substances that dramatically enhance (and sometimes damage) neurochemical mechanisms that serve psychological processes such as reward, reinforcement, or pleasure. Some therapeutic drugs are receptor agonists that are used to replace the neurochemical effects of the drug of addiction, to help wean the addict off of the addictive substance and to diminish the craving for the addictive drug in order to delay or prevent relapse. Other therapeutic drugs are receptor antagonists that diminish the pleasure induced by an addictive drug, or diminish the craving for that drug.

Therapeutic drugs cannot remedy all of the drug-induced abnormalities of addiction. The addict exhibits compulsive behavior intended to get pleasure from a drug, behavior that is enabled by a social context. Therapy for addiction must address all three parts of that biopsychosocial problem—behavior, social context, and the neurochemistry of pleasure. To reach that goal, addicts also require the support of nonpharmacological counseling or therapy. But even with a multimodal therapeutic approach, the treatment of addiction may not succeed in restoring the relationship between brain neurochemistry and behavior to its original, preaddiction state, because ingestion of addictive drugs induces enduring, sometimes permanent neuroadaptations in the brain that reorganize behavior. The possibility that addictive behavior is maintained by a permanent change in the brain and in behavior is perhaps most worrisome for the developing brain of an adolescent maturing under the influence of an addictive substance.

In short, no therapeutic drugs fix addiction. The best therapeutic drugs address only components of the problems the addict faces. Pharmacotherapy and behavior therapy for addiction have limited utility and must improve, because the incidence of use of addictive drugs continues to rise.

CHAPTER TEN

Major Depression and Bipolar Disorder

With each new choice along the way, Jon was never once convinced that his physician was confident that the next treatment for Jon's depression would be the solution. They began with venlafaxine, then tried fluoxetine, then bupropion, then buspirone, and now buspirone with citalopram. It always has been one side effect or another, and no lifting of his mood—over and over again. He has become afraid for himself. He has to do something. Will he submit to electroconvulsive therapy? Sure—anything that might work.

Pharmacotherapy for major depression or for bipolar disorder is characterized by successes and shortcomings that provide the opportunity for exploring a variety of issues regarding the use of psychotropic drugs as therapy. Among the successes is the fact that numerous classes of drugs provide relief of symptoms for depression or bipolar disorder. This provides limited assurance to a patient that if one drug is not effective for relief of symptoms, another one might be. In addition, it provides some assurance that if an effective drug proves to have side effects that become intolerable, another drug in the same class or from a different class might be equally effective without having a particular troubling adverse effect.

There are many options for drug therapy because the business of using pharmacotherapy to treat disordered mood has been going on for quite some time, producing a published literature of clinical drug trials so vast that meta-analyses of drugs' effects now are necessary to attempt to summarize the published findings (Nemeroff & Schatzberg, 2007; von Wolff et al., 2012). In addition, the lifetime prevalence of major depression is relatively high, affecting more than 30 million people in the United States (Kessler et al., 2003). Of those diagnosed and treated, most patients experience repeated episodes (Bresee, Gotto, & Rapaport, 2009), often requiring switching of medications. Thus, there are both a sizable market for drugs that treat disordered mood and a continuing demand for new and better medications.

Another element of success, related to having a variety of classes of drugs as options for treatment, is the opportunity for using one drug having one mechanism of action to augment a second drug having a different mechanism of action. While this kind of polypharmacy can have its drawbacks, it does provide a useful approach for treating a disorder for which many diagnosed patients are unresponsive to a variety of monotherapies (Bresee, Gotto, & Rapaport, 2009).

Among the shortcomings of pharmacotherapy for major depression is the fact that, despite the enormous volume of evidence-based support for various antidepressant medications, it is not possible to predict which patient will respond to which particular drug. The meta-analyses of clinical drug trials do not identify any single antidepressant drug as being more effective than all others (Nemeroff & Schatzberg, 2007). Therefore, the initiation of drug therapy for a patient represents essentially an educated guess in choosing among a variety of drugs in a preferred class of drugs at that particular point in time. If that first drug fails to be suitable, one of two approaches may then become useful: switch from that drug to another drug in the same class or in a different class, or use a second drug to augment continuing treatment with the first drug. Either approach may find some support in the growing published literature that attempts to identify preferred drug switches and preferred combinations of drugs for augmentation.

Another concern regarding the current use of pharmacotherapy is the fact that major depression and bipolar disorder are maladies that present serious peril when a patient fails to respond to therapy, because of the potential for suicide. The failure to treat successfully and swiftly can cost a patient's life, making the unpredictable outcome of choosing that first pharmacotherapy a serious problem. These facts support the wisdom of combining pharmacotherapy with some method of psychotherapy at the very outset of treatment.

Finally, it is quite disappointing that so many patients can be unresponsive to treatment—not only unresponsive to pharmacotherapy but also unresponsive to psychotherapy (Craighead, Sheets, Brosse, & Ilardi, 2007). These unresponsive patients become candidates for electroconvulsive shock therapy, a last-resort treatment that remains useful for treating major depression despite being a rather crude way to alter brain processes and despite the lack of understanding of how electroconvulsive therapy alters brain to lift depressed mood (Reininghaus et al., 2012). The facts that shock therapy remains useful and that so many depressed patients are unresponsive to a variety of treatments tell us something important about contemporary treatment of major depression: We remain considerably ignorant about what is going on in the brain of many depressed patients, despite our wealth of knowledge about the presumed mechanisms of action for the various classes of antidepressant medications. This ignorance is not altogether a bad thing. It leaves the door open for learning more about brain and depression, such that new drugs and novel therapeutics can be developed, prescribed, and sold.

HOW HAVE DRUGS BEEN USED TO TREAT MAJOR DEPRESSION AND BIPOLAR DISORDER?

> The antidepressant lifts Phil's depressed mood just fine. It is his inability to experience a lift elsewhere that he has started to worry about—he can't perform sexually, and he is certain it is because of the medication. He will demand that another drug be prescribed and will take his chances that a different medication will be as effective without presenting such a challenge to his manliness.

A consideration of the drugs used to treat disordered mood is perhaps most efficiently structured in two parts: drugs to treat major depression, and drugs to treat bipolar disorder.

Major depression. Four classes of drugs have emerged during the past 60 years as being useful for the treatment of major depression (Table 10.1). The monoamine oxidase (MAO) inhibitors arrived first when iproniazid was introduced in 1952; next came imipramine, the first of the tricyclic antidepressants (Jacobsen, 1986). In 1980 the FDA approved fluoxetine, the first selective serotonin reuptake inhibitor (SSRI). More recently, drugs with combined effects of serotonin and norepinephrine reuptake inhibition (SNRI) have become available.

Of these four classes of antidepressant medications, the tricyclic antidepressants were the first to become known as the preferred choice for initiating pharmacotherapy for depression. The tricyclic drugs were replaced by the SSRIs as the preferred choice, but now the SNRIs rival the SSRIs as the preferred class of antidepressant medications. This gradual shift from tricyclics to SSRIs to SNRIs is a shift based not on improved effectiveness for relieving symptoms of depression but, rather, a move to classes of drugs having some-

TABLE 10.1

Evolution of use of drugs over the decades to treat depression and bipolar disorder.

DRUG/DRUG CLASS	MECHANISM	1950s	1960s	1970s	1980s	1990s	2000s	2010s
Depression								
MAO inhibitors	NE/SER/DA/MEL	x	x	x	x	x	x	x
Tricyclics	NE/SER	x	x	x	x	x	x	x
SSRIs	SER				x	x	x	x
SNRIs	SER/NE					x	x	x
Bupropion	NE/DA/ACh/?				x	x	x	x
Bipolar disorder								
Lithium	?			x	x	x	x	x
Valproate (anticonvulsants)	?					x	x	x
Second-generation antipsychotics	SER/DA/?						x	x

Note: x indicates decade in which drug was prescribed. MAO, monoamine oxidase; SSRIs, selective serotonin reuptake inhibitors; SNRIs, serotonin and norepinephrine reuptake inhibitors; NE, norepinephrine; SER, serotonin; DA, dopamine; MEL, melatonin; ACh, acetylcholine; ?, unknown mechanism. This table illustrates that (a) the advent of newer drugs to treat depression or bipolar disorder has not rendered useless the older medications, and (b) the neurochemical processes enhanced by these drugs, that is, the presumed mechanisms of action, vary across drugs and classes. Although the tricyclics and the SNRIs both enhance neurotransmission of serotonin and norepinephrine, the SNRIs are generally characterized as having more balanced effects on serotonin and norepinephrine and relatively more tolerable side effects.

what improved side effect profiles, likely attributable to the more pharmacologically selective effects of the newer classes of medications. But this
generalization (i.e., similar effectiveness but differing side effect profiles) is a
bit misleading, because for an individual patient, a drug in any one of those
three classes can have intolerable side effects. Thus, a number of important
factors need to be considered when making a decision to initiate pharmacotherapy for major depression.

At the time of diagnosis of major depression, when considering whether
the patient fits a set of diagnostic criteria, it is also important to note the
characteristics the client shows that identify the patient as a unique case. For
example, is the patient depressed and also showing symptoms of anxiety, psychosis, insomnia, or hypersomnia? Does the patient present with comorbidity,
showing symptoms that fit two diagnostic categories? Various clinical characteristics may (Sobel, 2012) or may not (Rush et al., 2008) facilitate choosing
among medication options. But whether or not clinical characteristics are
useful predictors of effectiveness of a particular drug or class of drugs, the fact
that drugs in all classes are generally considered to be of equivalent effectiveness, having clinical diagnostic information that can only *presume* to predict
effectiveness may not be absolutely necessary. On the other hand, for the
patient presenting with diagnosed comorbidity, it may be important to use
that information to select the more appropriate antidepressant or combined
treatments (Berman et al., 2009). For example, when anxiety is comorbid
with major depression, an SSRI or an SNRI may be the best first-line treatment option, given the anxiolytic properties of those classes of drugs. When
a patient shows major depression with psychotic symptoms, monotherapy is
more likely to fail, and combined antipsychotic and antidepressant medications may be the best starting point.

When first considering the selection of a medication, it is important to
discuss the potential important advantages of integrating pharmacotherapy
with psychotherapy. Methods of psychotherapy with evidence-based support
for their effectiveness for treating major depression include interpersonal psychotherapy, cognitive behavioral therapy (CBT), and the cognitive behavioral analysis system of psychotherapy (Craighead et al., 2007). Combining
psychotherapy and pharmacotherapy from the outset realistically anticipates
the fact that many patients will fail to respond to pharmacotherapy alone
(Pies, 2012). Therefore, for the patient who is refractory to the first-line medication, psychotherapy will be valuable.

The evidence that combined pharmacotherapy and psychotherapy for
depression is more effective than either treatment given alone is based on
limited published research and is not compelling (von Wolff et al., 2012). For
example, a comparison of four evidence-based treatment conditions selected

by the subjects in the study—cognitive therapy, interpersonal psychotherapy, cognitive therapy plus pharmacotherapy, or interpersonal psychotherapy plus pharmacotherapy—demonstrated equivalent rates of remission through 26 weeks of treatment, with cognitive therapy alone showing the more rapid rate of improvement (Peeters et al., 2012). Despite this type of finding from clinical research, one decided advantage of combining psychotherapy with drug therapy is the fact that patients on combined therapies are less likely to discontinue taking their medication prematurely (Olfson, Marcus, Tedeschi, & Wan, 2006b).

The selection of antidepressant medication should be guided also by the patient's expressed concerns regarding desired outcomes and which particular side effects the patient would consider to be tolerable or intolerable. The older classes of antidepressant medications offer the advantage of being better-known commodities, and therefore they may present somewhat greater predictability regarding their benefits and risks.

Benefits and risks of medications will to some extent be determined by age, sex, gender, and ethnicity of the patient. Regarding the age of a patient, there is very little published evidence to support the use of antidepressant medications or psychotherapy in children or adolescents diagnosed with depression. Meta-analysis of the few studies that assess effectiveness of pharmacotherapy, psychotherapy, or the combination of the two reveals apparent equivalency of effectiveness and no clear advantage for combining medication with psychotherapy when treating adolescents (Cox et al., 2012). The practice of treating adolescents according to published findings from clinical trials in adults is common but does not represent evidence-based treatment.

The situation is similar for the treatment of the elderly suffering major depression. Little published work supports one approach over another, and risks associated with polypharmacy are a greater problem for treating the elderly. For example, the elderly, especially when being medicated for other conditions, are at increased risk of falling when being treated with a tricyclic antidepressant (Lindsey, 2009). The SSRIs have become the preferred choice for initiation of pharmacotherapy for the elderly, although the elderly do seem to be more sensitive to some of the adverse effects of this class of drugs (Lindsey, 2009).

There are also differences in sensitivity to antidepressant medications for various races and ethnicities. For example, African-Americans, Hispanics, and Asians are generally more sensitive to the antidepressant effects and to the adverse effects of tricyclic antidepressant drugs and SSRIs, a factor that can diminish adherence to the drug regimen (Chaudhry et al., 2008), as can other cultural factors (Diaz et al., 2005). In addition, Hispanic and African-American patients are less likely than Caucasian patients to find antidepressant medication to be an acceptable method of treatment (Cooper et al., 2003).

Relatively more is known regarding sex and gender differences for drugs used to treat major depression. There are numerous reports of sex differences in pharmacokinetics and pharmacodynamics of antidepressant medications in all classes (Bies, Bigos, & Pollock, 2003; Keers & Aitchison, 2010; Yonkers & Brawman-Mintzer, 2002; Yonkers et al., 1992). One of the more interesting examples is a demonstration that the SSRI sertraline can have a more favorable main effect than the tricyclic antidepressant imipramine in women than in men, whereas imipramine can have a more favorable effect than sertraline in men than in women (Kornstein et al., 2000). This benefit of sertraline is not apparent in postmenopausal women, however, suggesting that endogenous (and perhaps exogenous) estrogen might enhance the effectiveness of SSRIs through estrogen's interaction with serotonin neurotransmission (Keers & Aitchison, 2010). Also demonstrated in this study (Kornstein et al., 2000) is a gender difference between men and women regarding adverse events: Women taking imipramine were more likely to drop out of the study than were women taking sertraline, whereas men taking sertraline were more likely to drop out than men taking imipramine. These findings may not predict sex-related differences for other SSRI or tricyclic antidepressant drugs (Keers & Aitchison, 2010), but they do offer the potentially far-reaching lesson that differences related to sex or gender are likely to have an impact on the effectiveness of an antidepressant medication and on side effects that might diminish adherence to prescribed use of an antidepressant medication.

Given the considerable frequency of failure of medication to improve symptoms of major depression, it is important to consider when and how to move to an alternative treatment when the initial (or a subsequent) attempt at pharmacotherapy fails. Assuming that some method of psychotherapy continues, the options for a subsequent step for pharmacotherapy include (a) switching from one drug to another drug in the same class, (b) switching to a drug in a different class, or (c) augmenting the current drug with a second, usually from a different class.

When is it too soon or too late to make a decision to switch or to augment? Failure to respond to an SSRI antidepressant by the fourth week of treatment (Boyer & Feighner, 1994), or by as few as two weeks (Nierenberg et al., 1995), can be taken as an indicator that continued treatment with the same drug is not likely to be useful. These findings encourage making an early assessment of a drug's effectiveness, but very little published evidence guides choosing among the options of switching drugs or drug classes or augmenting one drug with another (Dupuy, Ostacher, Huffman, Perlis, & Nierenberg, 2012). For example, clinical information and the patient's treatment history

are not always useful in predicting a successful switch from an SSRI antidepressant drug to another SSRI, to an SNRI, or to bupropion (Rush et al.,
2006, 2008), although failure to respond to one drug in a class can justify selecting the subsequent antidepressant from a different class. In addition, augmentation (using bupropion or mirtazapine) of ineffective SSRI or SNRI
monotherapy will not always improve effectiveness compared with monotherapy alone (Rush et al., 2011). In contrast, the antipsychotic medication
olanzapine combined with the SSRI fluoxetine can produce greater improvement in treatment-resistant patients having major depression without psychotic features than can fluoxetine or olanzapine alone (Shelton et al., 2001).
In summary, there are published reports of successful drug-switching and
drug-augmentation strategies, some of which can be used to support the idea
that the better augmentation strategy is one that combines drugs from two
different classes of antidepressants having different mechanisms of action
(Richelson, 2013). However, there is insufficient evidence to provide comprehensive guidelines for drug-switching strategies pertinent to the large
number of drugs used for pharmacotherapy for major depression (Connolly &
Thase, 2011, 2012; Papakostas, 2009).

The assortment of drugs for treating depression offers more than clinical
options. The history of the use of antidepressant medications has facilitated
Another problem regarding the selection of medication for depression is
that the improved pharmacological selectivity of the newer classes of antidepressant drugs (i.e., the SSRIs and the SNRIs) and their generally improved
side effect profiles do not guarantee that the newer drugs will be more effective for the relief of symptoms. It is a bit of a trap to assume that the newer
drugs will be more effective because they are newer, more pharmacologically
selective, and therefore somehow improved compared with the older drugs,
because it takes only one intolerable side effect to render a drug unacceptable
and useless to an individual patient. In addition, less experience and less published evidence are available for the newer SNRIs compared with the older
tricyclic antidepressants and the SSRIs. This fact does provide some advantage for the use of the relatively older, more familiar SSRIs, whose effects may
be somewhat more predictable.

An older class of medications, the MAO inhibitors, has not become useless as newer drug options have been developed (Table 10.1). The major disadvantage to the MAO inhibitors has been the requirement for dietary
restraint necessary to avoid ingestion of foods rich in tyramine. This requirement no longer holds for one of the more recently developed MAO inhibitor
drugs, selegiline, which is administered through a patch instead of orally,
thereby decreasing the risk of a potentially lethal gastrointestinal interaction
between ingested tyramine and an orally ingested MAO inhibitor.

The assortment of drugs for treating depression offers more than clinical
options. The history of the use of antidepressant medications has facilitated

the development of both understanding regarding the neurochemical factors that contribute to depressed mood and novel antidepressant medications. For example, the realization that the tricyclic antidepressant drugs share the ability to inhibit reuptake of norepinephrine, thereby increasing norepinephrine neurotransmission, pointed to a role for that neurotransmitter in the etiology of depression and guided the development of new drugs that could enhance norepinephrine neurotransmission in various ways. In addition, realization that a tricyclic drug such as clomipramine can also inhibit reuptake of synaptic serotonin encouraged expanding a norepinephrine theory of depression to include serotonin. This newer, neurochemically more broad monoamine theory of depression preceded the discovery of the class of SSRI drugs. The clinical successes experienced with the SSRIs encouraged the development of drugs that combined the best attributes of the SSRIs and the tricyclics, resulting in the development of the SNRIs. The utility of the SNRIs further reinforces the view that depression is often an expression of combined serotonin and norepinephrine dysfunction.

One continuing frustration with the effectiveness of pharmacotherapy for depression is the somewhat delayed latency to respond to initiation of antidepressant medication. This delayed clinical response provoked the idea that depression has less to do with amounts or levels of neurotransmitters in synapses and more to do with the availability of receptors in synapses for these neurotransmitters. A relevant working hypothesis is that the delayed behavioral response to an antidepressant medication parallels the time frame for the development of antidepressant-drug-induced downregulation of synaptic receptors for serotonin, norepinephrine, or both and that it is this downregulation of receptors that is necessary for a positive clinical response. This kind of working hypothesis contributes to the evolution of theory for etiology of depression and to the development of new drugs. The genesis of such working hypotheses depends heavily upon both clinical findings (Dunlop et al., 2009) and research in animals (Duman, 2009; Sillaber, Holsboer, & Wotjak, 2009).

In summary, evidence-based consideration of use of antidepressant medications does not favor one drug or one class of drugs over another based on effectiveness in relief of symptoms of major depression. This fact permits making a decision, regarding which class and which particular drug, based on the patient's willingness to tolerate side effects and the patient's history with treatment for depression. The patient's willingness to tolerate discomforting adverse events to some extent will depend upon the degree to which the medication is providing relief of symptoms. Moreover, the use of pharmacotherapy combined with psychotherapy may evolve for an individual patient as that patient improves from the acute stage of treatment, to the continuing stage, and finally to the maintenance stage of treatment where ideally the goal of complete remission of symptoms is reached and sustained.

Bipolar disorder. Does it make logical sense that someone who is depressed for awhile, then manic for awhile, and then depressed again would best be treated with one of these three types of drugs: a toxic substance lacking clearly identified effects on neurotransmission, a substance having anticonvulsant properties, or an antipsychotic medication? No, it does not. But that is where we essentially are with options for the pharmacological treatment of bipolar disorder. Unlike the case for major depression, bipolar disorder lacks a unifying neurochemical theory, and it lacks an assortment of neurochemically related classes of pharmacological options for treatment (Table 10.1).

Bipolar disorder is not merely major depression alternating with mania. It is a complex, relapsing disorder that is poorly understood. Effective therapy must address the depression, the mania, the cycling between the two, the prevention of relapse, and the fact that approximately 25% of patients attempt suicide (Keck & McElroy, 2007). To make matters more complicated, bipolar disorder frequently presents with comorbidity, particularly for anxiety or substance dependence or abuse. These facts certainly complicate making decisions about the use of drugs as therapy and about the complementary roles of psychotherapy and pharmacotherapy.

Lithium carbonate is the drug with the longest history for treatment of bipolar disorder. The mechanism of action of lithium is unknown, a fact that offers no help for understanding the neurochemical basis of bipolar disorder. The additional fact that lithium treatment presents the problem of toxicity illustrates that some pharmacological treatments are established in the face of ignorance and are motivated by desperation to help patients in need. Despite these conceptual shortcomings, lithium is useful for treatment of bipolar disorder during the depression phase and during the manic phase, and, more important, lithium is useful for delaying or preventing relapse in patients who are free of symptoms (Taylor & Geddes, 2012).

A variety of drugs with anticonvulsant properties are used to treat bipolar disorder, valproate being the one with the longest history of use. Generally considered, valproate is as effective as lithium for treating mania but is less effective for treating bipolar depression. However, a patient with comorbid bipolar disorder and addiction to alcohol is likely to respond favorably to valproate (Azorin et al., 2010).

Among the antipsychotic medications that have been used to treat bipolar disorder (Keck & McElroy, 2007), the second-generation antipsychotic quetiapine is considered to be the drug most likely to show favorable effects and is generally viewed as being more effective than lithium for treating bipolar depression (Taylor & Geddes, 2012). In general, an antipsychotic medication might be most useful for treating a bipolar disorder patient who shows psychotic symptoms, and for use in augmenting another medication.

The bipolar disorder patient may enter into treatment while in a phase of depression or a phase of mania. The initiation of treatment of bipolar depression would typically not employ one of the drugs demonstrated to be effective in treating major depression, although an SSRI antidepressant might be used in combination with either a mood-stabilizing drug such as lithium or the second-generation antipsychotic olanzapine (Keck & McElroy, 2007).

The bipolar disorder patient entering treatment in a manic phase is most likely to be treated with lithium or valproate. Prevention of relapse following the acute treatment phase is most likely to benefit from long-term treatment with lithium, although an assortment of other drugs show some ability to prevent relapse (Taylor & Geddes, 2012). There is little published evidence to guide selection of a second-line drug treatment when switching drugs, or augmenting a drug therapy, in the face of treatment resistance. In addition, evidence for combining pharmacotherapy with psychotherapy for bipolar illness is too thin to be helpful (Keck & McElroy, 2007), although CBT and interpersonal psychotherapy have demonstrated their utility, and psychotherapy is important for increasing the likelihood of adherence to the prescribed medication regimen, especially during the maintenance phase of treatment (Miklowitz & Craighead, 2007).

In summary, the uses of lithium, an anticonvulsant, or an antipsychotic drug for treatment of bipolar disorder represent treatments that are used principally because they work. Those drugs do not fit a neurochemical theory of bipolar disorder, nor are they drugs that specifically repair an *identified* abnormality in brain neurochemistry. That situation reveals massive ignorance regarding our understanding of the etiology and pathophysiology of the constellation of behavioral symptoms that have been labeled as bipolar disorder. Finally, the treatment of bipolar disorder does have facets of success, but overall it does not represent a major success story for the use of psychotropic medication and deserves further preclinical research in animals and clinical research in humans.

CAN THE FDA ENSURE THAT AN APPROVED ANTIDEPRESSANT WILL BE EFFECTIVE?

(Drugs Can Be Demonstrated to Be Only Relatively Effective and Safe.)

Carl has been prescribed, at one time or another, at least six different medications to treat his depression. He has tried drugs in every class of antidepressant medications—moving from fluoxetine to paroxetine to venlafaxine to imipramine to phenelzine to combinations of several of those. Several of those medications have offered him some relief, but his unwillingness to tolerate particular side effects has contributed to his repeated switching from one medication to another. He knows that all of those drugs have earned FDA approval from the results of clinical trials, yet none of them seems to provide the kind of help that meets Carl's high hopes. Carl has wondered whether his expectations for successful pharmacotherapy are unrealistic. Or are the medications inadequate? And if so, how can that be? What is the FDA doing to help patients like him?

By the time the FDA approves a new antidepressant medication, thereby permitting its marketing and sale, substantial information is in hand regarding the drug's pharmacokinetics in humans, any evidence of toxicity in animals or humans, recommended dosages, expected benefits, and adverse events. This information would have been obtained in research in animals and in phase I, II, and III trials in humans following guidelines prepared by the FDA. The data obtained in such trials are sufficient to make a bet on the benefits and risks of the new drug when humans begin to use it in clinical settings. But the data are not sufficient to ensure effectiveness and safety for each and every patient, because the studies conducted to obtain the data have their limitations.

For a newly approved antidepressant medication, the consumer can expect that clinical trials have demonstrated that the new drug can be more effective than placebo for relief of symptoms in the acute phase of treatment for depression. In addition, the new drug is likely to compare favorably with an antidepressant medication that has been in clinical use for some time. Comparing favorably with an older drug usually means that the new drug is equally effective or more effective for relief of symptoms and probably better or no worse than the older medication regarding side effects. Such comparisons (and outcomes) are likely to have been observed in at least two drug trials in humans and are likely to have been limited in duration to several months of treatment. Because the duration of each study is likely to be relatively short, often there is little or no information helpful for predicting whether or not the new drug will be effective and well tolerated for continuing or maintenance treatment of depression.

There are other insufficiencies in the knowledge about the effectiveness and safety of a new drug at this early time in its clinical life:

- The data from these early clinical trials are likely obtained from the study of only a few dosages of the drug, and the doses are likely to be relatively small. The study of the effects of smaller doses would likely minimize the risk of adverse effects in clinical trials, enhancing the likelihood the data obtained would support the request for approval from the FDA.

- There are likely no data obtained from patients who show comorbidity; the early clinical drug trials would typically be conducted in humans who have a diagnosable disorder that is not complicated by other health issues, including comorbid psychiatric conditions.

- It is likely that the data were obtained from mostly adult male Caucasian subjects, precluding comparisons of the drug's effectiveness (and safety) between men and women or between different ethnic groups; there also would likely not be information pertinent for the use of the drug in adolescents or the elderly.

- The results of the clinical trials most likely would have demonstrated that the new drug produces statistically significant improvement in symptoms (compared with placebo treatment). For an antidepressant medication, this likely would mean improvement on measures of depression such as the Hamilton Rating Scale for Depression or the self-report Beck Depression Inventory. Finding statistically significant improvement in measures of depression using these ratings scales in a clinical trial cannot ensure that the medication will produce a meaningful improvement in the quality of life of a patient treated in a clinical setting. Moreover, it is not likely that the results of the study would demonstrate that the new drug can produce complete remission of symptoms of depression.

- There are likely no data for the use of the new drug in combination with another drug or with psychotherapy.

- Early published clinical trials may overestimate the antidepressant efficacy of a new drug: The status of the SNRI reboxetine exemplifies how "publication bias" can overestimate the clinical utility of a new drug (Eyding et al., 2010).

In summary, the results of these early clinical trials, although conceivably sufficient to convince the FDA that the new drug would be an important addition to the list of marketed antidepressant medications, would not be sufficient to ensure that the new drug would be effective and safe for all patients for whom the drug was prescribed. This means that for the individual patient prescribed the new antidepressant, it would be difficult or impossible to predict to what extent the drug would be helpful in relieving symptoms, which side effects would appear, and whether or not the side effects experienced would contribute to the patient not adhering to the recommended dosage regimen. But there are also reasons to be excited about the availability of a new antidepressant medication, even in the face of these limitations.

Once the antidepressant is on the market, patients who have been resistant to treatment can be offered some new hope for successful treatment. For them, the new drug may just be that new successful monotherapy, or it may be an effective agent to use in an augmentation strategy or in combination with a method of psychotherapy. In addition, for better or worse, the FDA approval for treatment of adults suffering major depression also makes the drug available for off-label use to treat adolescents suffering depression or to treat other disorders (when anecdotal clinical information suggests the idea).

The SSRI sertraline provides an example of the evolution toward the broad clinical utility of a drug originally approved for its antidepressant properties. The FDA approved sertraline in 1991 for the treatment of major depression in adults, adding a new drug to the list of pharmacological tools that inhibit the reuptake of serotonin. This kind of development, together with fact that clomipramine, a tricyclic antidepressant effective for inhibiting reuptake of both norepinephrine and serotonin, had become the treatment of choice for obsessive-compulsive disorder (OCD), encouraged consideration of the use of SSRIs to treat OCD (Lydiard, 1994). The successful off-label use of sertraline to treat OCD confirmed this idea. Then in 1996 sertraline received formal approval for treatment of OCD in adults, and in 1997 for treatment of pediatric OCD, panic disorder, and posttraumatic stress disorder (PTSD). In 2002 it was approved for treatment of premenstrual dysphoric disorder, and in 2003 for treatment of social anxiety. Thus, within 12 years of its initial FDA approval for treatment of major depression, sertraline had demonstrated its effectiveness for treatment of OCD in adults, children, and adolescents and for a variety of anxiety disorders. This evolution of sertraline's utility for treating depression and anxiety disorders encouraged further off-label treatment for additional subcategories of depression and anxiety and for other behavioral problems in children and adolescents. And so sertraline's clinical service continued to expand (Block, Yonkers, & Carpenter, 2009): it now has been used off-label with some success to treat Alzheimer's dementia, depression associated with Parkinson disease, depression linked to fatigue in multiple sclerosis, depression in schizophrenic patients, generalized anxiety disorder, impulse-control disorder, trichotillomania, anorexia nervosa, bulimia nervosa, binge-eating disorder, night-eating syndrome, aggressive behaviors associated with personality disorders or Huntington disease, pathological crying, hot flashes associated with menopause, major depression in children and adolescents, and pervasive development disorder. Sertraline has failed to show its effectiveness in the off-label treatment of substance use disorders and pathological gambling.

These off-label benefits of sertraline for various conditions can come with side effects, including gastrointestinal disturbances, sleep disturbances, headache, dry mouth, sexual dysfunctions, palpitations, asthenia, weight gain, myalgia, rhinitis, and tinnitus (Block et al., 2009). And sertraline carries a black box warning for increased risk of suicidal ideation in children and adolescents, as do other antidepressant medications.

In summary, what can be said about the effectiveness and safety of the SSRI sertraline when used for these various purposes? Although originally heralded as one of the newer SSRI drugs having antidepressant properties, sertraline has since demonstrated its utility for treating a variety of categories of depression and anxiety: it is likely to be useful for some (but not all) patients diagnosed with major depression, OCD in adults and children, PTSD, panic disorder, premenstrual dysphoric disorder, and social anxiety disorder. The fact that sertraline has FDA approval for these conditions means that published evidence supports these various purposes. In other words, the FDA has certified that sertraline can be effective and relatively safe when used to treat these conditions. Whether or not an *individual patient* finds sertraline to be effective and finds its side effects to be tolerable is an open question. Moreover, whether or not an individual patient will experience complete remission of symptoms or a significantly improved quality of life is an open question. Finally, sertraline frequently has been used off-label for a long list of conditions, among them conditions accompanied by symptoms of depression or anxiety. The published evidence supporting the off-label use of sertraline for these purposes is meager, so the likelihood that an individual patient finds sertraline to be effective and finds its side effects to be tolerable is uncertain.

Despite the uncertainty of the outcome when using sertraline or any other antidepressant for off-label treatment, off-label use can open the door to advances in treatment. This can be illustrated by considering a situation in which sertraline *fails* to help patients diagnosed with OCD—a condition for which it has FDA approval: Prior to its FDA approval in 1991 for treatment of major depression, sertraline's ability to treat OCD produced mixed results in studies, including reports that it was ineffective for treating OCD (Jenike et al., 1990). Such negative findings are to be expected, even though ultimately evidence was sufficient for the FDA to approve sertraline in 1996 for treatment of OCD. Remember that FDA approval for treating OCD will not ensure that each OCD patient will respond favorably; there will be OCD patients who are resistant to sertraline. One such adolescent male patient unresponsive to sertraline monotherapy became the subject of a published case study reporting that the second-generation antipsychotic aripiprazole successfully augmented sertraline for this patient (Storch, Lehmkuhl, Geffken, Touchton, & Murphy, 2008). This case study was followed by an open-label clinical trial demonstrating successful aripiprazole augmentation in some patients (Ak, Bulut, Bozkurt, & Ozsahin, 2011) and then a double-blind clinical trial demonstrating successful aripiprazole augmentation (Sayyah, Sayyah, Boostani, Ghaffari, & Hoseini, 2012)—both studies in patients for whom OCD had been resistant to SSRI monotherapy. The use of aripiprazole for augmentation of SSRIs in the treatment of OCD remains an off-label use, but aripiprazole has received FDA approval as monotherapy or as an adjunct for treatment of bipolar disorder and as an adjunct for treatment of major depression.

In conclusion, FDA approval cannot ensure effectiveness and safety for a drug being used for its approved purpose or for that same drug being used off-label. Despite the imperfect ability to predict success, the occasional failures for individual patients, and the reasonable worries over excessive off-label use, unexpected good consequences can result that advance the clinical utility of psychotropic medications.

HOW DOES LITHIUM FORESTALL RELAPSE OF BIPOLAR DISORDER?

(A Therapeutic Drug Is Used Because It Works.)

Lithium treatment has relieved Marko of his mania, and it has relieved him of his depression. Better still, when Marko is symptom-free and taking his lithium, many months can go by with no symptoms of his bipolar disorder. Marko asked his physician why lithium could do all of those various things and heard the reply, "We don't know." Marko thought that was pretty hilarious.

When the FDA in 1974 approved the use of lithium to treat bipolar disorder, lithium's mechanism of action was unknown. Forty years later, lithium remains the drug of choice to treat the acute manic-phase bipolar depression and for the maintenance phase for a bipolar patient who is symptom-free (Freeman et al., 2009). Lithium is cost-effective, and its side effects are well tolerated. Lithium has been measured to alter synaptic processes for numerous neurotransmitters, including norepinephrine and serotonin, and lithium alters numerous intracellular processes. However, over 40 years later, the mechanism of action of lithium remains unknown. Knowing the mechanism of action of lithium's effects on the various components of bipolar disorder would be quite useful. Such knowledge would facilitate understanding what is going on in the brain of a patient suffering bipolar disorder, which in turn could facilitate the development of new drugs to treat bipolar disorder. But knowing the mechanism of action of lithium is not necessary for the successful treatment of bipolar disorder. It is enough to know that lithium can be effective. Lithium is used because it works.

Lithium is not the only drug used to treat disordered mood that has a somewhat mysterious mechanism of action (Table 10.1). Bupropion has effects on a variety of neurotransmitter processes, including norepinephrine, dopamine, and acetylcholine, but its pharmacological profile does not place it in any of the classes of tricyclic, MAO inhibitor, SSRI, or SNRI antidepressants (Clayton & Gillespie, 2009). Bupropion's antidepressant mechanism of action remains unknown, despite it being approved in 1989 for use in treating depression.

IS IT WISE TO USE DIETARY SUPPLEMENTS TO TREAT DEPRESSION?

(Dietary Supplements May or May Not Be Effective and Safe.)

Samantha is depressed yet again. And she knows that again it will be expensive to have to pay for a prescription for an antidepressant medication, because her copayment obligation has increased again and is fairly sizable. She also knows that St. John's wort is less expensive and might work just as well. Her physician does not agree, but she suspects that it is because he and the drug company representative are in cahoots, encouraging people to use expensive medications rather than readily available and inexpensive homegrown remedies that have stood the test of time. So, she'll let him write the prescription, but she'll be buying St. John's wort.

The FDA cannot assure each individual patient that an approved medication will be effective and tolerable. There is even less assurance that dietary supplements and herbaceuticals will be effective and cause no harm, given that the FDA has no role in regulating the chemicals that enter the market as dietary supplements. Does this mean that such products are not likely to be used in productive ways to treat depression or bipolar disorder?

Consumers exhibit a healthy appetite for what are viewed as natural remedies such as dietary supplements and herbaceuticals to treat a wide variety of ailments, including mood disorders (Carpenter, 2011; Howland, 2012a; Mischoulon, 2009). The sale of these products would be difficult to sustain if their use by consumers was marked by years of complete disappointment and failure. But for the most part, the heavy use of these products is not based on the kind of evidence that the FDA expects to see when considering the approval of a new drug. Absent FDA regulation of the dietary supplement industry, there is little incentive for the manufacturers of supplements to pay for expensive clinical trials to evaluate the effectiveness and safety of their products. Thus, the published evidence that might support use of dietary supplements is meager and not particularly convincing. But there may be some hope on the horizon.

Three products have at least some evidence suggesting their effectiveness for the treatment of major depression: St. John's wort, S-adenosyl-L-methionine (SAMe), and omega-3 fatty acids (Carpenter, 2011; Deligiannidis & Freeman, 2010; Freeman et al., 2010; Mischoulon, 2009). The results of published studies evaluating the effectiveness and safety of these substances are mixed, but there is just enough evidence to suggest that further research—studies having sound methodological design—should be conducted. Is there enough evidence for a professional mental health clinician to recommend the use of such treatments? No, but many patients are not waiting for a professional recommendation to use these products.

There should be conversations that raise the following issues with patients regarding the use of dietary supplements and herbal remedies:

- The use of dietary supplements is not evidence-based use, and there is very little if any scientific evidence to support their use.
- If a dietary supplement is being used instead of recommended antidepressant medication or psychotherapy, the patient runs the risk of delaying active and aggressive treatment, a situation that could result in worsening of symptoms.
- Dietary supplements will have side effects, although omega-3 fatty acids appear to have few if any.
- Dietary supplements can present harmful drug-drug interactions. Therefore, patients must be candid regarding their use of all such products.
- The quality control that would guarantee consistency of dietary supplements (e.g., across batches, between products made by different companies) is relatively deficient. Patients should be warned to attempt to purchase only from reputable sources.
- Although dietary supplements sold as having antidepressant properties may have fewer side effects than prescription antidepressant medications, it does not mean that the supplements are more effective for treating depression. In fact, quite the opposite may be true—the lack of side effects may indicate a lack of biological activity.

Dietary supplements and herbal remedies should not be viewed as acceptable alternatives to prescription medications for the treatment of major depression (Carpenter, 2011; Mischoulon, 2009). Their use should be limited to mild or moderate depression, and their proper role might be as an adjunct to psychotherapy or antidepressant medication.

The use of dietary supplements and herbal remedies to treat bipolar disorder is even more suspect. There is nothing more than preliminary evidence that a few substances (e.g., omega-3 fatty acids, N-acetylcysteine, branch-chain amino acids, inositol, folic acid, choline, magnesium, tryptophan) might have slight benefit in treating some aspects of bipolar disorder. The scientific evidence is weak and mixed but is of sufficient interest to encourage methodologically sound clinical trials to evaluate effectiveness and safety of some of these chemicals (Sarris, Lake, & Hoenders, 2011; Sarris, Mischoulon, & Schweitzer, 2011; Sylvia, Peters, Deckersbach, & Nierenberg, 2013).

CAN PLACEBO HAVE A ROLE IN THE TREATMENT OF DEPRESSION?

(Placebo Can Have Drug-Like Effects.)

Peter believes that taking daily doses of omega-3 fatty acids and frequently eating omega-3-rich fish are preventing a relapse of his bipolar disorder. His physician knows of no convincing evidence that this could be true. But Peter believes that those capsules and that mackerel are effective medications, and that belief might just be good medicine.

In clinical trials evaluating the effects of antidepressant medication on depression, placebo treatment can have pronounced effects (Walsh et al., 2002). For example, between 10% and 50% of subjects can show remission (e.g., >50% reduction in Hamilton Rating Scale scores). These are only *presumed* effects of placebo, because the measured improvement in symptoms may incorporate the benefits of other factors common to the structure of clinical trials, including regular supportive consultations with the personnel conducting the trials, group therapeutic activities available to in-patients, spontaneous remission, fluctuations in the course of depression, and the passage of time. Characteristics of a patient's depression that increase the likelihood that placebo will be effective include short duration of illness, mild or moderate depression, a precipitating event, and a previous positive response to antidepressant medication (Sonawalla & Rosenbaum, 2002).

The magnitude of these effects for a placebo treatment condition in a clinical trial presents a problem for interpretation of the clinical significance or potency of a drug's effect, because the placebo treatment condition is the typical control condition providing a reference point against which to measure an effect of the drug being investigated (Sonawalla & Rosenbaum, 2002). In other words, if 50% of people receiving placebo show remission, and 65% of people receiving drug show remission, then how many patients in a clinical setting really *need* the drug to improve—only 15%?

Although it is difficult to disentangle the true placebo effect from the effects of other factors present in a placebo treatment condition in a clinical trial, there is accumulating evidence that placebo treatment in the context of clinical trials can produce changes in the human brain that can be measured using neuroimaging (Beauregard, 2009; Benedetti et al., 2005; Mayberg et al., 2002) or electrophysiological techniques (Hunter et al., 2006; Leuchter et al., 2002). Whether these changes in the brain are the result of a true placebo effect and are not confounded by other factors such as supportive counseling is not clear, but there are interesting and provocative findings regarding the effects of placebo on the brain. For example, some of the changes in glucose metabolism in the brain that correlate with placebo treatment are dissimilar and appear in different sites in the brain than do those correlated with treatment by fluoxetine for major depression (Mayberg et al., 2002). Moreover, placebo-induced changes in the brain are different from those induced by CBT (Goldapple et al., 2004) or interpersonal psychotherapy for major depression (Brody et al., 2001; Martin, Martin, Rai, Richardson, & Royall, 2001). Overall, these findings suggest that placebo can be an active treatment for major depression, capable of inducing changes in the brain while contributing to the relief of symptoms. Despite the demonstrated ability of placebo to induce changes in the brain that are unique yet similar to those induced by antidepressant medication or by psychotherapy, it remains to be seen whether such findings are sufficiently compelling to overcome ethical concerns regarding the use of placebo as therapy.

Although placebo treatment is not likely to be useful for the maintenance phase of treatment for depression (Stewart et al., 1998), there may be ways to use placebo for short-term, early treatment. One reasonable suggestion (Dago & Quitkin, 1995) for use of placebo as therapy is to initiate short-term placebo treatment for depression including close observation and psychotherapy to determine which depressed patients demonstrate improvement without medication; patients who do not respond sufficiently to placebo would then be prescribed antidepressant medication (Sonawalla & Rosenbaum, 2002). Such an approach may become more realistic with the ability to use neurophysiological techniques that can identify which patients diagnosed with major depression are more likely to be responsive to placebo or to antidepressant medication (Hunter et al., 2006; Leuchter et al., 2002).

In conclusion, placebo is not doing nothing to behavior and to the brain when administered in clinical trials to patients diagnosed with major depression, but it is not yet clear how to most effectively use placebo in a clinical setting.

CAN AN ANTIDEPRESSANT ALONE SUCCESSFULLY TREAT DEPRESSION?

(Pharmacotherapy Is Best Used as One Among Several Tools.)

Susan has been assured that she will not be taking antidepressant medication forever—that the plan is to wean her off of the drug once her symptoms of depression have essentially disappeared. At that point she will continue with a version of interpersonal psychotherapy at regular intervals for as long as it seems to be useful. The purpose of the continuing psychotherapy is to prevent relapse, which is an important consideration for Susan given that this is now her fifth bout with debilitating depression.

A comparison between the effects of CBT and the SSRI paroxetine reveals that, while either treatment improves symptoms of major depression, each of the treatments can produce some changes in the brain that are similar and some that are unique to the modality of treatment (Goldapple et al., 2004; Kennedy et al., 2001). The same can be said for the effects of CBT and the SNRI venlafaxine (Kennedy et al., 2007). What, if anything, do these results of neuroimaging studies predict about the utility of combining psychotherapy with pharmacotherapy to treat major depression?

These findings permit speculation that therapeutically effective talk or drug treatments may be altering brain processes in a similar way, or in a complementary manner, or doing a bit of each:

- When psychotherapy and medication are measured to be acting on the *same sites in the brain in the same way*, one could argue that when talk and drug are used together it represents either (a) a waste of resources because the two methods are somewhat redundant, or (b) a way that one method can enhance the impact of the other method, similar to doubling a dose of treatment. This speculation supports the prediction that combining talk and drug will produce (a) no enhancement of therapeutic outcome or (b) greater therapeutic outcome than talk alone or drug alone.

- When psychotherapy and medication are measured to be acting on *different sites in the brain in a different manner,* one could argue that when talk and drug are used together it represents a way for one method to enhance the impact of the other method, as if the two methods were invoking two different mechanisms of action. This speculation supports the prediction that combined talk and drug therapy will produce greater therapeutic benefit than talk alone or drug alone.

One can add another consideration to these speculations—the idea that psychotherapy also has effects on major depression that will not appear as measurable changes in the brain, and that these effects on behavior will add to any impact on therapeutic outcome that drug therapy can provide. This idea supports the prediction that combined talk and drug therapy will produce greater therapeutic outcome than talk alone or drug alone. Which of these predictions regarding the impact of combined pharmacotherapy and psychotherapy on major depression are supported by the results of clinical trials?

There is no convincing published evidence that any combination of psychotherapy and antidepressant medication is better than monotherapy for the treatment of major depression. There are examples of modest benefit for combined drug and talk therapies for depression (Blom et al., 2007; Bottino et al., 2012; Fava, Grandi, Zielezny, Rafanelli, & Canestrari, 1996; Keller et al., 2000; Kocsis et al., 2003; Lynch et al., 2011; Pampallona, Bollini, Tibaldi, Kupelnick, & Munizza, 2004; Peeters et al., 2012; Schramm et al., 2007) and for bipolar disorder (Berk et al., 2010). There also are examples of little or no benefit for combined drug and talk therapies for major depression (Kocsis et al., 2009; Thase et al., 2007). Meta-analyses of published work also report modest or no benefit for combined drug and talk treatments for major depression (von Wolff et al., 2012).

Thus, the literature on the question of the superior effectiveness of combined drug and talk treatments is unconvincing, but guidelines emerge out of clinical experience and common sense. First, given the relatively high risk of suicide in major depression and in bipolar disorder, together with the fact that it is not uncommon for first-line antidepressant medication to fail to show benefit, the combination of some method of psychotherapy with pharmacotherapy makes good sense for the acute phase of treatment. Second, given that chronic maintenance on an antidepressant medication has its disadvantages (e.g., adverse advents), weaning a patient off medication while maintaining psychotherapy to prevent relapse makes good sense. In addition, maintenance pharmacotherapy for preventing relapse of bipolar disorder is important and does benefit from psychotherapy or counseling focused on encouraging adherence to using the prescribed medication (Berk et al., 2010).

Nothing more definitive can be said regarding evidence-based use of combined drug and talk therapies until clinical trials evaluating various combinations of the different effective methods of psychotherapy plus antidepressant medications are more numerous and their results are more convincing.

CAN ANIMAL MODELS TEACH US ABOUT PHARMACOTHERAPY FOR DEPRESSION?

Ronnie the Rat is forced to play every day with that bully Freddy the Ferret. He dreads going over to Freddy's place. For one thing, Freddy's place is a tiny one-room flat—nothing but four walls, with a water fountain on one wall and a food trough on another. And Freddy just seems to want to bash Ronnie around, and when he isn't whacking on Ronnie, Freddy just stands there very still, staring that killer stare. That daily experience just presses the starch out of Ronnie, so much so that when he gets home at the end of the day even his freshly prepared sugar solution does not taste very good to Ronnie. Talk about depressing!

Although animal models for depression are generally known for their reasonably good predictive validity despite their poor construct validity, the models have had relatively little success in identifying novel pharmacotherapeutic approaches (Berton, Hahn, & Thase, 2012). Many of the models utilize chronic, inescapable exposure to mild stress. The more recent animal models include those that attempt to incorporate pathophysiology as well as behavioral symptoms of depression (Sillaber et al., 2009). Examples of useful animal models for depression include (Edwards & Koob, 2012; Fernando & Robbins, 2011) the following.

Methods for exposure to sustained stress:
- Chronic social stress in rodents (e.g., exposure of an intruder rat to an aggressive resident rat)
- Forced long-duration swimming by rodents
- Various models of learned helplessness in the face of unpredictable, unavoidable, and inescapable stress
- Maternal deprivation in young animals

- Tail suspension testing in rodents—measuring latency to surrender in the face of sustained stress

  Measures of consequences of exposure to sustained stress:
- Changes in preference for sweet solutions in rodents
- Changes in threshold values for electrical stimulation of the brain in rats

Here are recent examples of the use of some of these animal models that include assessments of the effects of medications used clinically:

- Rats exposed to daily social stress for five weeks in a resident/intruder paradigm exhibit reduced locomotor activity, reduced exploration measured by rearing and sniffing, and diminished preference for sucrose solution; these depressive-like behaviors are ameliorated by the SSRI fluoxetine (Rygula, Abumaria, Domenici, Hiemke, & Fuchs, 2006a).
- Rats exposed to daily social stress for five weeks in a resident/intruder paradigm exhibit reduced locomotor activity, reduced exploration measured by rearing and sniffing, diminished preference for sucrose solution, and increased duration of immobility in a forced swimming test. The SSRI citalopram abolishes each of these depressive-like behaviors (Rygula et al., 2006b). The SNRI reboxetine ameliorates all of these effects, whereas the antipsychotic haloperidol and the antianxiety drug diazepam do not (Rygula et al., 2008). Despite these effects of reboxetine in an animal model for depression, the clinical utility of reboxetine is unsatisfactory (Eyding et al., 2010), an inconsistency that challenges the predictive validity of animal models of depression.
- Chronic daily treatment with the SSRI fluoxetine fails to diminish depressive-like behaviors of rats in a forced swimming test (Bouet et al., 2012).
- Immobility in rats in a forced swimming test is reduced by administration of the SNRI venlafaxine or the tricyclic antidepressant imipramine, with venlafaxine being slightly more effective than imipramine (Nowakowska, Kus, & Chodera, 2003).

In summary, the recent history of the use of animal models for depression mainly involves measurement of behavioral changes induced by sustained stress. Some of these experimental paradigms have predictive value for the clinical utility of drugs for treatment of depression in humans.

TIDBITS ON PSYCHOPHARMACOLOGY LEARNED FROM THE TREATMENT OF MOOD DISORDERS

The following are brief examples illustrating other principles of pharmacology or recommendations from Part I of this book, taken from the clinical treatment of mood disorders or from basic research on mood disorders:

- *No drug has only one effect.* Tricyclic antidepressants relieve symptoms of depression presumably due to their ability to inhibit reuptake of synaptic norepinephrine and serotonin, but side effects such as dry mouth, blurry vision, constipation, urinary hesitancy, and memory difficulties are likely attributable to the drugs' ability to act as antagonists to receptors for acetylcholine (Nemeroff & Schatzberg, 2007).
- *Compromise on benefits and risks is a realistic goal for pharmacotherapy.* The controversy over whether the data unequivocally support the FDA warning that adolescents perhaps should not be treated with antidepressant medications due to their risk of suicide remains unresolved (Sobel, 2012). This controversy is important given the finding that combined CBT and fluoxetine appears to be more effective for treatment of major depression in adolescents than is cognitive-behavioral monotherapy or fluoxetine monotherapy (March & Vitiello, 2009).
- *Desired effects and unwanted effects are related to dosage.* The tricyclic antidepressant nortriptyline relieves symptoms of depression when given in dosages between 50 and 150 mg/day; doses lower or higher than this range are usually ineffective (Nemeroff & Schatzberg, 2007).
- *Drug interactions can be potent and unpredictable.* Fluoxetine plus the second-generation antipsychotic olanzapine can have greater than additive effects for improving symptoms of major depression in treatment resistant patients (Shelton et al., 2001).
- *Sensitivity to a drug varies from one individual to another.* The effectiveness of psychotherapy for major depression, using interpersonal psychotherapy, CBT, or behavior therapy, is quite variable from patient to patient (Craighead et al., 2007), as are the patient-to-patient responses to various classes of antidepressant medications (Nemeroff & Schatzberg, 2007).
- *Sex, age, and genetics can determine the magnitude of effects of a drug.* A pharmacogenetic marker in elderly patients having major de-

pression may predict early discontinuation of paroxetine, and perhaps other SSRI antidepressant medications (Murphy et al., 2004).

- *A person's drug history can affect a drug's effectiveness.* Substance-dependent patients are less likely to adhere to an antipsychotic medication regimen for bipolar disorder (Sajatovic et al., 2007).

- *Culture and community can affect the utility of pharmacotherapy.* Many Aboriginal Australians do not view depression as a disorder that warrants treatment. Depression is seen as a characteristic of an individual's personality, often going unnoticed, and therefore does not activate traditional Aboriginal customs of treatment (Vicary & Westerman, 2004).

- *Drugs can mimic endogenous neurochemicals.* Agomelatine, an agonist for MT1 and MT2 melatonin receptor subtypes, shows potential for development as a novel antidepressant medication (Holsboer, 2009).

- *Drugs can block endogenous neurochemicals.* Mirtazapine is useful for treatment of major depression. Its presumed mechanism of action is antagonism for alpha-2-adrenergic receptors, and 5-HT2 and 5-HT3 serotonin receptor subtypes (Schatzberg, 2009).

- *Pharmacological effects on brain neurochemistry can be enduring.* Downregulation of receptors for serotonin and norepinephrine are measured following treatment with various antidepressant medications (Dunlop et al., 2009; Gillespie et al., 2009).

- *Drugs differ in their potential for addiction.* Despite the fact that antidepressant medications elevate mood in people suffering depression, antidepressant medications are not drugs that are abused recreationally.

- *Drugs can alter the organization of a developing brain.* The off-label use of antidepressant drugs in children and adolescents is common despite limited evidence for their effectiveness and safety in children and adolescents, and despite black-box warnings regarding suicidal ideation (Jensen et al., 1999).

- *The role of pharmacotherapy varies for different people and disorders.* The best approach for use of antidepressant medication and psychotherapy is to construct an individualized treatment program (Berman et al., 2009).

- *Serendipity can bring new opportunities for pharmacotherapy.* Development of iproniazid for its utility in treating tuberculosis unexpectedly led to development of MAO-inhibiting drugs for their antidepressant properties; the search for better antipsychotic medications revealed the antidepressant properties of imipramine (Sobel, 2012).

- *Consumers demand new and better drugs.* The SSRI drugs have captured enough of the market for antidepressant medications that it is limiting the potential for commercial success for newer drugs that might be developed (Connolly & Thase, 2012).
- *Successful use encourages increased use, for better or worse.* Successful use of SSRI antidepressants in adults has increased use of these drugs in adolescents and the elderly despite limited evidence supporting this off-label use (Nemeroff & Schatzberg, 2007).
- *The FDA attempts to approve new and better drugs.* There is no clear drug of choice for first-line treatment of major depression (Nemeroff & Schatzberg, 2007).
- *Off-label use has its advantages and disadvantages.* From 2001 to 2004, the SSRI drugs sertraline and paroxetine were the two most frequent off-label prescribed central-nervous-system–altering drugs in outpatient pediatric settings (Bazzano et al., 2009).
- *Health insurance practices can determine accessibility to a drug.* The short-term costs of antidepressant medications are less than short-term costs of psychotherapy (Barrett, Byford, & Knapp, 2005), although premature discontinuation of medication probably accounts for some portion of those reduced costs (Hodgkin, Merrick, & Hiatt, 2012).
- *Diagnosis guides choice of pharmacotherapy.* Tricyclic antidepressants are generally less effective in depressed patients showing psychotic symptoms than in depressed patients without psychotic symptoms (Nemeroff & Schatzberg, 2007).
- *Clients should be active participants in their pharmacotherapy.* The effective use of a drug for maintenance therapy during remission for bipolar disorder depends upon the willingness and ability of patients to take their medication reliably (Keck & McElroy, 2009).

SUMMARY AND PERSPECTIVE

The state of the contemporary use of psychoactive drugs to treat depression and bipolar disorder reveals five points of perspective. First, despite the availability of various classes of effective antidepressant medications, and multiple pharmacotherapy options for bipolar disorder, approximately one-third of people who suffer depression or bipolar disorder fail to benefit from pharmacotherapy. Second, despite 50 years of using psychotropic medications for depression and for bipolar disorder, there is no clear drug of choice for first-line treatment for either disorder. Third, the near equivalence of effectiveness of antidepressant drugs in the various classes emphasizes the importance of looking to potential side effects as decisive factors when choosing among medication options. Fourth, owing to the potentially severe consequences of failure to successfully treat depression or bipolar disorder, together with the lack of confidence that the first choice of medication will be helpful for any individual patient, a significant role for psychotherapy for treating mood disorders is undeniable. Fifth, clinical trials are only beginning to provide evidence that identifies the most effective ways to combine pharmacotherapy and psychotherapy, to switch from an ineffective medication to another drug, and to use one drug to augment the effectiveness of another medication.

Thus, there is much room for more progress in the development of new drugs to treat disordered mood. Such progress will be aided by further development of neurobiological theories of major depression and bipolar disorder—new theories that have greater explanatory power. New theories should broaden the neurochemical angles of approach for developing novel therapeutic mood-normalizing drugs. Progress will also depend upon the investment in clinical trials that evaluate the effectiveness of novel drugs and combinations of therapeutic methods.

Finally, there is abundant opportunity and need for the artful application of clinical skills to negotiate choices of pharmacotherapy and psychotherapy, especially for patients at risk, because it is not at all obvious what will be the optimal therapeutic program for each different patient.

CHAPTER ELEVEN

Attention Deficit Hyperactivity Disorder

Felix's math teacher complains that Felix cannot seem to sit still in class and, by "talking all the time," is constantly distracting fellow students all around him. His teacher tells Felix's parents to consider that their son has ADHD and that they should probably have him medicated. When pressed with a few questions, the teacher admits that their son is doing very well academically and in fact is the top-performing student in her math class. The parents suggest that in light of his fine academic performance, perhaps he is bored in class and therefore is doing what he can to turn the classroom into an entertaining carnival. Although Felix's parents wish the young lad would be better behaved and more compliant, they also are determined that their child will not be medicated principally to make it easier for a teacher to keep control of her classroom. They will not solve the teacher's problem by medicating their son.

Pharmacotherapy to treat attention deficit hyperactivity disorder (ADHD) has proven its utility. Many published clinical trials collectively establish four comprehensive findings regarding pharmacotherapy for properly diagnosed ADHD (Paykina, Greenhill, & Gorman, 2007)—a serious debilitating disorder that warrants treatment.

First, more than 70% of children diagnosed with ADHD respond favorably to the first attempt to medicate the disorder (Plessen & Peterson, 2009), and between 80% and 90% respond to pharmacotherapy overall (Vaughan, March, & Kratochvil, 2012; Wigal, 2009). This represents an impressive rate of response to medication, when considered in the context of rates of response to pharmacotherapy for depression, bipolar disorder, schizophrenia, or addiction. This notable utility of medications opposes the fact that the pathophysiology of ADHD remains poorly understood.

Second, psychomotor stimulant drugs remain the most frequently used class of drugs to treat ADHD (Garfield et al., 2012), although there are now nonstimulant alternatives for pharmacotherapy (Dziegielewski, 2006; Vaughan et al., 2012). The most frequently used stimulant drug for treating ADHD is the stimulant methylphenidate (Garfield et al., 2012), first used in 1955. Many published studies document the effectiveness and tolerability of methylphenidate (Paykina et al., 2007).

Third, although the short-term effectiveness and tolerability of pharmacotherapy for ADHD are well documented, what remains poorly understood is whether or not chronic exposure of the developing human brain to therapeutic doses of a stimulant drug has deleterious long-term consequences (Plessen & Peterson, 2009).

Finally, combined pharmacotherapy and psychotherapy is generally more effective than psychotherapy alone for ADHD but is no more effective than pharmacotherapy alone (Paykina et al., 2007; Plessen & Peterson, 2009; Vaughan et al., 2012; Wigal, 2009). Moreover, behavior therapy or psychotherapy usually is not sufficient to treat ADHD when offered without pharmacotherapy (Vaughan et al., 2012). This makes pharmacotherapy appear to be the treatment of choice for ADHD.

HOW HAVE DRUGS BEEN USED TO TREAT ADHD?

It had been virtually impossible for Sam to function in school. His behavior annoyed everyone around him—students, teachers, and staff—making it nearly impossible for him to be well liked or to function academically or socially. Methylphenidate changed it all for Sam. He is still a bit of a nuisance while medicated, but the edge is off so that his behavior is now regarded more as a reflection of his personality rather than a symptom of a troubling disorder that is out of control. Everyone can now see that he is bright, inquisitive, energetic, and an interesting person with strong academic potential, rather than a major irritant.

The history of pharmacotherapy for ADHD begins and continues for decades with psychomotor stimulant medication. Although the designations given to what has now become known as ADHD have evolved over the past 50 years from "hyperkinetic impulse disorder" to "minimal brain dysfunction" to "hyperkinetic reaction of childhood" to "attention deficit disorder" to "attention deficit hyperactivity disorder" (including subtypes in *DSM-5*), the principal pharmacotherapeutic tactic has remained the use of various formulations of psychomotor stimulant drugs (Table 11.1).

Amphetamine was used in the 1940s and 1950s to treat children with various emotional and behavioral problems, ultimately leading to the use of another psychomotor stimulant—methylphenidate—to treat "hyperkinetic impulse disorder" beginning in 1956 (Strohl, 2011). Two significant developments mark the history of pharmacotherapy for ADHD since the mid-1950s. First, concern about exposing the brains of children and adolescents to the potent effects of stimulant drugs has led to the successful use of drugs that do not have stimulant properties. Second, the effectiveness of stimulant drugs has been so convincing that a variety of stimulant drugs and formulations of those drugs have been developed and used clinically, including racemic amphetamine, D-amphetamine, L-amphetamine, mixed-enantiomer/mixed-salt amphetamine, and the FDA-approved prodrug lisdexamfetamine (Heal et al., 2013). The various formulations of the stimulant drugs present alternatives for the rate and duration at which a drug reaches and maintains a therapeutic level in the blood. Several of these formulations present the advantage of requiring only once-daily dosing, which can facilitate the administration of the drugs for children attending school.

Although stimulant drugs are viewed as the first-line therapy for ADHD, the use of pharmacotherapy is not without its complexities:

- Properly diagnosing ADHD is not easy—it should require the collaboration of the clinician, parents, teachers, and the child (Pliszka & AACAP Work Group on Quality Issues, 2007). Proper diagnosis is essential, because it is important to avoid unnecessarily exposing a child to chronic administration of a psychomotor stimulant drug, and because treatment of the child diagnosed with comorbidity requires special consideration.
- Many but not all children with ADHD respond to medication, and it is not possible to predict which children will not respond (Paykina et al., 2007).
- As many as two-thirds of children diagnosed with ADHD have a co-occurring psychiatric condition complicating their treatment (Pliszka & AACAP Work Group on Quality Issues, 2007; Vaughan et al., 2012).

TABLE 11.1

Evolution of use of drugs over the decades to treat ADHD.

DRUG	MECHANISM	1950s	1960s	1970s	1980s	1990s	2000s	2010s
Amphetamine formulations	DA/NE/?	x	x	x	x	x	x	x
Methylphenidate	DA/NE/?	x	x	x	x	x	x	x
Atomoxetine	NE						x	x
Guanfacine	NE							x
Clonidine	NE							x

Note: x indicates decade in which drug was prescribed. DA, dopamine; NE, norepinephrine; ?, unknown mechanism. This table illustrates the presumed mechanisms of action and the relatively slow pace of development of FDA-approved medications for treatment of ADHD. This slow pace is partially attributable to the lack of knowledge of etiology and pathophysiology for ADHD, the lack of clarity regarding the therapeutic mechanism of action of effective medications, and the fact that various formulations of amphetamine and methylphenidate have been fairly effective.

- Children or adolescents with ADHD who present the more common comorbidities, such as oppositional defiant disorder, conduct disorder, pervasive development disorder, autism, anxiety, depression, psychosis, substance dependence, or Tourette syndrome, are more difficult to treat with only stimulant medication (Chen, Gerhard, & Winterstein, 2009a), and relatively little evidence supports using combinations of psychotropic medications (Wigal, 2009).
- The use of pharmacotherapy for ADHD in very young, preschool children presents special difficulties; despite the lack of a broad base of published evidence, there are helpful treatment guidelines (Gleason et al., 2007).
- Patients using pharmacotherapy for ADHD benefit from frequent consultations to assess progress with therapy and counseling regarding the use of medication for the particular set of circumstances that the child presents (Hinshaw, Klein, & Abikoff, 2007).
- Stimulant medications can slow the growth (height and weight) of some children (Vaughan et al., 2012).
- Between 60% and 85% of children treated for ADHD will meet diagnostic criteria for ADHD as adults (Vaughan et al., 2012), indicating that treatment of ADHD during childhood does not usually lead to full and enduring remission.

Despite their widespread and evidence-based use, and the fact that stimulant drugs generally appear to be more effective than nonstimulant drugs for treating ADHD (Biederman & Spencer, 2008), chronically medicating a child with a stimulant drug is not an ideal approach. An alternative tactic can select among nonstimulant medications (Wood, Crager, Delap, & Heiskell, 2007), such as the norepinephrine reuptake inhibitor atomoxetine, the alpha-2-adrenergic agonists guanfacine or clonidine, or bupropion used off-label. Each of these alternatives is listed in recent guidelines for considering pharmacotherapeutic options for ADHD, which recommends the following stages of sequential options (Pliszka et al., 2006; Wagner & Pliszka, 2009): (1) a psychomotor stimulant medication, (2) an alternative stimulant drug, (3) atomoxetine, (4) a stimulant drug plus low-dose atomoxetine, (5) bupropion or a tricyclic antidepressant, (6) an alternative tricyclic antidepressant or bupropion, (7) guanfacine or clonidine. This algorithm takes into account evidence regarding effectiveness of each of the drugs, as well as their potential for adverse effects.

Among the pharmacological alternatives (Table 11.1), stimulant drugs do have the advantage of years of results from clinical trials to draw upon, providing considerable helpful information regarding effective dose ranges, duration of action for different formulations, and anticipated adverse effects (e.g., Paykina et al., 2007; Pliszka & AACAP Work Group on Quality Issues, 2007). For parents or clients concerned about the chronic use of stimulant medications, the various nonstimulant alternatives are useful and nearly as effective. There also are off-label options for monotherapy or for augmenting drug therapy (Dziegielewski, 2006), although these are burdened with the disadvantage that off-label use is not evidence-based use.

In summary, the state of the art regarding pharmacological treatment of properly diagnosed ADHD is better than the circumstances for treating numerous other psychiatric disorders (Paykina et al., 2007): There is much published evidence and clinical experience to support the use of medications for ADHD and to establish evidence-based treatment guidelines for ADHD and for ADHD with comorbidity (Pliszka et al., 2006); many of the medications have a long history of effective clinical use; many of the patients are responsive to the first-line medications; the side effects of the medications tend to be well tolerated; and the medications are generally more effective and less expensive than behavior therapy or psychotherapy.

WHY WOULD A STIMULANT DRUG DIMINISH HYPERACTIVITY IN ADHD?

(Serendipity Can Bring New Opportunities for Pharmacotherapy.)

Kevin is not sure why one street name for amphetamine is "speed," because when he takes his prescription amphetamine for his ADHD, it certainly does not speed him up. In fact, he feels calmed by the drug—more tranquil, less frantic, and better able to keep his focus on the task at hand. He rather likes the effects of the drug during the daytime. It helps him to function better, but he feels no euphoria associated with the use of his medication. His restlessness at night sometimes makes it difficult for him to fall asleep, but he has learned ways to cope with that.

Investigation in the 1930s of the potential for amphetamine to treat headache led to an appreciation of its ability to improve behaviors of children with emotional and behavioral disorders, including some children who displayed chronic restlessness and inattentiveness (Strohl, 2011). Somewhat paradoxically, whereas amphetamine was observed to energize some children and make them more animated, the drug also subdued children who were having difficulties performing in social situations because they were too rambunctious and disruptive (Bradley, 1950). Continuing research on psychomotor stimulant drugs led in 1956 to the use of methylphenidate to treat what was soon to be known as hyperkinetic impulse disorder (Laufer, Denhoff, & Solomons, 1957).

Methylphenidate and all other psychomotor stimulant drugs used to treat ADHD are known to enhance synaptic transmission of catecholamine neurotransmitters, thereby *increasing* alertness, vigor, and stamina in healthy adults and children (Iversen et al., 2009). But children and adults diagnosed with ADHD, exhibiting hyperactivity and impulsiveness, certainly do not leave the impression of needing any increase in their ability to move about. Yet the behavioral effects of methylphenidate, amphetamine, and methamphetamine can be beneficial to children and adults with ADHD (Wigal, 2009). How does this make sense?

As of yet there is no thorough explanation of the mechanism by which stimulant (or nonstimulant) drugs improve symptoms of ADHD. One way to examine stimulant drug therapeutic mechanisms of action is to measure in the human brain the neurochemical consequences of acute and of chronic stimulant drug administration. Methylphenidate and amphetamines share the ability to increase dopamine and norepinephrine in synapses in the brain (Iversen et al., 2009), and therapeutic doses of methylphenidate increase extracellular dopamine in the striatum of the human brain (Volkow et al., 2001), but whether or not this enhanced synaptic availability of dopamine is the single cause of improvement of symptoms of ADHD has not been demonstrated.

A recent finding provides a step toward understanding the mechanism of action of stimulant drugs for relief of symptoms of ADHD: Humans treated for 12 months with methylphenidate showed improvement in various symptoms of ADHD that correlated with the amount of dopamine released into synapses in the striatum, prefrontal cortex, and temporal cortex (Volkow et al., 2012). Exactly how this contributes to improvement in symptoms of inattentiveness and impulsivity remains to be determined. It also remains unclear whether it is *only* the stimulant drugs' effects on dopamine neurotransmission that is important for their therapeutic benefits. It seems unlikely that ADHD is only a dopamine-related disorder, because some of the drugs that are useful clinically affect other neurochemicals, most notably norepinephrine (Table 11.1).

IS ATOMOXETINE A BETTER OPTION THAN METHYLPHENIDATE?

(Consumers Demand New and Better Drugs.)

Nick's parents do not want their 10-year-old son swallowing stimulant medication every day for years. They cannot imagine how in the long run the chronic use of a powerful drug will be a good thing for his still developing brain and nervous system. They know that relief of his ADHD symptoms is necessary and good for his ability to perform and to get along with classmates and teachers in school, but they want a better drug for Nick, one without the reputation for being used illicitly on the street.

Psychomotor stimulant drugs have demonstrated their effectiveness for improving symptoms of ADHD in children, adolescents, and adults (Wigal, 2009), but these potent drugs are also well known for their addictive potential (Nestler, 2009). Many parents of children treated with these medications are understandably concerned about exposing the brain and nervous system of their child to drugs that could potentially increase the vulnerability for addiction.

Thus, the development of the first nonstimulant drug treatment for ADHD was greatly anticipated (Michelson et al., 2002), with atomoxetine receiving FDA approval in 2002. Whereas various stimulant drugs can enhance the availability of synaptic dopamine, norepinephrine, and serotonin, atomoxetine's effects are relatively selective for enhancing the availability of norepinephrine by inhibiting its presynaptic transport (Iversen et al., 2009). This essentially means that atomoxetine's pharmacological properties only partially resemble those of methylphenidate and the amphetamines, raising the possibility that atomoxetine might have some of the effectiveness of those stimulant drugs, have fewer side effects, and not bear the addictive potential that is presumably related to the stimulant drugs' ability to enhance neurotransmission of dopamine.

So how has the development of atomoxetine played out regarding its utility for treating ADHD? There are three reasons that atomoxetine has not yet become the obvious better alternative than stimulant drugs for treatment of ADHD. First, a direct comparison of the effectiveness of atomoxetine to methylphenidate at the end of a six-week treatment period reveals methylphenidate to be more effective than atomoxetine (Newcorn et al., 2008), but this does not mean that atomoxetine is not a clinically important option. For one, there are patients who may wish to avoid stimulant medication altogether, regardless of whether or not that means using an alternative medication that is somewhat less effective. In addition, some patients who are unresponsive to methylphenidate can be responsive to atomoxetine (Newcorn et al., 2008). Moreover, a recent meta-analysis of effectiveness and safety of atomoxetine reveals that atomoxetine's relief of symptoms continues to increase for at least 12 weeks, suggesting that the comparison of atomoxetine to methylphenidate in a six-week trial (Newcorn et al., 2008) may underestimate the ultimate longer-term effectiveness of atomoxetine (Bushe & Saville, 2013).

Second, the worry that long-term treatment with stimulant medication will increase the likelihood of later development of substance dependence or abuse has been a legitimate concern. It may not be well founded, however, for several reasons: It is possible that the effects of a stimulant drug on the brain that are relevant for developing substance use disorders are different for people with ADHD than for people who do not have ADHD (Volkow & Insel, 2003). Stimulant medication for ADHD is being used in a context in which a presumably abnormal brain is being exposed to a substance that ideally brings relief of symptoms. In contrast, a stimulant drug is used recreationally in a context in which a brain is being exposed to a substance that is expected to induce intense euphoria. The two contexts are meaningfully different in numerous ways, only some of which may be important for establishing vulnerability to addiction (Badiani & Robinson, 2004). Moreover, although the nonmedicinal use of stimulant drugs before 18 years of age can increase the likelihood of later development of dependence-like symptoms (Chen et al., 2009b), adolescents with ADHD who are *not treated* with pharmacotherapy appear to be at *greater risk* of developing a substance use problem than are adolescents who have been treated with pharmacotherapy for ADHD (Wilens, Faraone, Biederman, & Gunawardene, 2003). This suggests that the risk for not treating ADHD is greater than the risk for treating ADHD with stimulant medications. A more recent study, however, produced equivocal results: Pharmacotherapy for ADHD neither increased nor decreased the risk for subsequent substance use (Biederman et al., 2008b).

Third, although early clinical trials of atomoxetine revealed the side effects to be relatively tolerable and less worrisome than the side effects presented by stimulant drugs (Michelson et al., 2002), within three years of the FDA approval of atomoxetine the manufacturer was required to display a black box warning on its label.

WHY WOULD A NEWLY APPROVED MEDICATION HAVE A BLACK BOX WARNING?

(*The FDA Attempts to Approve New and Better Drugs.*)

The warning on the label is frightening to Ralph and to his parents. Why would his physician prescribe a medication that could make Ralph consider suicide? Merely thinking about the concept of suicide frightens Ralph. How worried should he be? He will need to trust that his parents and his doctor have his best interests in mind.

Within one year of the FDA requiring a black box warning on labeling for a number of antidepressant medications, the FDA acted promptly and assertively to require a similar warning on the packaging for atomoxetine. This decision was influenced by the fact that atomoxetine shares pharmacological properties with some antidepressant medications that already carried black box warnings, and the decision was based on limited data from clinical trials studying the effects of atomoxetine on ADHD: Examination of data from approximately 2,200 children and adolescents given either atomoxetine or placebo revealed that 0.4% of children (i.e., 1 in 250) taking atomoxetine exhibited suicidal ideation, but none of the children taking placebo exhibited such ideation (Miller, 2005; Wooltorton, 2005).

Subsequent meta-analysis of clinical trials for atomoxetine revealed that the limited data that originally led to the warning on atomoxetine may have been equivocal, but at the time of the issuing of the warning, doing so may have been a suitably cautious action. Analysis of more recent data pooled from 13 clinical trials reveals 1.5% frequency of suicidal ideation, 0.3% suicide attempts, 0.1% suicidal behaviors, and zero completed suicides by patients treated with atomoxetine (Bushe & Saville, 2013). The warning regarding the potential for atomoxetine to induce thoughts of suicide probably should be interpreted as a way to foster vigilance for suicidal ideation, but not to discourage considering the use of atomoxetine as a suitable option for treatment of ADHD (Garnock-Jones & Keating, 2010).

IS OFF-LABEL PRESCRIBING OF DRUGS A GOOD IDEA FOR TREATING ADHD?

(Off-Label Usage Has Advantages and Disadvantages.)

It just doesn't seem to make sense to Ryan's parents that most children respond to the stimulant medications or to one of the nonstimulant drugs but that Ryan does not. Why not? He seems like the typical ADHD child to them. Why are they being advised to try a so-called off-label prescription drug for him? Why make him a test case for some unproven, unapproved drug? Why not use behavior therapy instead?

If two-thirds of children diagnosed with ADHD respond favorably to a first-line pharmacotherapy, and if nearly 90% are responsive to either a first or a second attempt at medication (Vaughan et al., 2012), then there should be relatively little need for off-label pharmacotherapy for ADHD. But untreated ADHD is likely to result in limited functionality and reduced quality of life into adulthood (Shaw et al., 2012). Therefore, for those relatively few who do not respond to the most frequently administered medications, it would seem to be best to search for an effective off-label treatment or to employ one or another method of nonpharmacological therapy (Hodgson, Hutchinson, & Denson, 2012).

Off-label use of medication for ADHD does occur. For example, off-label use of relatively expensive second-generation antipsychotic medications to treat ADHD has increased recently, contributing to increased spending on pharmaceuticals for treating ADHD in the state of Florida (Fullerton et al., 2012). Despite lack of supporting evidence for effectiveness and safety of off-label use of antipsychotic drugs for ADHD, such use is consistent with one of the recommendations of the published practice parameters for treatment of ADHD in children and adolescents (Pliszka & AACAP Work Group on Quality Issues, 2007). Recommendation 8 suggests a review of the appropriateness of the diagnosis of ADHD when the standard treatments for ADHD have failed for a patient, a consideration of the use of behavior therapy, and the off-label use of one of a number of drugs that have not yet been approved by the FDA specifically for treatment of ADHD, including bupropion, clonidine (subsequently approved in 2010), guanfacine (subsequently approved in 2009), or a tricyclic antidepressant such as imipramine or nortriptyline. The alpha-adrenergic agonists clonidine and guanfacine are also recommended (when other options have failed) for treatment of ADHD in preschool children (Gleason et al., 2007).

In summary, when other highly recommended treatments have failed, off-label use of psychotropic medication to treat ADHD is recommended to be considered, because choosing no treatment is not viewed as an acceptable option (Shaw et al., 2012), and because nonpharmacological treatments for ADHD are likely to be less cost-effective than pharmacotherapy (Wu et al., 2012).

WHY IS THE USE OF MEDICATIONS FOR ADHD INCREASING?

(Successful Usage Encourages Increased Usage, for Better or Worse.)

Kara's father thinks that if 20% of the children in school are taking stimulant drugs by prescription to improve their academic performance, then they'd best get Kara to their physician for a prescription, because she will someday need to compete with those other children for awards and scholarships. It will not be such a big problem to make a case for Kara needing a prescription. They will describe her restlessness, talkativeness, high level of activity, limited attention span—the usual things that can get you a diagnosis.

Various sources of data (Akinbami, Liu, Pastor, & Reuben, 2011; Getahun et al., 2013) reveal that over the past decade the prevalence of diagnosis of ADHD in the United States has increased from approximately 7% to 9%; prevalence has increased for Caucasians, African-Americans, Hispanics, and Puerto Ricans in similar proportions between approximately 2000 and 2010 (Akinbami et al., 2011). Concurrent with this increase in prevalence has come an increase in the use of various psychotropic medications for treatment of ADHD (Castle, Aubert, Verbrugge, Khalid, & Epstein, 2007; Garfield et al., 2012; Winterstein et al., 2008). Stimulant drugs remain the leading class of drugs being used to treat ADHD, with approximately 90% of patients being prescribed one or another stimulant drug over the past decade (Garfield et al., 2012). Such a high rate of prescription stimulant drug use surely speaks to the fact that the drugs are effective and relatively safe treatments for what is considered to be a serious, debilitating, chronic disorder. There are a variety of interesting facts about the pattern of use of medications for ADHD over the period from 2000 to 2010 in the United States (Garfield et al., 2012):

- There is a trend for declining use of stimulant medications from 2000 to 2010; the percentage of outpatient visits during which a prescription was dispensed for stimulant medication declined from 96% to 87%.
- This decline in use of stimulant medications was apparently compensated for by the increased use of guanfacine, which received FDA approval in 2009.
- A decline in the use of atomoxetine followed its black box warning, which was issued in 2005.
- The use of methylphenidate (as a proportion of all stimulant drugs used) increased from 50% in 2000 to 52% in 2010.
- The introduction of stimulant drug formulations having longer duration of action resulted in an increase in the use of long-acting stimulant drugs from 14% in 2000 to 87% in 2010, and a proportional decrease in the use of short-acting stimulant drugs.
- Across this decade, there was an increase in the number of diagnoses of ADHD made by psychiatrists rather than by nonspecialist physicians.
- The number of outpatient visits to a physician that included a diagnosis of ADHD increased by 66% from 2000 to 2010.

From 2000 to 2010, the increase in prevalence of diagnosis of ADHD has been accompanied by an increase in the number of prescriptions recommended for psychotropic medications for ADHD (Garfield et al., 2012). It is not likely that the measured increase in prevalence is attributable entirely to an increase in true prevalence of ADHD, because other factors very likely would have had an impact on frequency of diagnosis. For example, increased awareness of the nature of ADHD and the importance of treatment of the disorder may have encouraged more parents to seek treatment for their children. In addition, the publication of clinical guidelines for treatment of ADHD, and the growing reputation for success of pharmacotherapy for ADHD, may have encouraged the seeking of treatment and the use of pharmacotherapy specifically. The appearance of new, heralded as improved, options for pharmacotherapy (e.g., atomoxetine, guanfacine, clonidine) and the introduction of drugs with longer duration of action that facilitate the daily treatment of children may have encouraged more clients to seek pharmacotherapy and to adhere to its use for a sustained period of time.

In summary, there are very good, though imperfect, drug treatments for ADHD. There is increased knowledge of the availability of successful treatments and of the importance of treatment for the disorder. All of this inspires hope for successful treatment of ADHD using pharmacotherapy, which has the advantage of being more convenient and less costly than behavior therapy.

WHY WILL MY INSURER PAY FOR MEDICATION BUT NOT PSYCHOTHERAPY?

(Health Insurance Practices Can Determine Accessibility to a Drug.)

It will cost Dan's parents a lot less money if they agree to medication for Dan's ADHD rather than insisting upon behavior therapy. They very much do not want to be medicating their son for years and years, but their physician tells them the medications are effective and that it is likely that their insurance will cover most of the cost. They are philosophically opposed to medicating for what they believe to be "nonmedical" problems—for psychological problems. Maybe they need to rethink their position on that issue—rethink it for what is in Dan's best interests.

Practice parameters and guidelines do urge consideration of the use of behavior therapy or psychotherapy as the initial treatment for children and adolescents with ADHD (Pliszka & AACAP Work Group on Quality Issues, 2007; Pliszka et al., 2006). Even stronger advice to first consider nonpharmacological therapy is offered in guidelines for treating preschool children (Gleason et al., 2007). Despite these recommendations to at least begin by considering nonpharmacological therapy, the evidence convincingly supports the successful use of medications for treating ADHD. This fact plays to the preferences of the pharmaceutical industry and health insurers.

Insurers and health managers establish policies that favor the use of successful treatments that are cost-effective. These policies often, but not always, are consistent with the needs and desires of patients, practitioners, and families of patients. For the most part there is a nice fit between policies that encourage cost-effective choices among options for treatment of ADHD and options for treatment that are preferred by clinicians and patients. Nonetheless, there is some awkwardness and tension in that fit. For example, the concluding recommendation of the practice parameters for treating ADHD prepared by the American Academy of Child and Adolescent Psychiatry emphasizes the need to resist attempts by third-party payers to limit the patient's access to frequent visits with the clinician (Pliszka & AACAP Work Group on Quality Issues, 2007). Moreover, some policies that determine the patient's payment obligation for pharmaceuticals can impose subtle constraints upon access to specific drugs.

Because the money spent on drugs to treat ADHD has increased over the past decade or more (Fullerton et al., 2012; Garfield et al., 2012), it has become increasingly important for health plans to keep the spending on drugs at acceptable levels. One device for managing spending on drugs is the tiered formulary—an increasingly common approach for minimizing spending on drugs by the third party, accomplished by placing drugs in different tiers that establish different cost obligations to the client. There are various ways in which the use of a tiered formulary strategy can have an impact on the use of pharmacotherapy for ADHD (Huskamp et al., 2005):

- Implementing for the first time a tiered formulary system can decrease the likelihood of a patient using medication for ADHD, can reduce expenditures on medication by as much as 20%, and can shift an appreciable portion of expenditures from the health plan to the patient.
- Implementing a tiered formulary system can increase the likelihood that a patient will change to a different medication for ADHD; this change appears to be incentivized by reducing the cost of the copayment.
- A patient can make a change in medication from a drug in one tier to a drug in a different tier in the formulary in a manner that increases spending by the third party while reducing spending by the patient, without having an impact on the patient continuing pharmacotherapy for ADHD.

- Increases in copayment obligation for a patient can lower overall spending on drugs, can substantially increase spending by the patient, and therefore can have an impact on the patient's choice of medication for ADHD.

Thus, a tiered formulary can be structured in such a way as to have an impact on selection of options for pharmacotherapy for ADHD. When cost to the patient is a significant issue, the tiered formulary can impose constraints on the ability to choose the drug treatment that may be in the best interests of the patient, thereby hampering the ability to provide the patient with the most appropriate individualized treatment program.

Properly creating an individualized treatment program would certainly consider the combined use of pharmacotherapy and behavior therapy or psychotherapy. The decision to use pharmacotherapy, psychotherapy, or both can be influenced by the imposition of constraints related to cost. Fortunately for the treatment of ADHD, pharmacotherapy appears on average to be the more effective treatment approach (Vaughan et al., 2012), and it appears to be the more cost-effective approach based on a meta-analysis comparing *outcomes and costs* of various treatment methods (Wu et al., 2012):

- Pharmacotherapy is cost-effective compared with no treatment and compared with behavior therapy for ADHD with or without comorbidities.
- Pharmacotherapy for ADHD is cost-effective compared with combined pharmacotherapy plus behavior therapy.
- It is not clear whether use of stimulant drugs is more or less cost-effective compared with use of nonstimulant drugs.
- Long-acting methylphenidate formulation is cost-effective compared with short-acting methylphenidate.

These kinds of findings predict that patients generally would likely find their health plans providing incentives to choose pharmacotherapy alone and to choose the long-acting formulation of methylphenidate as the drug treatment option. Recent documented use of treatment options lines up rather well with these predictions: Data for the year 2010 (from a nationally representative audit) show that 87% of visits to a physician resulted in a prescription for a stimulant drug to treat ADHD; 83% of patients used pharmacotherapy alone; 52% of patients using a stimulant medication selected methylphenidate; and 87% of those using stimulant medication were using long-acting medication (Garfield et al., 2012). It is perhaps a happy coincidence that the more effective evidence-based treatments for ADHD are the treatments that are the more cost-effective and therefore more likely to be incentivized.

CAN ANIMAL MODELS TEACH US ABOUT PHARMACOTHERAPY FOR ADHD?

Ronnie the Rat falls for the trick nearly every single time. He always presses the one lever to immediately get the tiny morsel of food, instead of pressing the other lever to get the big piece of chocolate cake 20 minutes later. Pretty much 90% of the time, he just cannot inhibit his tendency to go for the quick tiny snack. So he gets that quick tasty morsel, eats it, and then sits there wondering how good that cake might taste if he could only be less impulsive. When he complains to Dr. Model about this problem, the good Dr. assures Ronnie that it can be fixed with a little methylphenidate.

Not knowing the causes and the pathophysiology of ADHD as well as the likelihood that ADHD is a collection of multiple subtypes, has hindered the development of animal models. Animal models for ADHD can attempt to represent all or some of the behavioral characteristics displayed by humans diagnosed with ADHD, including inappropriate levels of impulsivity, inattentiveness, and hyperactivity. But none of the models has proven its ability to predict clinical effectiveness of drugs for treating ADHD in humans (Wickens, Hyland, & Tripp, 2011). Examples of potentially useful animal models for ADHD include methods of inducing behavioral abnormalities that resemble those of ADHD, and behavioral paradigms that measure in normal rats features of behaviors in ADHD.

Genetic models or induced models:
- The spontaneously hypertensive rat (SHR), a genetic model that spontaneously exhibits motor impulsiveness, deficits in attentiveness, and hyperactivity
- A Wistar Kyoto rat substrain, identified as WKY/NCrl, considered to be a possible model for the inattentive subtype of ADHD
- The dopamine transporter knockout mouse and various other mutant mouse models.
- Prenatal or early postnatal exposure of rodents to alcohol, nicotine, 6-hydroxydopamine, or polychlorinated biphenyls
- Rat pups reared in social isolation

Behavioral paradigms used to model component abnormalities
of ADHD in normal animals:

- Performance in a T-maze task that requires choosing between a quickly acquired smaller reward versus a later-arriving larger reward—that is, a delay-discounting paradigm that measures impulsivity
- Performance in a task that requires attention to a brief visual stimulus indicating when to make the proper choice to gain a food reward—for example, the five-choice serial reaction time (5-CSRT) test that measures attentiveness
- Performance in a task that requires inhibiting a prepotent motor response—for example, the stop signal reaction time (SSRT) task that measures impulsivity

Among these examples of animal models for ADHD (Kostrzewa, Kostrzewa, Kostrzewa, Nowak, & Brus, 2008; Russell, 2011; Tripp & Wickens, 2012), the spontaneously hypertensive rat is considered by some to be the best-validated model of ADHD (Sagvolden, Dasbanerjee, Zhang-James, Middleton, & Faraone, 2008; Sagvolden & Johansen, 2011), although its predictive validity remains to be determined (Wickens et al., 2011).

Here are recent examples of the use of animal models for ADHD:

- Juvenile rats trained in a T-maze delay-discounting paradigm exhibit diminished impulsivity following administration of methylphenidate, atomoxetine, amphetamine, and the tricyclic desipramine (Bizot, David, & Trovero, 2011).
- Rats that perform poorly (i.e., show high levels of impulsivity) in a 5CSRT test have their performance improved by methylphenidate (Navarra et al., 2008).
- Atomoxetine decreases impulsivity of rats performing in an SSRT task (Robinson et al., 2008).
- Lesions created by 6-hydroxydopamine in neonatal rats induce hyperactivity when those rats are juveniles; methylphenidate decreases this hyperactivity (Davids, Zhang, Tarazi, & Baldessarini, 2002).
- Lower (but not higher) doses of methylphenidate improve performance of spontaneously hypertensive rats on an attentional set-shifting paradigm intended to assess impulsivity, perseverative responding, and inattentiveness (Cao et al., 2012).

In summary, animal models for ADHD have demonstrated that several different drugs currently used to medicate for ADHD can improve performance on measures of behaviors characteristic of ADHD. It remains to be seen whether these animal models will prove to be useful for predicting therapeutic effectiveness of new drugs for treatment of ADHD in humans.

TIDBITS ON PSYCHOPHARMACOLOGY LEARNED FROM THE TREATMENT OF ADHD

The following are brief examples illustrating other principles of pharmacology or recommendations from Part I of this book, taken from the clinical treatment of ADHD or from basic research on ADHD:

- *No drug has only one effect.* Amphetamine enhances synaptic neurotransmission for dopamine, norepinephrine, and serotonin. These amphetamine-induced effects on brain neurochemistry are massive and are accompanied by numerous effects on psychological processes and behaviors.
- *Compromise on benefits and risks is a realistic goal for pharmacotherapy.* Insomnia can be worsened in ADHD patients successfully treated with psychomotor stimulant drugs (Kratochvil, Lake, Pliszka, & Walkup, 2005).
- *Desired effects and unwanted effects are related to dosage.* The transdermal delivery (skin patch) of methylphenidate can provide consistent, extended duration of bioavailability of drug with benefits for behavior for as long as 12 hours during the day, but that mode of drug delivery can also produce insomnia at night (Biederman & Spencer, 2008).
- *Drug interactions can be potent and unpredictable.* Combined treatment of ADHD using atomoxetine plus methylphenidate is accompanied by significantly greater adverse events, including insomnia, decreased appetite, and heightened irritability (Bushe & Savill, 2013).
- *Sensitivity to a drug varies from one individual to another.* The ability of methylphenidate to increase extracellular dopamine varies considerably across different individual humans (Volkow et al., 2001).
- *Sex, age, and genetics can determine the magnitude of effects of a drug.* The ratio of boys to girls diagnosed with ADHD is approximately 3:1. Although the therapeutic effects of stimulant medication do not seem to differ between sexes, nonpharmacological treatments for ADHD tend to benefit girls more so than boys (Hodgson et al., 2012).

- *A person's drug history can affect a drug's effectiveness.* Previous exposure to stimulant medication can improve the effectiveness of a stimulant drug for treating ADHD (Newcorn et al., 2008).
- *Culture and community can affect the utility of pharmacotherapy.* For the years 1996–1997 and 2004–2005, comparisons of the incidence of diagnosis of ADHD differed significantly among Caucasians (50% and 40%), African-Americans (31% and 24%), and Hispanics (9% and 19%) in the state of Florida (Fullerton et al., 2012); across those two time periods, incidence declined for Caucasians and African-Americans, but increased for Hispanics.
- *Drugs can mimic endogenous neurochemicals.* Guanfacine, a selective agonist for the alpha-2A receptor for norepinephrine, has demonstrated effectiveness for treatment of ADHD (Biederman et al., 2008a; Sallee et al., 2009).
- *Drugs can block endogenous neurochemicals.* Although preclinical experiments in animals suggest the possibility that antagonist drugs for H3 receptors for histamine may provide useful alternative nonstimulant medications for ADHD, a clinical trial in humans shows no benefit of three different doses of the H3 antagonist bavisant (Weisler et al., 2012).
- *Pharmacological effects on brain neurochemistry can be enduring.* Maintenance on medication for ADHD for an average of five years had a modest benefit on academic performance assessed at nine years, but academic performance was not normalized (Powers, Marks, Miller, Newcorn, & Halperin, 2008). Whether or not this enduring improvement in behavior reflects enduring drug-induced changes in brain neurochemistry is not known.
- *Drugs differ in their potential for addiction.* Pharmacotherapy using potentially addictive stimulant drugs for ADHD may have no effect on the likelihood of developing substance dependence during adulthood (Biederman et al., 2008b; Volkow & Swanson, 2008).
- *Drugs can alter the organization of a developing brain.* Methylphenidate administered chronically during adolescence produces a variety of enduring changes in the brain and in the behavior of adult animals, but methylphenidate produces fewer neuroadaptations than does amphetamine or cocaine (Marco et al., 2011).
- *Drugs can be demonstrated to be only relatively effective and safe.* All drugs that have ever been approved to treat ADHD have side effects.
- *A therapeutic drug is used because it works.* Stimulant and nonstimulant medications for treating ADHD have different acute and

long-term effects on brain neurochemistry (Marco et al., 2011), but there is insufficient knowledge of those effects to provide explanations for the mechanisms of action by which stimulant and nonstimulant drugs improve symptoms of ADHD. Drugs to treat ADHD are used because they work, not because their mechanisms of action are known.

- *Dietary supplements may or may not be effective and safe.* Various complementary and alternative medical therapies for ADHD have been considered, but the evidence for their utility is slim; among the possibly useful dietary supplements are omega-3-fatty acids, vitamin B6, magnesium, S-adenosyl-L-methionine (SAMe), melatonin, and St. John's wort (Pellow, Solomon, & Barnard, 2011).

- *Placebo can have drug-like effects.* Augmenting amphetamine pharmacotherapy with a placebo pill presents an advantage for maintaining effective relief of symptoms of ADHD; 50% of the original dose of amphetamine combined with placebo can sustain effective treatment (Sandler, Glesne, & Bodfish, 2010).

- *Pharmacotherapy is best used as one among several tools.* Although this is a tenet worth taking seriously, there is little published evidence for treatments of ADHD that a particular method of behavior therapy or psychotherapy combined with a specific medication improves the outcome compared with pharmacotherapy alone. This is a topic that would benefit from further research (Hodgson et al., 2012).

- *Diagnosis guides choice of pharmacotherapy.* Diagnosis of ADHD increased dramatically by 66% from 2000 to 2010. This increase probably reflects not an increase in true incidence of the disorder but, more likely, greater public awareness, availability of new treatments, and marketing by pharmaceutical companies (Garfield et al., 2012).

- *The role of pharmacotherapy varies for different people and disorders.* Despite the demonstrated effectiveness of stimulant drugs for treating ADHD in children and adolescents, the nonstimulant drug atomoxetine was the first drug approved by the FDA for treatment of ADHD in adults (De Sousa & Kalra, 2012).

- *Clients should be active participants in their pharmacotherapy.* Children who expresses concern regarding embarrassment or stigma associated with being required to take their medication for ADHD during the school day can now benefit from the introduction of extended-release or longer-acting formulations of stimulant and nonstimulant medications.

SUMMARY AND PERSPECTIVE

Psychotropic medication for ADHD in children, adolescents, and adults generally is effective, and side effects are well tolerated. There are a variety of evidence-based options for drug therapy, including the relatively recent introduction of long-acting stimulant and nonstimulant drug formulations. Most patients who select pharmacotherapy for ADHD are responsive to it. While there are advantages to adjunctive behavior therapy or psychotherapy, properly selected and closely supervised use of medication alone is often sufficient therapy. Practice guidelines for implementing pharmacotherapy within a treatment program are evidence based. Thus, despite lack of a satisfactory understanding of what exactly is the problem in the brain of a person with ADHD, and without complete understanding of which drug-induced alterations in brain neurochemistry are mediating the relief of symptoms, psychotropic medications are helpful and cost-effective for treating ADHD.

There are issues regarding the use of drugs to treat ADHD that warrant further attention or investigation. Perhaps most important among these is the lack of sufficient knowledge regarding the enduring effects of chronic exposure of the developing brain to powerful addictive psychomotor stimulant drugs. Although it certainly is difficult to study that issue in humans, because it would require expensive longitudinal studies replete with ethical concerns, it is important to continue to pursue the research in humans, taking the lead from the research findings in animals. Other related problems follow from the fact that drug therapy is quite effective for treating ADHD: The success of current options for pharmacotherapy can easily breed complacency that can stunt the development of newer, safer drugs for treating children and adolescents diagnosed with ADHD. Overconfidence in the success of pharmacotherapy also can diminish the use of effective nonpharmacological methods of treatment.

CHAPTER TWELVE

Anxiety

Raylan signed a contract to write a book and deliver it to the publisher by a deadline. As soon as he signed on, he began to worry that he just couldn't do it. The anxiety helped to motivate him to get cracking on the work; it was a good anxiety that marshaled the resources to get up to the challenge—resources including focus, discipline, dog-walk breaks, and an anxiolytic glass of wine at night. But, for a short time, his worry was perilously close to a destructive worry—an anxiety beyond the reality of the situation that could have brought on the dreaded writer's block. That kind of debilitating anxiety might have sent him begging to the physician for a prescription for lorazepam.

Fear and anxiety are useful normal feelings that humans can have when facing stressful situations. But the magnitude of anxiety at times can be out of proportion to the reality of the situation. That intense anxiety can be debilitating, leading to difficulty performing the basic behaviors necessary for being a self-assured, capable, productive spouse, parent, employee, student, or t-ball player. The factors contributing to the development of a debilitating anxiety disorder can include inherited vulnerability, poor coping skills, stress, trauma, disease, or more likely some combination of those factors. The unique characteristics of each factor, and the dynamics of how those factors interact, may determine the specific behavioral features of anxiety that are determined at diagnosis as fitting into one category or another—generalized anxiety disorder, panic disorder, social anxiety disorder, obsessive-compulsive disorder

(OCD), posttraumatic stress disorder (PTSD), or phobia (Wehrenberg & Prinz, 2007). Whatever the causative factors, it is likely that the best therapy for disproportionate worrying about real events or eventualities includes a drug-induced change in the physiological correlates of feeling anxious, together with nondrug therapy that teaches methods to effectively cope with real stressors in order to diminish their impact.

Despite that commonsense dual approach for treating various anxiety disorders, medicating for anxiety is often recommended as a first-line treatment with the goal of quickly getting the patient functioning and productive (Sobel, 2012). Do the various categories of diagnosed anxiety disorders benefit equally from pharmacotherapy or from behavior therapy? Do the various classes of drugs having demonstrated clinical utility better serve one category of anxiety disorder than another? Has there been meaningful progress in the use of psychotropic medications for treatment of anxiety disorders?

WHICH DRUGS ARE USED FOR TREATING DIFFERENT ANXIETY DISORDERS?

> Lorazepam seems to be the answer—lorazepam on demand. Cate knows that the problem is the size of her workload. She is attempting to do too much for a constraining 24 hours in a day and a measly seven days in a week. The anxiety is not constant; it comes in waves. Alcohol can take the edge off of it, but she has been advised to use a prescribed medication instead. Lorazepam can have anxiolytic effects similar to alcohol, but medicating with a prescription drug would give the impression that she is working while sober. An alternative remedy is to reduce the workload, but somehow Cate views this idea as an unacceptable solution.

Barbiturates, known for their sedative, tranquilizing properties, were the first psychoactive drugs used clinically to treat anxiety in the 1950s (Table 12.1). Meprobamate was introduced soon after as being equally effective and safer than the barbiturates. Meprobamate was popular until the benzodiazepines chlordiazepoxide and diazepam were introduced in 1963, heralded for their anxiolytic properties (Jacobsen, 1986). The benzodiazepines also carry reduced risk of death from overdose compared with the barbiturates or meprobamate, and consequently chlordiazepoxide and diazepam were often recommended to treat anxiety in the 1970s. These various drugs—the barbiturates, meprobamate, the benzodiazepines—and alcohol share the ability to enhance the activity of the GABA-A receptor subtype, and they share the potential for addiction. Perhaps more than any other negative attribute of these drugs, the

TABLE 12.1

Evolution of use of preferred drugs over the decades to treat various anxiety disorders.

DRUG/DRUG CLASS	MECHANISM	1950s	1960s	1970s	1980s	1990s	2000s	2010s
Barbiturates	GABA	x						
Meprobamate	GABA	x						
Benzodiazepines	GABA		x					
MAO inhibitors	NE/SER/DA	x	x	x	x	x	x	x
Clomipramine	SER/NE		x	x				
Buspirone	SER/DA/NE				x	x	x	x
Tricyclics	NE/SER				x	x	x	x
SSRIs	SER				x	x	x	x
SNRIs	SER/NE					x	x	x

Note: x indicates decade in which drug was prescribed. MAO, monoamine oxidase; SSRIs, selective serotonin reuptake inhibitors; SNRIs, serotonin and nor-epinephrine reuptake inhibitors; GABA, gamma-aminobutyric acid; NE, norepinephrine; SER, serotonin; DA, dopamine. This table illustrates that (a) a wide variety of drugs have been used to treat various anxiety disorders, and (b) the drugs currently used share the ability to alter neurotransmission for one or several monoamine neurotransmitters. Although the MAO inhibitors have been used since the 1950s, their current use is quite limited (see Table 12.2) potential for addiction has prompted the continuing search for more effective and safer options for treating anxiety disorders. At present, benzodiazepines are still a reasonable option for treating several categories of anxiety, but benzodiazepines are no longer considered to be the first-line drug treatment option.

The class of drugs most often used as a first-line treatment for a variety of anxiety disorders is the selective serotonin reuptake inhibitors (SSRIs; Table 12.2) (Mathew, Hoffman, & Charney, 2009). This fact does not follow from evidence that SSRI drugs are always more effective than other medications for treating anxiety disorders but instead more from clinical experience that the side effect profiles for SSRI drugs tend to be more favorable compared with many other medications having anxiolytic properties.

The SSRI drugs were first used for their antidepressant properties. How have they come to be the most frequently used drugs to treat the variety of anxiety disorders? Patients showing symptoms of depression and anxiety were observed to respond well to tricyclic antidepressant medication (Johnstone et al., 1980), suggesting that some tricyclic medications might have anxiolytic properties. This was an important clinical observation in light of the fact that tricyclic drugs do not have the potential for addiction, whereas the benzodi-

TABLE 12.2
Rank-ordering of drugs currently used to treat various anxiety disorders.

DRUG/DRUG CLASS	DECADE INTRODUCED	ANXIETY DISORDER				
		PANIC	SOCIAL	GAD	OCD	PTSD
MAO inhibitors	1950s	5	4	—	—	—
Benzodiazepines	1960s	4	3	4	—	—
Clomipramine	1960s	—	—	—	2	—
Buspirone	1980s	—	—	3	—	—
Tricyclics	1980s	3	—	4	—	—
SSRIs	1980s	1	1	1	1	1
SNRIs	1990s	1	2	2	—	2

Note: 1 indicates typically first-line option for medication, 2 indicates second-line option, and so forth. GAD, generalized anxiety disorder; OCD, obsessive-compulsive disorder; PTSD, posttraumatic stress disorder; MAO, monoamine oxidase; SSRIs, selective serotonin reuptake inhibitors; SNRIs, serotonin and norepinephrine reuptake inhibitors. This table illustrates (a) the current status of SSRI drugs as first-line medications for a variety of anxiety disorders, followed most often by SNRI drugs as likely second-line medication; (b) the relatively fewer medication options for treatment of OCD and PTSD compared with options available for other anxiety disorders; and (c) the fact that the older medications have been relegated to somewhat lesser utility (with the exception of clomipramine for treatment of OCD).

azepines do. Tricyclic medications subsequently came to be useful for managing the discontinuation of long-term use of benzodiazepines to treat anxiety (Rickels et al., 2000)—weaning a patient off of an addictive drug having anxiolytic properties by substituting a nonaddictive tricyclic medication having anxiolytic properties. But tricyclic medications do have their own adverse effects—they are not the ideal medication for anxiety or any other disorder.

Along came the development of SSRI drugs with their antidepressant properties, and the availability of this class of drugs provided three common-sense reasons to consider them for the treatment of anxiety. First, if a few drugs in one class of antidepressant medications (i.e., the tricyclics) can relieve symptoms of anxiety, why not consider drugs from another class of antidepressant medications for their potential anxiolytic effects? Second, patients showing symptoms of depression often also show symptoms of anxiety, providing further justification to examine the ability of a novel antidepressant medication for its potential anxiolytic properties. Third, the side effect profiles for SSRIs are generally better than those for the tricyclic drugs.

Direct comparisons of the effectiveness of an SSRI against tricyclic or benzodiazepine drugs have been particularly telling regarding the utility of SSRIs for treating anxiety. For example, the SSRI paroxetine or the tricyclic imipramine can be more effective than the benzodiazepine diazepam for treating generalized anxiety (Rocca, Fonzo, Scotta, Zanalda, & Ravizza, 1997), and paroxetine has the best side effect profile of the three. The SSRI drugs ultimately received a very close look for their potential for treating each of the categories of anxiety disorders, and they have proved to be quite effective in many instances (Mathew, Hoffman, & Charney, 2009). In fact, at present (Table 12.2), the SSRI drugs can be considered to be first-line medication for generalized anxiety disorder (Baldwin, Waldman, & Allgulander, 2012), panic disorder (Batelaan, Van Balkom, & Stein, 2012), social anxiety disorder (Blanco, Bragdon, Schneier, & Liebowitz, 2012), OCD (Fineberg, Brown, & Pampaloni, 2012a), and PTSD (Ipser & Stein, 2012). This qualifies the SSRI drugs as broadly effective antianxiety agents, expanding their effectiveness beyond their initial renown as antidepressants.

Perhaps the principal utility of pharmacotherapy for anxiety is the ability of anxiolytic drugs to reduce physiological and behavioral expressions of anxiety (e.g., heart palpitations, compulsive behaviors), but the drugs themselves are not able to teach coping skills that might serve to diminish the ability of a stressor to induce anxiety. Thus, the best treatments for anxiety would seem to combine pharmacotherapy and some amount of supporting behavior therapy or psychotherapy. Moreover, different categories of anxiety have somewhat different preferred treatments when employing nonpharmacological methods and different classes of psychoactive drugs.

SSRIs and SNRIs.   The SSRIs represent the first-line pharmacotherapy for the range of the anxiety disorders—panic disorder, social anxiety disorder, generalized anxiety disorder, PTSD, and OCD (Table 12.2). The SNRI ven-lafaxine shares first-line medication status with the SSRIs for panic disorder (Batelaan et al., 2012) and can be considered the second-line option for so-cial anxiety disorder (Blanco et al., 2012), generalized anxiety disorder (Bald-win et al., 2012), and PTSD (Ipser & Stein, 2012). The statuses of the SSRIs and SNRIs are based on published evidence from clinical trials assessing their effectiveness, coupled with their relatively favorable side effect profiles. The SSRIs (and SNRIs) are not always convincingly determined to be more effec-tive than other classes of drugs, but they offer two advantages: They tend to be more tolerable or safer and are able to relieve symptoms of anxiety and of depression (Mathew, Hoffman, & Charney, 2009) in patients who present this rather common comorbidity (Kessler, Chiu, Demler, Merikangas, & Wal-ters, 2005).

Finally, the SSRIs can benefit from some help from other therapeutic op-tions: They share their first-line treatment status with cognitive behavioral therapy (CBT) for the treatment of OCD (Fineberg et al., 2012a). And be-cause SSRI-induced relief of anxiety can have a latency of several weeks, an SSRI drug may be augmented with a benzodiazepine drug for the first four weeks of treatment for panic disorder, in order to capitalize on the shorter-latency anxiolytic effect of the benzodiazepine (Sobel, 2012).

Benzodiazepines.   Although benzodiazepines are sometimes prescribed to treat panic disorder, social anxiety disorder, and generalized anxiety disorder, their status in the sequence of pharmacotherapeutic options has declined to third or fourth in line (Table 12.2), principally due to the addictive potential of benzodiazepines. Benzodiazepines should only rarely be recommended for treatment of OCD or PTSD.

Tricyclic antidepressants.   Tricyclic antidepressants continue to be useful for treatment of panic disorder and generalized anxiety disorder, but their place in the sequence of options is now third or fourth. Tricyclics are gener-ally considered not useful for treating social anxiety, OCD, or PTSD (Table 12.2).

Clomipramine.   Clomipramine performs as an exceptional tricyclic med-ication, apparently owing to its ability to inhibit reuptake of both serotonin and norepinephrine. The drug's effect on serotonin neurotransmission is therefore somewhat similar to that of the SSRI or SNRI drugs. The fact that clomipramine appears to be as effective as the SSRIs but with less tolerable side effects when used to treat OCD (Fineberg et al., 2012a) places it second to the SSRIs as a treatment option (Table 12.2).

Buspirone. Buspirone, which offers a mix of agonist and antagonist effects on receptors for serotonin, dopamine, and norepinephrine, is useful (behind the SSRIs and the SNRI venlafaxine) for the treatment of generalized anxiety disorder (Table 12.2).

In summary, the 50-year history of pharmacotherapy for anxiety disorders can be described as moving from effective but relatively unsafe drugs to equally effective but safer drugs. The SSRI medications now tend to dominate the field as the best options, supplemented by the SNRI venlafaxine for social anxiety, generalized anxiety, and PTSD, and supplemented by clomipramine for treatment of OCD. Having alternative medications for treating anxiety disorders is important because (a) none of the medication options are able to diminish anxiety in all diagnosed patients and (b) anxiety disorders generally are chronic and not fully remitting. Finally, anxiolytic medications are not sufficiently effective to put behavior therapy, particularly CBT, out of business.

CAN A THERAPIST BE CERTAIN THAT A SPECIFIC DRUG WILL SUCCESSFULLY TREAT PANIC DISORDER FOR A PATIENT?

(Diagnosis Can Guide Choice of Pharmacotherapy.)

Rick is fearful of many, many things, and he is anxious every day. He is often afraid to leave the house, because he knows he will need to interact with people once he enters the neighborhood or the grocery store. He is afraid people will think less of him, because he is an Army veteran recently returned from a war zone. And he believes they will know this just by looking at him, their eyes meeting his. And then they will ask questions, forcing him to chat about things he'd rather not speak about. So he avoids going out, and when he must go out, he takes a route that decreases the likelihood of meeting someone. When he does meet anyone, his heart races, he begins to sweat, he feels panicked. Consequently, he has learned how to avoid meeting people, and he works to avoid making eye contact. But he returns home emotionally exhausted, including on those days when he has successfully avoided any conversations.

Upon Rick's first appointment with his physician, after two years of agonizing, it is not clear what ultimately will be his diagnosis. Social anxiety? Agoraphobia? Generalized anxiety disorder? Is his malady a consequence of wartime trauma? Is a panic attack on the way? Without a definitive diagnosis, how will his physician be able to consider options for the best treatment?

Approximately only one-third of people seek help within the first year of showing symptoms of panic disorder, and of those seeking help, fewer than half are likely to receive treatment that is evidence based (Batelaan et al., 2012). Even with treatment, panic disorder is likely to be chronic, relapse is common, and the prospect of development of comorbidity is high. Thus, it is in the patient's best interests to seek treatment soon and to receive evidence-based treatment that is appropriate for a formal diagnosis with or without comorbidity. Will a diagnosis of panic disorder find an initial treatment that is effective?

There is published evidence for the effectiveness of a variety of drugs for treating panic disorder, including the SSRIs, the SNRI venlafaxine, several of the tricyclic antidepressants, the MAO inhibitor phenelzine, and the benzodiazepines (Batelaan et al., 2012). Thus, a broad range of drugs from different classes, most of them also having antidepressant properties, can be effective for panic disorder (Table 12.2). But these medications bring their characteristic long latency of treatment response (i.e., several weeks following initiation of medicating). They also bring advantages and disadvantages that are specific to each class of drugs, to individual drugs from a class, and to particular characteristics of the patient's situation. Given the lack of published results identifying one or another drug as being the most effective for relief of symptoms, the decision regarding which medication to choose to initiate treatment may as well begin with considering potential adverse effects and the preferences and attitude of the patient.

Advantages of specific drugs and classes of drugs, together with attributes of a patient identified at diagnosis or during treatment, can guide selection of treatment for panic disorder:

- A rank ordering of classes of drugs based on their overall effectiveness and tolerability (Batelaan et al., 2012) is (1) an SSRI or an SNRI (most likely venlafaxine), (2) tricyclic antidepressant (most likely clomipramine or imipramine), (3) benzodiazepine, (4) MAO inhibitor (most likely phenelzine).
- Effective dosages of antidepressant medications used to treat panic disorder are similar to dosages effective for treating major depression (Batelaan et al., 2012); this knowledge provides some limited degree of predictability for expected side effects.

- Although the extended-release formulation of the SNRI venlafaxine appears to be no more effective than the SSRI paroxetine when administered for 12 weeks (Pollack et al., 2007), an ability to delay relapse after discontinuation of pharmacotherapy may favor the use of venlafaxine (Ferguson, Khan, Mangano, Entsuah, & Tzanis, 2007). Problems associated with discontinuation of drug therapy can be lessened by CBT (Davidson, Connor, & Zhang, 2009).
- Benzodiazepines have a short latency for their effectiveness in treating symptoms of panic disorder (Batelaan et al., 2012), making them more useful for initiating therapy when a patient is at particular risk; a benzodiazepine can be useful when combined with an antidepressant at the initiation of treatment through the first several weeks, compensating for the longer-latency anxiolytic response to the antidepressant medication (Davidson et al., 2009).
- Benzodiazepines can be useful for treating the increased anxiety that can be caused by treatment with an SSRI or venlafaxine (Davidson et al., 2009), although this tactic introduces the problem of polypharmacy.
- SSRIs and tricyclic drugs can be useful and tolerable for up to two years for treatment of panic disorder (Batelaan et al., 2012; Davidson et al., 2009). This is important for treating a chronic, relapsing disorder.
- Drugs having antidepressant properties are useful for treatment of panic disorder that is comorbid with depression (Batelaan et al., 2012).

Disadvantages of specific drugs and classes of drugs, together with attributes of a patient identified at diagnosis or during treatment, also can guide selection of treatment for panic disorder:

- Benzodiazepine drugs present risks for addiction and overdose, especially when a patient continues use of alcohol.
- Elderly patients medicated with benzodiazepines (Landi et al., 2005) or tricyclic drugs (Hilmer et al., 2007) are particularly prone to falling.
- Benzodiazepines are not useful for treatment of panic disorder comorbid with depression (Batelaan et al., 2012).
- Premature discontinuation of treatment is most likely for MAO-inhibiting drugs, principally owing to the requirement to adhere to a tyramine-free diet (Batelaan et al., 2012).

- Considerable effective off-label use that is not evidence based does occur for treating the patient whose panic disorder is not resolved by other drugs or behavior therapy. Off-label drugs that have been used include the norepinephrine reuptake inhibitor reboxetine, the GABA agonists vigabatrin and tiagabine, the MAO inhibitor moclobemide, the antipsychotic olanzapine, bupropion, various anticonvulsants, antihypertensive drugs, and other SNRIs (Batelaan et al., 2012).

Despite the variety of medication options for panic disorder, as many as one-third of treated patients may be unresponsive, and as many as half who do respond may not experience complete remission (Pollack et al., 2007). Panic disorder patients showing incomplete remission of symptoms are at considerable risk of relapse. What are the best options for treatment of panic disorder that is not responsive to initial pharmacotherapy?

Options for next-step treatment include increasing the dose of first-line medication, augmenting the first-line drug with a second medication, switching to a second-line medication, or combining CBT with a first- or second-line medication. Little published evidence facilitates deciding among these alternatives (Batelaan et al., 2012; Ravindran & Stein, 2010), although augmentation of first-line medication with CBT (Rodrigues et al., 2011) or augmentation with a second medication can be equally effective next-step options for treatment of panic disorder (Simon et al., 2009). In addition, switching from one medication to another has been recommended to proceed in the following sequence (Batelaan et al., 2012): (1) SSRI or venlafaxine, (2) different SSRI or venlafaxine, (3) clomipramine or imipramine, (4) benzodiazepine, (5) MAO inhibitor.

In summary, it can be difficult to assess symptoms of anxiety and confidently diagnose a patient as having a specific category of anxiety disorder that is unmistakably different from other categories and also is lacking comorbidity. However, this kind of difficulty should not hinder the selection of a first-line medication for panic disorder (or other categories of anxiety), because the SSRI drugs are currently viewed as being acceptable first-line medications for treatment of all varieties of anxiety disorders (Mathew, Hoffman, & Charney, 2009). Difficulty regarding choosing among treatments is more serious for the patient who presents panic disorder with comorbidity, or the patient who fails to respond to first-line medication. These situations demand of the therapist and the client some collaborative agility in using the limited published evidence together with an assessment of the benefits and risks associated with alternative medications. Finally, panic disorder has the advantage (compared with social anxiety disorder or generalized anxiety disorder) that combined pharmacotherapy and psychotherapy may be more effective than either pharmacotherapy or psychotherapy alone (Bandelow, Seidler-Brandler, Becker, Wedekind, & Ruther, 2007).

IS PHARMACOTHERAPY A BETTER OPTION THAN PSYCHOTHERAPY FOR SOCIAL ANXIETY?

(The Proper Role of Pharmacotherapy May Vary for Different People and Disorders.)

> There is nothing Jennifer likes better than going to a party to discover that she is the only one there—because being in a room full of people is terribly frightening to her, giving her the feeling that she is being continually gawked at, judged, and mocked and that ultimately she will be humiliated. She avoids attending events that will be attended by others. She feels safe when alone or at some distance from others, so she stays to herself whenever possible. That is how she copes with the stress. That is how she can control the anxiety. But she does miss some pretty good parties.

The significance of choosing between pharmacotherapy and psychotherapy for the treatment of social anxiety was apparent from the time that the utility of MAO-inhibiting drugs began to be studied in clinical trials in the 1990s (Blanco et al., 2012), because the use of a drug such as phenelzine requires the patient to adhere to a diet that eliminates foods containing tyramine. The need to avoid ingesting tyramine when ingesting a MAO-inhibiting drug is a serious inconvenience that, if not sustained, can result in hypertensive crisis and death. The very thought of that potential scenario is itself anxiety provoking, providing good reason for not adhering to the medication regimen, for preferring a different medication, or for preferring psychotherapy instead of medication. Therefore, despite the demonstrated effectiveness of an MAO inhibitor such as phenelzine, a social anxiety patient and that patient's therapist likely would be looking for a better alternative.

The better alternative pharmacotherapy is now known to include a number of the SSRI drugs—fluvoxamine, paroxetine, sertraline, fluoxetine, and escitalopram (Blanco, Bragdon, Schneier, & Liebowitz, 2013). The SSRIs (or the SNRI venlafaxine) are considered to be the first-line pharmacotherapy option because clinical trials have demonstrated that SSRIs are effective for treating social anxiety disorder, patients tolerate SSRIs better than most other drugs that are also effective, and SSRIs are relatively effective for treating the symptoms of social anxiety disorder together with comorbid conditions that are common, including major depression and other anxiety disorders

(Blanco et al., 2013). Although benzodiazepine drugs are considered to be equally effective to the SSRIs, the potential for addiction presented by the benzodiazepines seriously diminishes their appeal, especially for those patients who present social anxiety with a comorbid substance use disorder.

Any enthusiasm for the utility of SSRIs to treat social anxiety disorder cannot dismiss the fact that CBT is considered to be equally useful as a first-line therapeutic option (Blanco et al., 2013; Fedoroff & Taylor, 2001). Moreover, CBT has been examined for its effectiveness when combined with pharmacotherapy to treat social anxiety: Combined CBT plus the MAO inhibitor phenelzine can be more effective than either phenelzine alone or CBT alone (Blanco et al., 2010), whereas earlier studies of CBT combined with other drugs have shown no greater benefit than monotherapy (Aaronson, Katzman, & Gorman, 2007).

Where do these various facts leave the patient facing choices regarding options for individualized evidence-based treatment for social anxiety disorder? The first-line pharmacotherapy offered probably should be an SSRI or the SNRI venlafaxine. But if a patient asks which drug treatment would benefit most from being combined with a nondrug therapy, the advice based on published evidence might be to combine CBT with phenelzine, not an SSRI or venlafaxine. But once the patient learns the dietary restriction required of phenelzine medication, the phenelzine plus behavioral therapy option would appear less attractive. The clinician then might offer the knowledge that newer, reversible MAO-inhibiting drugs do not require the tyramine dietary restraint but that those drugs appear not to be as effective as phenelzine and there is no evidence for their additional benefit when combined with behavioral therapy. At that point, the original recommendation of an SSRI or venlafaxine would begin to look like a better idea, and the patient would likely be advised to also consider CBT as an adjunctive therapy. A different patient might be more willing to commit to the demands of the combination of phenelzine plus CBT. The treatment program that will work best may be the one that the patient is best prepared to accept and to endure.

AM I CONFIDENT THAT I AM RECEIVING THE BEST TREATMENT FOR MY PTSD?

(Clients Should Be Active Participants in Their Own Pharmacotherapy.)

Eileen is plagued by the nightmares, and further exhausted by the fitful sleep and inadequate rest. She is difficult to live with when her mood and demeanor are so affected by being tired, and when she is so frequently reminded of the trauma experienced during much of her six months on duty overseas. Something has to be done if her marriage is to survive—for that matter, if she is to survive.

The SSRIs sertraline and paroxetine and the SNRI venlafaxine have replaced tricyclic antidepressants and MAO inhibitors as recommended first-line medications for PTSD (Davidson et al., 2009; Ipser & Stein, 2012). Despite this fact, the off-label use of benzodiazepine drugs to treat PTSD in war veterans had become increasingly common (Hawkins, Malte, Imel, Saxon, & Kivlahan, 2012) over the past decade (2003–2008). Although this somewhat undeserved popularity has begun to decline as the use of SSRIs and SNRIs has increased (Bernardy, Lund, Alexander, & Friedman, 2012), benzodiazepines continue to be prescribed off-label for approximately 30% of war veterans diagnosed with PTSD (Lund, Bernardy, Alexander, & Friedman, 2012). Thus, the relatively recent patterns of use of medications for PTSD does not appear to adequately comply with treatment guidelines (Bandelow et al., 2012; Jeffreys, Capehart, & Friedman, 2012; Stein, Ipser, & McAnda, 2009).

Can a patient with PTSD be confident that the recommended medication represents the best evidence-based treatment that can be had? The patient seeking reassurance on this point should be able to gain it through conversations with the prescribing clinician. Those conversations can benefit the patient in multiple ways, including increased understanding about the patient's situation; greater appreciation that patients are contributing partners in decisions about their treatment; increased confidence that the treatment is based on sound evidence; and additional resolve to make the sacrifices necessary to give the treatment program a reasonable chance to be successful. The therapist also stands to gain from those conversations and the patient's questioning, because the conversation is likely to provide the therapist with additional information that can instill confidence that the correct diagnosis has been made, that the appropriate treatment is being offered, and whether or not the patient is faithfully following recommendations. Toward those ends, here are questions the patient with PTSD might ask regarding pharmacotherapy (or that clinicians might ask of themselves), followed by reasonably appropriate answers (in italics):

- Based on the scientific evidence, which medications for PTSD are most likely to be helpful and least likely to be harmful? *The SSRIs paroxetine and sertraline and the SNRI venlafaxine.*
- What will those drugs do to my brain? *They should increase the availability of the neurotransmitter serotonin, and to a lesser extent they should increase the availability of the neurotransmitter norepinephrine.*

- Based on the scientific evidence, how long should I continue taking one of those drugs? *In the interests of experiencing a maximum improvement in symptoms, and preventing relapse, you should maintain recommended use of your medication for at least one year* (Ipser & Stein, 2012).

- Will I experience side effects when using one of those drugs? *As for any drug, yes, you will experience side effects. We might be able to predict what some of those could be. Let's have a conversation about potential side effects, so that you can tell me which ones might be difficult for you to tolerate. That conversation will help me to recommend a medication for you that you would more likely find to be helpful and tolerable.*

- I can tell you now that I won't tolerate any sexual dysfunction as a side effect, so what can we do if that begins to happen to me? *We can switch you to a different medication and hope for the best.*

- Exactly how might drug therapy help me? *Well, ideally a medication will help to alleviate all of your symptoms. And some of those symptoms you are now experiencing—your difficulty concentrating, memory problems, wishing to avoid others, irritability—may actually be making it more difficult for you to benefit from our conversations or from psychotherapy. A medication that diminishes some of those symptoms could help to maximize the benefit you receive from counseling or psychotherapy* (Jeffreys et al., 2012).

- If the drug that you recommend does not help me, are there other options for medication? *Yes, there are several other drugs that we could try, but none of the other drugs have scientific evidence that supports their use for the treatment of PTSD. That means that those drugs are somewhat less likely to be helpful than are the SSRIs or venlafaxine.*

- A friend who has PTSD is using a benzodiazepine drug. Why not prescribe a benzodiazepine for me? *For two reasons: There is no scientific evidence that a benzodiazepine will improve symptoms of PTSD, and benzodiazepine drugs are addictive.*

- You say it is fortunate that I don't have a comorbid condition. If I did develop something, what would we do about that? *Here are two examples: If it were comorbid depression, the SSRI or SNRI medication would be helpful for both the PTSD and the depression. If you were having nightmares, we could add the alpha-1 adrenergic antagonist prazosin to your prescribed medication* (Jeffreys et al., 2012).

- Are there any talk therapies that might help me? *Yes. At the very least you and I will be talking about how you are feeling as the weeks progress. And I will give you advice regarding how to better cope with some of the troubling symptoms that you are experiencing and how to lesson the impact of the daily reminders of the trauma you experienced. We will also talk about how you are feeling about the drug therapy.*

- Is there a more formal, structured psychotherapy that could help me? *Well, there is some evidence that trauma-focused cognitive behavioral therapy can be beneficial* (Shalev, 2009), *but very little is known about the effectiveness of other methods of psychotherapy for PTSD. In fact, for combat-related PTSD there is evidence that medication is more effective than a variety of methods of behavior therapy* (Stewart & Wrobel, 2009).

- Will I get better? *Let's hope so. Approximately half of patients treated for PTSD get better. You and I together will do everything we can to make it happen.*

In summary, the recommended options for pharmacotherapy and for psychotherapy for evidence-based treatment for PTSD are relatively fewer than for other anxiety disorders. This is unfortunate given the enduring nature of PTSD, the negative impact that the relatively unremitting disorder has on patients and their families, and the increased likelihood of comorbidity for depression, other anxiety disorders, and substance use disorders (Ipser & Stein, 2012). Taken together, these factors serve to emphasize the significance of an open, trusting relationship between client and clinician in which they can learn from one another as collaborators working toward the goal of creating a successful individualized treatment program.

WHERE CAN I LEARN MORE ABOUT OCD TO BECOME A MORE SUCCESSFUL PATIENT?

(There Are Sources of Trustworthy Advice.)

Rhonda seems to be spending half of her life wearing rubber gloves. She can hardly reach for the box of rubber gloves without first putting on a pair of rubber gloves. But she has learned that wearing the gloves is a better problem than the need to wash her hands dozens or a hundred times per day.

Things have gotten a bit better recently. The medication appears to have taken some of the edge off of her anxiety, saving her the cost of a few pairs of gloves each day. But she knows she is not living a normal life, and realizing that is beginning to make her feel depressed.

Obsessive-compulsive disorder was considered virtually untreatable until the 1960s when clomipramine began to be used to medicate for the disorder. Since then clomipramine has slipped slightly to become the second-line medication for OCD, replaced by the SSRI drugs as the first-line recommended pharmacotherapy (Fineberg, Brown, Reghunandanan, & Pampaloni, 2012b). Among the SSRIs, paroxetine, sertraline, fluvoxamine, and fluoxetine have been approved by the FDA to treat OCD, and although they appear to be no more effective than clomipramine, their side effect profiles give the SSRIs a slight but meaningful advantage over clomipramine (Dougherty, Rauch, & Jenike, 2007).

In addition to, or in place of, pharmacotherapy, CBT is recommended as a first-line therapy for OCD (Koran et al., 2007), and there is evidence that combined CBT plus medication can have greater benefit for treating OCD than medication alone (Aaronson et al., 2007; Eddy, Dutra, Bradley, & Westen, 2004; Franklin & Foa, 2007). Moreover, long-term maintenance SSRI pharmacotherapy can be effective for preventing relapse (Fineberg et al., 2012b), as can CBT (Dougherty et al., 2007).

That profile of treatments for OCD appears more optimistic than the reality of the situation, because approximately one-half of patients do not respond to SSRI medication (Fineberg et al., 2012a). Failure to respond or failure to reach full remission is a serious problem for the following reasons. First, OCD is an enduring illness with peaks for incidence of diagnosis between 12–14 and 20–22 years of age. It can exact a high cost on social effectiveness and quality of life for patients and their families. Second, although there are a variety of strategies for next-step treatments following failure to respond to first-line medication, other than clomipramine the various options for alternative or augmenting pharmacotherapy represent off-label, not evidence-based, use of medications (Fineberg et al., 2012b). Third, comorbidity is common for OCD, including major depression in two-thirds of patients, specific phobia, social anxiety disorder, eating disorder, alcohol dependence, panic disorder, Tourette syndrome, and increased likelihood of suicide (Fineberg et al., 2012a).

In addition to the problems for treatment presented by the frequency of comorbidity, many people suffering obsessions and compulsive behaviors do not seek treatment (Rasmussen & Eisen, 1990). For those not seeking treatment who do have some awareness of their issues, for those seeking treatment who are not experiencing sufficient relief of symptoms, and for families of those afflicted, resources are available to learn more about OCD. Use of these resources may encourage patients or their families to take further steps toward getting appropriate and effective therapy and may improve their ability to take an active role in the design and implementation of their treatment program. The following are examples of some of the types of useful resources:

Internet resources for trustworthy information:

- A brief online booklet for children (and their families) that can help to better understand OCD, and what they might do about it (http://www.ocdkids.org)
- A website established by an international foundation that provides a broad range of opportunities for learning about OCD for children, adolescents, parents, and teachers with links for advice, books to read, and a wide variety of other resources (http://www .ocfoundation.org)
- A site established by the Mayo Clinic that provides advice and information regarding a broad range of topics, encouraging the seeking of professional treatment (http://www.mayoclinic.com/ health/obsessive-compulsive-disorder/DS00189)
- A site within the National Institute of Mental Health website that provides information regarding a broad range of topics, encourages seeking professional guidance and treatment, and provides links to relevant pamphlets and published clinical trials
- (http://www.nimh.nih.gov/health/topics/obsessive-compulsive-disorder-ocd/index.shtml)
- The "Drugs" site within the FDA website, which provides access to recent information regarding drugs, including those used to treat OCD, including alerts, news regarding adverse effects, drug recalls, and mechanisms of action (http://www.fda.gov/Drugs/default .htm)

Books

If you search a bookseller website for "obsessive-compulsive disorder," you will pull up well over 500 titles. Here are several suggestions that have been recommended to me:

- *What to Do When Your Brain Gets Stuck: A Kid's Guide for Overcoming OCD* (Huebner, 2007).
- *Freeing Your Child From Obsessive-Compulsive Disorder: A Powerful, Practical Program for Parents of Children and Adolescents* (Chansky, 2001).

- *What to Do When Your Child Has Obsessive-Compulsive Disorder: Strategies and Solutions* (Wagner, 2002).
- *If Your Adolescent Has an Anxiety Disorder: An Essential Resource for Parents* (Foa and Wasmer Andrews, 2006).
- *Anxiety Disorders: The Go-To Guide for Clients and Therapists* (Daitch, 2011).

CAN ANIMAL MODELS TEACH US ABOUT PHARMACOTHERAPY FOR ANXIETY?

Ronnie the Rat likes to party—well, he used to, anyway, but something has changed. He has become more and more fearful of leaving his flat. He worries there will be trouble out there, although he's never run into any himself. But he reads the newspapers lining the floor of his cage and knows from them that bad things do happen. His unfounded fears have come to be so debilitating that Ronnie will not leave his flat even though the door occasionally is left ajar. He just stays in there where he feels safe, because when he does venture out his feet get clammy, his mouth gets dry, and his heart races and pounds in his chest. Ronnie is happiest when just stretched out on the floor at home, or on those days when Dr. Model drops by and gives Ronnie a dose of paroxetine. Dr. Model has told Ronnie the Rat that the paroxetine is so very useful for helping agoraphobic rats that Doc recommended that it be used to treat agoraphobic humans.

Animal models for anxiety must span a heterogeneous group of disorders that likely have a variety of causes and neurochemical and behavioral abnormalities. Many of the animal models for anxiety measure behaviors in situations created to instill fear or anxiety in an animal, but most of these models cannot claim to model one specific type of anxiety disorder—that is, a model that can completely and decisively discriminate among different anxiety disorders (Sullivan, Debiec, Bush, Lyons, & LeDoux, 2009). Examples of useful animal models for anxiety include the following.

Behavioral assessments of situation-induced anxiety:
- Operant conflict test in which a rat has learned that performing a lever press can bring reward but that the reward sometimes is accompanied by punishment
- Social interaction with an unfamiliar animal of the same species
- Measuring the latency to initiate eating or the amount eaten in a potentially threatening situation

- Elevated plus maze in which a rodent can choose to spend time in an open, well-lit area or in a darkened, enclosed area presumed to be more safe
- Open field test in which the rodent can spend more or less time in relatively more safe places (e.g., adjacent to a wall) or can exhibit more or less exploration as measured by movement and rearing on its hind legs
- Hole board test in which the rodent puts its nose at risk by poking it into holes in the floor
- Defensive burying, a rodent's reaction to an object that appears to be threatening
- Ultrasonic distress calls emitted by infant rodents when separated from their mothers
- Conditioned fear test that measures the tendency of an animal to freeze in an aversive environment

Models of OCD:
- Naturally occurring (ethological) models, including alopecia in cats, feather picking in birds, cribbing in horses, schedule-induced polydipsia in rats, and food-deprivation-induced hyperactivity
- Drug-induced models, for example, quinpirole-induced compulsive checking, and neonatal clomipramine-induced perseveration, hoarding, impaired memory, and abnormalities in elevated plus maze and marble burying (Andersen, Greene-Colozzi, & Sonntag, 2010)
- Stop-signal reaction time (SSRT) test, requiring inhibiting a pre-potent motor response
- Genetic mutant mouse models

These examples of animal models for anxiety (Cryan & Sweeney, 2011; Haller & Alicki, 2012; Sullivan et al., 2009) and for OCD (Albelda & Joel, 2012; Fineberg et al., 2011) have been validated by demonstrating that drugs with known clinical utility for diminishing anxiety can produce the predicted effects on behaviors in animals. But these models have demonstrated only limited predictive value for development of new drugs for treatment of anxiety. Here are examples of the use of animal models for anxiety:

- The SSRI fluvoxamine, the tricyclic drug clomipramine, and the novel tachykinin NK-1 receptor antagonist RP67580 each produce dose-related inhibition of marble burying in mice (Millan, Girardon, Mullot, Brocco, & Dekeyne, 2002).

- Pregabalin induces dose-related anxiolytic effects in rats tested in a social conflict test and in an elevated X-maze (Field, Oles, & Singh, 2001).
- Agomelatine induces anxiolytic effects in rats in three test conditions: an operant conflict test, an elevated plus maze, and a conditioned ultrasonic vocalization test (Papp, Litwa, Gruca, & Mocaer, 2006).
- The SNRIs milnacipran and venlafaxine and the benzodiazepines diazepam and chlordiazepoxide produce anxiolytic effects on performance of mice in an elevated plus maze, whereas the SSRIs paroxetine and fluvoxamine and the tricyclics imipramine and amitriptyline do not (Takeuchi, Owa, Nishino, & Kamei, 2010).
- The tricyclic clomipramine attenuates the compulsive checking induced by quinpirole in rats (Szechtman, Sulis, & Eilam, 1998).
- Schedule-induced polydipsia in rats can be inhibited by chronic administration of the SSRIs fluoxetine or fluvoxamine or the tricyclic clomipramine, but not by the antipsychotic haloperidol or the benzodiazepine diazepam (Woods et al., 1993).

In summary, there are numerous clever ways to attempt to measure the effects of drugs on animals made anxious, and there are other animal models for anxiety disorders, including attempts to model OCD. Some of these experimental paradigms have limited predictive value for the clinical utility of drugs for treatment of anxiety in humans (Haller & Alicki, 2012), but genetic mouse models have yet to demonstrate their predictive validity (Fineberg et al., 2011).

TIDBITS ON PSYCHOPHARMACOLOGY LEARNED FROM THE TREATMENT OF ANXIETY

The following are brief examples illustrating other principles of pharmacology or recommendations from Part I of this book, taken from the clinical treatment of anxiety disorders or from basic research on anxiety:

- *No drug has only one effect.* Among the tricyclic drugs having antidepressant properties, clomipramine is relatively unique in that it inhibits the reuptake of norepinephrine and serotonin; the latter effect distinguishes clomipramine from other tricyclic drugs and presumably provides clomipramine its ability to be useful also for the treatment of OCD (Davidson et al., 2009).

- *Compromise on benefits and risks is a realistic goal for pharmacotherapy.* The benefit of SSRI drugs to diminish symptoms of OCD in children appears to outweigh the risk those drugs present for inducing suicidal ideation (Fineberg et al., 2012b).

- *Desired effects and unwanted effects are related to dosage.* The ability of SSRIs to improve symptoms of OCD and the ability of those same drugs to cause side effects are related to dosage (Fineberg et al., 2012b).

- *Drug interactions can be potent and unpredictable.* The second-generation antipsychotic risperidone effectively augments SSRI medication in obsessive-compulsive patients who have been resistant to SSRI monotherapy (Fineberg et al., 2012b).

- *Sensitivity to a drug varies from one individual to another.* The SSRI escitalopram is less effective for improving symptoms of OCD in patients who score high on the hoarding/symmetry symptom dimension of the Yale-Brown Obsessive Compulsive Scale (Fineberg et al., 2012b).

- *Sex, age, and genetics can determine the magnitude of effects of a drug.* There are reports of differences between sexes for the pharmacokinetics and pharmacodynamics of various benzodiazepine drugs (Yonkers et al., 1992).

- *A person's drug history can affect a drug's effectiveness.* Previous or current substance dependence or abuse essentially invalidates prudent use of benzodiazepine drugs to treat an anxiety disorder for that patient.

- *Culture and community can affect the utility of pharmacotherapy.* Hispanics are more likely than Caucasians to believe that medications for treating anxiety disorders will not be effective (Hunt et al., 2013).

- *Drugs can mimic endogenous neurochemicals.* Agomelatine, an agonist for MT1 and MT2 receptors for melatonin, appears to be effective for treatment of generalized anxiety disorder, and there is anecdotal evidence that it may be effective for treating other anxiety disorders (Levitan et al., 2012).

- *Drugs can block endogenous neurochemicals.* Quetiapine, an antagonist for D2 dopamine, 5HT-2 serotonin, alpha-1 noradrenergic, and H1 histamine receptors, is effective and well tolerated as monotherapy for generalized anxiety disorder (Katzman et al., 2010).

- *Pharmacological effects on brain neurochemistry can be enduring.* A variety of neuroadaptations in serotonin neurotransmission in the brain follow chronic administration of SSRIs and some tricyclic drugs (Markou, Kosten, & Koob, 1998).

- *Drugs differ in their potential for addiction.* The only class of drugs that has the potential for addiction that remains used to treat panic disorder, social anxiety disorder, or generalized anxiety disorder is the benzodiazepines.

- *Drugs can alter the organization of a developing brain.* The SSRI fluoxetine produces opposite effects (measured by magnetic resonance imaging) in the adult rat brain for rats chronically administered fluoxetine as juveniles compared with rats chronically administered fluoxetine during adulthood (Klomp et al., 2012).

- *Drugs can be demonstrated to be only relatively effective and safe.* The MAO inhibitors are approved for treatment of depression and anxiety, despite the requirement to maintain a tyramine-free diet and the risk of hypertensive crisis if that requirement is violated.

- *A therapeutic drug is used because it works, and off-label use has its advantages and disadvantages.* Pregabalin is approved by the FDA for treatment of seizures, diabetic peripheral neuropathy, postherpetic neuralgia, and fibromyalgia; pregabalin has demonstrated successful off-label use for treatment of generalized anxiety disorder (Mathew, Hoffman, & Charney, 2009).

- *Dietary supplements may or may not be effective and safe.* Studies evaluating the effectiveness of St. John's wort for improving symptoms of OCD have produced mixed results (Davidson et al., 2009). In contrast, omega-3 fatty acids appear to reduce anxiety in medical students who do *not* yet have a diagnosed anxiety disorder (Kiecolt-Glaser, Belury, Andridge, Malarkey, & Glaser, 2011).

- *Placebo can have drug-like effects.* Placebo has very little effect on symptoms of OCD in clinical trials (Mavissakalian, Jones, & Olson, 1990), unlike the appreciable effect of placebo on symptoms of other categories of anxiety disorders (Mathew et al., 2009).

- *Pharmacotherapy is best used as one among several tools.* Combined CBT plus the SSRI sertraline for 12 weeks can produce better improvement than either monotherapy alone in children (7–17 years of age) diagnosed with separation anxiety, generalized anxiety disorder, or social anxiety disorder (Walkup et al., 2008).

- *Serendipity can bring new opportunities for pharmacotherapy.* Finding that clomipramine was the only tricyclic antidepressant to have appreciable anxiolytic properties eventually led to the understanding that clomipramine was the only tricyclic to have considerable potency for inhibiting the reuptake of serotonin, and eventually also led to considering that the SSRIs might have anxiolytic properties.

- *Consumers demand new and better drugs, and the FDA attempts to approve new and better drugs.* The MAO-inhibiting drugs have had the disadvantage of requiring the patient to maintain a diet free of tyramine. The more recent reversible MAO-inhibiting drugs do not require the elimination of tyramine from the diet, but unfortunately these drugs are less effective than the older, irreversible MAO inhibitors. The FDA has not approved the newer, safer, but less effective reversible MAO inhibitors (Mathew et al., 2009).

- *Successful use encourages increased use, for better or worse.* The use of benzodiazepine drugs to treat PTSD in war veterans increased from 2003 to 2010, despite guidelines recommending against their use. This apparent inappropriate increase in use may be attributable to the recognized ability of benzodiazepines to rapidly relieve anxiety in extremely stressful situations (Hawkins et al., 2012).

- *Health insurance practices can determine accessibility to a drug.* As for any diagnosed psychiatric condition, the cost of a psychotropic medication being used off-label to treat anxiety is less likely to be fully supported by a third-party payer (Frank et al, 2005).

SUMMARY AND PERSPECTIVE

Anxiety disorders are a diverse collection of disabling and enduring disorders that are known to respond to pharmacotherapy when SSRI drugs are used as first-line medications. This does not mean that the use of psychotropic medications to treat anxiety disorders has reached its pinnacle, for several reasons. First, many who suffer an anxiety disorder do not improve in response to SSRIs (or other medications). Second, despite the hypothesis that SSRIs diminish anxiety because SSRIs (and SNRIs and clomipramine) enhance serotonin neurotransmission, the mechanism by which these drugs relieve symptoms has not been definitively demonstrated. Third, some patients respond favorably to drugs that do not demonstrably alter serotonin neurotransmission, raising the possibility that various categories of anxiety disorders, or component symptoms of a specific disorder, may result from nonserotonergic pathophysiology. That possibility continues to fuel the development of novel medications for anxiety. Fourth, the fact that not all patients who receive the same specific diagnosis respond favorably to the same psychotropic medication reveals that the diagnostic categories of anxiety disorders are somewhat rudimentary and can be improved through continued study and reformulation.

The diagnosis of a specific anxiety disorder (or any other psychiatric condition) is merely the formulation of a hypothesis that can guide the selection of treatment options. Those options will continue to include psychotherapy as well as pharmacotherapy, because there is no evidence that medication alone (i.e., doing *nothing* more than ingesting medication) can achieve complete and enduring remission of anxiety in all patients. The selection of drug and talk treatments among the evidence-based and the off-label options will achieve the greatest success when well-informed clients and clinicians effectively collaborate while constructing and executing an individualized treatment program.

Ten Continuing Challenges
to Getting It Right

When he walked out of my office just now, I felt that what I had just told him was a bit of a fabrication. I had just written the fourth different prescription for a medication to treat his major depression, without having any confidence that this drug would help him. The first three drugs we tried did not lift his depression. Why would I be confident that the next drug would work? This was the first time that I thought, If I cannot be confident that my best advice will be helpful, maybe I should be in a different business.

Or was I simply making some mistakes? Had I been too hasty in making a diagnosis? Did I miss a comorbid condition? If there is comorbidity, it might have guided me toward different ideas for treatment. Is my patient not telling me everything I should know about his situation? If he were more candid, would I learn something useful for thinking about his diagnosis and treatment? Should we move more slowly, be more deliberate, more patient—have longer conversations, more seriously consider electroconvulsive therapy for sooner rather than for later, wait longer for a positive effect of medication?

Or is it the way we clinicians tend to do our business of treating for psychopathology that is the problem? I've had success using psychotropic medications to treat most of my patients, but now I'm thinking maybe we know less than we think we know about

the brain and about what drugs are doing to the brain. Are we leaning too heavily on psychopharmacology? Are we simply overly confident that we can offer successful treatment?

Serious challenges will continue to confront clinicians and patients, making it difficult to be confident that psychotropic medications are being used judiciously to treat psychopathology.

THE CHALLENGE OF DIAGNOSIS

Making an appropriate diagnosis is the first challenge facing the effective use of psychotropic medication to treat psychopathology. Establishing diagnosis is an imperfect endeavor: It represents the formulation of a hypothesis based on limited data, clinical experience, generalizations, and educated guesswork. But a diagnosis is necessary to provide a guide toward specific options that are generally considered suitable treatment for a particular disorder. Therefore, it would be best if we got the diagnosis right.

The determination of diagnosis for decades has relied on the *Diagnostic and Statistical Manual of Mental Disorders* (or similar handbooks) to establish criteria for diagnostic categories—criteria that have been based principally on behavioral symptoms. This heavy reliance on behavioral data incited criticism of the most recent revision of the manual (i.e., *DSM-5*) many months before its date of publication. One important criticism is that criteria for diagnosis ideally should consider pathophysiology, genetic features, and perhaps etiology, as well as behavior. That is a very nice idea, but it is premature. This is because, despite advances made in behavioral neuroscience for understanding the functional organization of the human brain, too much remains unknown about the causes of psychopathology and the pathophysiology supporting behavioral symptoms. It is simply not yet possible to meaningfully incorporate sufficient information on genetics, etiology, and pathophysiology, together with behavioral symptoms, to enable reconsideration and significant revision of diagnostic categories and subcategories of psychopathology. That revision is necessary work, but it requires more knowledge about the relation of brain and genetics to behavior for that work to get done properly.

For the time being, we will continue to rely principally on behavioral symptoms for establishing diagnosis—an approach that will continue to inadequately dissociate subcategories of illness, contributing to familiar difficulties for predicting effectiveness of psychotropic medications. This inadequacy for determining diagnoses ultimately will be resolved by further advances in behavioral neuroscience and behavioral genetics that eventually can support the development of a transformed *DSM*.

THE CHALLENGE OF IGNORANCE

Ignorance hinders the judicious use of psychotropic medications in several ways. First, our limited understanding of the relation between neurochemistry of the brain and behavior is a problem. Not knowing enough about how the normal brain organizes normal behavior and about how the abnormal brain organizes psychopathology hinders the development of animal models that are more valid and useful than current models, stunting the ability to improve upon current medications and to create new drugs that constitute novel tactics for pharmacotherapy. Further advances in behavioral neuroscience will alleviate this problem.

Second, limited knowledge about principles of pharmacology hampers the ability of clinicians and patients to work together toward the best use of psychotropic medications. As long as it is possible for a clinician to be cavalier about the disadvantages of off-label prescribing, polypharmacy, or failure to consider nondrug therapy, and as long as a patient is comfortable being unaware of the benefits and risks of the recommended psychotropic medication, ignorance about pharmacology can jeopardize the effectiveness of treatment. Gaining an appreciation for general principles of psychopharmacology can address that problem.

THE CHALLENGE OF MOMENTUM

Experiencing success despite not really knowing what you are doing is risky business. Successful use of psychotropic medications, despite limited knowledge about principles of psychopharmacology, has created misplaced confidence in the effectiveness of psychotropic medications. This overconfidence, this extraordinary trust in the utility and safety of psychotropic medications, contributes to the increasing use of such drugs, accompanied by the trend for decreasing use of methods of psychotherapy.

This extraordinary trust in drugs is inconsistent with some facts about the evolution of psychopharmacology. For one, although new drugs and new pharmacotherapeutic tactics have appeared consistently over the past five decades, the fact remains that considerable proportions of patients treated for psychopathology do not respond favorably to psychotropic medication; this is certainly the case for treatment of schizophrenia, depression, bipolar disorder, anorexia nervosa, bulimia nervosa, drug addiction, and various anxiety disorders. In addition, the newer drugs have generally improved upon the older drugs *not* by being more potent for having a main effect but, rather, by having fewer side effects. Although it is a good thing that newer drugs may be more tolerable, it would be an even better thing if the newer drugs were also more effective while being more tolerable. Those better newer drugs may be more slowly discovered and developed, however, when perception of the successful use of psychotropic medications is so sunny that it encourages a complacency that retards the expensive efforts required for drug development.

Extraordinary trust in the effectiveness and safety of psychotropic drugs also can create new problems, such as neuroenhancement—that is, the use of psychotropic drugs or dietary supplements to alter the brain in a manner that enhances cognitive performance or mood (Schermer, Bolt, de Jongh, & Olivier, 2009). This use of psychotropic drugs blurs the line between medicating to correct dysfunction for diagnosed psychopathology and doping to improve functioning in healthy adults and children. If and when neuroenhancement becomes the norm, we will be "medicating" both the dysfunctional and the fully functional. The arrival of that day would confirm a misplaced faith in drugs.

THE CHALLENGE OF OFF-LABEL USAGE

Off-label use of psychotropic medication is a good option gone out of control. The increasing off-label treatment for many diagnosed psychological disorders, including the apparent increased level of acceptance of off-label treatment for children and adolescents, has become a problem that can be ameliorated by greater effort to conduct clinical drug trials in children, adolescents, and adults. Reasons for not conducting this research are predominantly excuses indicating acceptance of the use of therapies that are not supported by scientific evidence. The less we demand that scientific evidence supports the use of therapeutic options, the closer we get to using any therapeutic method that appears to be a good idea based on intuition or clinical experience. That would be a move away from evidence-based therapy toward therapy based on dogma or, worse, fashion.

THE CHALLENGE OF NARROW PERSPECTIVE

The proper role for psychotropic medication is to contribute to the success of multifaceted approaches to treat psychopathology. It is reasonable to consider all instances of psychopathology as representing the unhealthy product of brain, behavior, and social context—that is, as biopsychosocial problems. Therefore, to enhance or support the effectiveness of a medication, it should be combined with nondrug therapeutic methods that facilitate changes in behavior and social context that are important components of the diagnosed condition. Those combinations of therapeutic drug and talk methods should be chosen based on scientific investigations evaluating the effectiveness of various combinations of therapeutic methods. There are too few of those studies. They are difficult and expensive to conduct, but there is no suitable substitute for data that address the question of a treatment's effectiveness.

THE CHALLENGE OF INDIVIDUALIZED TREATMENT

Patients bring unique characteristics related to their age, gender, genetics, ethnicity, history of drug use, socioeconomic status, history of diagnosis and treatment, goals for treatment, biases, and commitment for a treatment program. It is reasonable to expect that a multifaceted treatment program—including the choice of psychotropic medication or nondrug therapy—should be tailored to a patient's genetic and physiological distinctiveness and individual needs and expectations. But the successful construction of an individualized treatment program can be opposed by some factors external to the patient.

One such factor is the published literature reporting the results of clinical drug trials. Results from published trials report the average response to treatments. But the majority of patients are not the average patient, making it difficult to predict from the results of clinical trials whether or how an individual patient will respond to the treatment studied in the trial. Moreover, the results of clinical trials typically report whether or not a drug treatment can produce a statistically significant improvement on several select measures for a group of patients. The treatment that produces a statistically significant improvement in a carefully conducted clinical trial will not necessarily produce a meaningful improvement in the quality of life of an individual patient. These problems to some extent can be addressed by conducting clinical trials of extended duration and by analysis of dependent variables that assesses for clinically meaningful change.

A second factor is the constraint that can be imposed upon a treatment program by policies for insurance coverage or managed care. Those policies are not constructed with the unique individual patient in mind. Those policies are established more in keeping with published results and statistics regarding costs and outcomes (i.e., cost-effectiveness) for groups of patients and therefore may not represent what is in the best interests of an individual patient presenting a unique set of characteristics and circumstances.

Those policies can conspire to limit the choices of treatments when the policies have an impact on decisions regarding which drug to choose, whether or not to combine drug therapy with behavior therapy or psychotherapy, the duration of treatments, the number of follow-up visits to assess for progress or problems, and the proportion of the costs of those treatments assigned to the patient and to the third party. Those decisions can hinder the ability of clinician and client to assemble an individualized treatment program that fully provides for the best interests of the patient. These challenges will be difficult to overcome if cost-effectiveness is a higher priority than is treatment outcome.

THE CHALLENGE OF DEVELOPMENT OF NEW INTRUDER CHEMICALS

The very *idea* of psychotropic medication presents a continuing challenge. A psychotropic drug is an unwelcome intruder chemical introduced into the brain by well-intentioned and somewhat overly eager people. Is that a good idea or a bad idea? It is both.

Psychotropic medication is a good idea because when something needs to be done, taking a drug is doing something that may be effective. It is a good idea also because in many instances there is scientific evidence that the medication can help.

Psychotropic medication is also a bad idea because there are always side effects, and no patient ever asks to have those. It is also a bad idea because a medication can induce enduring effects on the brain and may alter the development of a maturing brain of a child or adolescent, which are considerable prices to pay for a medication that offers, at best, an incomplete solution to a biopsychosocial problem.

The fact that we accept the bad with the good when using psychotropic medications indicates the extent to which such drugs are indeed helpful and also the extent to which we can at times be desperate to find ways to help. Maximizing the good while minimizing the bad consequences of psychotropic medication will depend on vigilance regarding judicious use and on the development of newer, better drugs.

But helpful chemicals are intrusive to a brain that is not designed to comfortably accept the challenge of being chemically probed. Helpful chemicals also produce adverse effects, and we therefore can reasonably expect them to be replaced one day by better chemicals. The development of those better chemicals will be facilitated by a variety of newer rational approaches to drug development that take advantage of recent technological advances in genomics, molecular biology, and informatics and of collaborative partnerships among the biotechnology, academic, and pharmaceutical industries (Tollefson, 2009).

Regardless of the methods used to design and develop newer psychotropic medications, those new drugs remain substances exogenous to the brain and body. They may be improved invasive substances, and by some measure more brain-friendly, but they will continue to be intruders bringing benefits and risks.

THE CHALLENGE OF ANIMAL MODELS

The development of new psychotropic medications will continue to require the use of animal models, because psychopathology is only evident through human behavior, and human behavior is most reasonably modeled in living organisms that behave. But the development of animal models for psychopathology must break free of the constraint imposed by the influence of the *DSM*: As long as descriptions of psychopathology in the *DSM* are characterized principally by behavioral symptoms, there will be the expectation that an animal model principally models behaviors (and not underlying pathophysiology) that resemble symptoms of the particular human malady. Therefore, the inadequacies of the *DSM* sustain the limitations of animal models, often failing to incorporate pathophysiology and failing to adequately discriminate among subcategories of psychopathology. This can be resolved as research in behavioral neuroscience produces sufficient knowledge of the relation between brain and behavior to contribute to a transformative revision of the *DSM*, which then will better guide the creation of new animal models. Those newer animal models should improve upon the use of models to search for new drugs that have the same or similar mechanisms of action as current effective psychotropic medications, and they should enhance the ability to develop novel pharmacotherapies.

THE CHALLENGE OF PREVENTING RELAPSE

Keeping a chemical intruder in a brain for an extended visit is not an ideal situation, but removing a drug prematurely can increase the likelihood of relapse. Not enough is known from the results of clinical trials to know how to maximize the use of psychotropic medication together with nondrug therapy in the prevention of relapse. This is because most clinical trials are limited in duration and therefore evaluate the effectiveness of a psychotropic medication principally for its short-term effects on relief of symptoms and its short-term ability to produce partial or complete remission. More research is needed to determine the ideal ways to use psychotropic medications in long-term treatment programs, including programs that combine drug and talk therapies and programs that combine multiple medications. Such studies also need to determine which nondrug therapies maximize prevention of relapse once pharmacotherapy is discontinued.

THE CHALLENGE OF ANY TOOL

Psychotropic medications are powerful chemical tools that we are fortunate to have in hand to facilitate treatment of psychopathology. As for any powerful tool, psychotropic medications need to be understood for their strengths and their limitations, and they need to be used prudently such that they help more than they harm. Judicious use requires working knowledge of fundamental principles of psychopharmacology, the wisdom and humility to use the tool properly to achieve realistic expectations for success, and the patience to tailor the use of the treatment tool to the unique characteristics of each patient's situation.

THIS BOOK REDUCED TO A SENTENCE

After making an appropriate diagnosis, use published evidence and clinical experience to choose a medication carefully and to maximize its effectiveness when used with supportive behavior therapy or psychotherapy, while respecting the unique physiological, personal, social, and cultural characteristics of the individual patient, with the goal of achieving a sustained full remission of symptoms accompanied by risks that are tolerable to the patient.

Appendix: Table of Generic and Trade Names

GENERIC	TRADE	GENERIC	TRADE
acamprosate	Campral	imipramine	Tofranil
agomelatine	Valdoxan	iproniazid	Marsilid
alprazolam	Xanax	ketamine	Ketanest
amitriptyline	Elavil	lamotrigine	Lamictal
amphetamine	Adderal	lisdexamfetamine	Vyvanse
aripiprazole	Abilify	lithium carbonate	Eskalith
atomoxetine	Strattera	lorazepam	Ativan
baclofen	Kemstro	lorcaserin	Belviq
bavisant	—	mecamylamine	Inversine
buprenorphine	Subutex	mephedrone	—
bupropion	Wellbutrin	meprobamate	Miltown
buspirone	Buspar	methadone	Dolophine
chlordiazepoxide	Librium	methamphetamine	Desoxyn
chlorpromazine	Thorazine	methylphenidate	Ritalin
citalopram	Celexa	metreleptin	—
clomipramine	Anafranil	milnacipran	Savella
clonidine	Catapres	mirtazapine	Remeron
clozapine	Clozaril	moclobemide	Aurorix
desipramine	Norpramin	modafinil	Provigil
dexfenfluramine	Redux	morphine	Avinza
diazepam	Valium	nalmefene	Revex
disulfiram	Antabuse	naloxone	Narcan
ephedrine	Ephedra	naltrexone	Revia
escitalopram	Lexapro	nicotine	Nicoderm
fenfluramine	Podimin	nortriptyline	Pamelor
fluoxetine	Prozac	ondansetron	Zofran
flurazepam	Dalmane	olanzapine	Zyprexa
fluvoxamine	Luvox	orlistat	Xenical
guanfacine	Tenex	oxycodone	Oxycontin
haloperidol	Haldol	paroxetine	Paxil
hydrocodone	Vicodin	phencyclidine	Sernyl

GENERIC	TRADE	GENERIC	TRADE
phenelzine	Nardil	sertraline	Zoloft
phentermine	Adipex-P	sibutramine	Meridia
phenylpropanolamine	Accutrim	St. John's wort	—
pramlintide	Symlin	tesofensine	—
prazosin	Minipress	theophylline	Theolair
pregabalin	Lyrica	thionisoxetine	—
propranolol	Inderal	tiagabine	Gabitril
quetiapine	Seroquel	topiramate	Topamax
quinpirole	—	valproate	Depakote
raclopride	—	varenicline	Chantix
reboxetine	Edronax	venlafaxine	Effexor
rimonabant	Accomplia	vigabatrin	Sabril
risperidone	Risperdal	vilazodone	Viibryd
SAMe	—	zonisamide	Zonegran
selegiline	Emsam		

Note: Generic names of drugs are used throughout this book. This table provides what is likely to be the best-known trade name for each drug. An Internet search will provide alternative trade names for many of these drugs. —, no trade name.

References

Aaronson, C. J., Katzman, G. P., & Gorman, J. M. (2007). Combination pharmacotherapy and psychotherapy for the treatment of major depressive and anxiety disorders. In P. E. Nathan & J. M. Gorman (Eds.), *A guide to treatments that work* (3rd ed., pp. 681–710). New York, NY: Oxford University Press.

Abel, K. M., Drake, R., & Goldstein, J. M. (2010). Sex differences in schizophrenia. *International Review of Psychiatry, 22*(5), 417–428.

Abenhaim, L., Moride, Y., Brenot, F., Rich, S., Benichou, J., Kurz, X., . . . Begaud, B. (1996). Appetite-suppressant drugs and the risk of primary pulmonary hypertension. International Primary Pulmonary Hypertension Study Group. *New England Journal of Medicine, 335*(9), 609–616.

Adan, R. A. (2013). Mechanisms underlying current and future anti-obesity drugs. *Trends in Neurosciences, 36*(2), 133–140.

Addolorato, G., Caputo, F., Capristo, E., Domenicali, M., Bernardi, M., Janiri, L., . . . Gasbarrini, G. (2002). Baclofen efficacy in reducing alcohol craving and intake: A preliminary double-blind randomized controlled study. *Alcohol and Alcoholism, 37*(5), 504–508.

Adler, R. H. (2009). Engel's biopsychosocial model is still relevant today. *Journal of Psychosomatic Research, 67*(6), 607–611.

Adriani, W., Spijker, S., Deroche-Gamonet, V., Laviola, G., Le Moal, M., Smit, A. B., & Piazza, P. V. (2003). Evidence for enhanced neurobehavioral vulnerability to nicotine during periadolescence in rats. *Journal of Neuroscience, 23*(11), 4712–4716.

Adriani, W., Zoratto, F., & Laviola, G. (2012). Brain processes in discounting: Consequences of adolescent methylphenidate exposure. *Current Topics in Behavioral Neurosciences, 9*, 113–143.

Agras, W. S., Rossiter, E. M., Arnow, B., Schneider, J. A., Telch, C. F., Raeburn, S. D., . . . Koran, L. M. (1992). Pharmacologic and cognitive-behavioral treatment for bulimia nervosa: A controlled comparison. *American Journal of Psychiatry, 149*(1), 82–87.

Ak, M., Bulut, S. D., Bozkurt, A., & Ozsahin, A. (2011). Aripiprazole augmentation of serotonin reuptake inhibitors in treatment-resistant obsessive-compulsive disorder: A 10-week open-label study. *Advances in Therapy, 28*(4), 341–348.

Akinbami, L. J., Liu, X., Pastor, P. N., & Reuben, C. A. (2011). Attention deficit hyperactivity disorder among children aged 5–17 years in the United States, 1998–2009. *NCHS Data Brief, (70)*, 1–8.

Akincigil, A., Olfson, M., Siegel, M., Zurlo, K. A., Walkup, J. T., & Crystal, S. (2012). Racial and ethnic disparities in depression care in community-dwelling elderly in the United States. *American Journal of Public Health, 102*(2), 319–328.

Albelda, N., & Joel, D. (2012). Current animal models of obsessive compulsive disorder: An update. *Neuroscience, 211*, 83–106.

Ally, G. A. (2010). Nuts and bolts of prescriptive practice. In R. E. McGrath & B. A. Moore (Eds.), *Pharmacotherapy for psychologists: Prescribing and collaborative roles* (pp. 71–87). Washington, DC: American Psychological Association.

Alvarez, A. S., Pagani, M., & Meucci, P. (2012). The clinical application of the biopsychosocial model in mental health: A research critique. *American Journal of Physical Medicine and Rehabilitation, 91*(13 Suppl. 1), S173–S180.

Ampadu, E. (2011). The impact of immigration on the development of adolescent schizophrenia. *Journal of Child and Adolescent Psychiatric Nursing, 24*(3), 161–167.

Andersen, S. L. (2003). Trajectories of brain development: Point of vulnerability or window of opportunity? *Neuroscience and Biobehavioral Reviews, 27*(1–2), 3–18.

Andersen, S. L., Greene-Colozzi, E. A., & Sonntag, K. C. (2010). A novel, multiple symptom model of obsessive-compulsive-like behaviors in animals. *Biological Psychiatry, 68*(8), 741–747.

Andersen, S. L., & Navalta, C. P. (2004). Altering the course of neurodevelopment: A framework for understanding the enduring effects of psychotropic drugs. *International Journal of Developmental Neuroscience, 22*(5–6), 423–440.

Aparasu, R. R., & Bhatara, V. (2007). Patterns and determinants of antipsychotic prescribing in children and adolescents, 2003–2004. *Current Medical Research and Opinion, 23*(1), 49–56.

Aparasu, R. R., Mort, J. R., & Sitzman, S. (1998). Psychotropic prescribing for the elderly in office-based practice. *Clinical Therapeutics, 20*(3), 603–616.

Austvoll-Dahlgren, A., Aaserud, M., Vist, G., Ramsay, C., Oxman, A. D., Sturm, H., . . . Vernby, A. (2008). Pharmaceutical policies: Effects of cap and co-payment on rational drug use. *Cochrane Database of Systematic Reviews,* (1):CD007017.

Azorin, J. M., Bowden, C. L., Garay, R. P., Perugi, G., Vieta, E., & Young, A. H. (2010). Possible new ways in the pharmacological treatment of bipolar disorder and comorbid alcoholism. *Neuropsychiatric Disease and Treatment, 6*, 37–46.

Badiani, A., & Robinson, T. E. (2004). Drug-induced neurobehavioral plasticity: The role of environmental context. *Behavioural Pharmacology, 15*(5–6), 327–339.

Bai, B., & Wang, Y. (2010). The use of lorcaserin in the management of obesity: A critical appraisal. *Drug Design, Development and Therapy, 5*, 1–7.

Bakare, M. O. (2008). Effective therapeutic dosage of antipsychotic medications in patients with psychotic symptoms: Is there a racial difference? *BMC Research Notes, 1*, 25.

Baker, F. M., & Bell, C. C. (1999). Issues in the psychiatric treatment of African Americans. *Psychiatric Services, 50*(3), 362–368.

Baldwin, D. S., Waldman, S., & Allgulander, C. (2012). Evidence-based pharmacotherapy of generalized anxiety disorder. In D. J. Stein, B. Lerer, & S. M. Stahl (Eds.), *Essential evidence-based psychopharmacology* (2nd ed., pp. 110–127). New York, NY: Cambridge University Press.

Ban, T. A. (2001). Pharmacotherapy of mental illness—a historical analysis. *Progress in Neuro-psychopharmacology and Biological Psychiatry, 25*(4), 709–727.

Bandelow, B., Seidler-Brandler, U., Becker, A., Wedekind, D., & Ruther, E. (2007). Meta-analysis of randomized controlled comparisons of psychopharmacological and psychological treatments for anxiety disorders. *World Journal of Biological Psychiatry, 8*(3), 175–187.

Bandelow, B., Sher, L., Bunevicius, R., Hollander, E., Kasper, S., Zohar, J., . . . WFSBP Task Force on Anxiety Disorders, OCD and PTSD. (2012). Guidelines for the pharmacological treatment of anxiety disorders, obsessive-compulsive disorder and posttraumatic stress disorder in primary care. *International Journal of Psychiatry in Clinical Practice, 16*(2), 77–84.

Barak, Y., Shamir, E., Zemishlani, H., Mirecki, I., Toren, P., & Weizman, R. (2002). Olanzapine vs. haloperidol in the treatment of elderly chronic schizophrenia patients. *Progress in Neuro-psychopharmacology and Biological Psychiatry, 26*(6), 1199–1202.

Barrett, B., Byford, S., & Knapp, M. (2005). Evidence of cost-effective treatments for depression: A systematic review. *Journal of Affective Disorders, 84*(1), 1–13.

Bart, G. (2012). Maintenance medication for opiate addiction: The foundation of recovery. *Journal of Addictive Diseases, 31*(3), 207–225.

Batelaan, N. M., Van Balkom, A. J. L. M., & Stein, D. J. (2012). Evidence-based pharmacotherapy of panic disorder. In D. J. Stein, B. Lerer, & S. M. Stahl (Eds.), *Essential evidence-based psychopharmacology* (2nd ed., pp. 73–89). New York, NY: Cambridge University Press.

Bays, H. E. (2011). Lorcaserin: Drug profile and illustrative model of the regulatory challenges of weight-loss drug development. *Expert Review of Cardiovascular Therapy, 9*(3), 265–277.

Bazzano, A. T., Mangione-Smith, R., Schonlau, M., Suttorp, M. J., & Brook, R. H. (2009). Off-label prescribing to children in the United States outpatient setting. *Academic Pediatrics, 9*(2), 81–88.

Beauregard, M. (2009). Effect of mind on brain activity: Evidence from neuroimaging studies of psychotherapy and placebo effect. *Nordic Journal of Psychiatry, 63*(1), 5–16.

Beglinger, C., Degen, L., Matzinger, D., D'Amato, M., & Drewe, J. (2001). Loxiglumide, a CCK-A receptor antagonist, stimulates calorie intake and hunger feelings in humans. *American Journal of Physiology. Regulatory, Integrative and Comparative Physiology, 280*(4), R1149–R1154.

Beierle, I., Meibohm, B., & Derendorf, H. (1999). Gender differences in pharmacokinetics and pharmacodynamics. *International Journal of Clinical Pharmacology and Therapeutics, 37*(11), 529–547.

Beitman, B. D., Blinder, B. J., Thase, M. E., Riba, M., & Safer, D. L. (2003). *Integrating psychotherapy and pharmacotherapy: Dissolving the mind-brain barrier.* New York, NY: Norton.

Benedetti, F., Carlino, E., & Pollo, A. (2011). How placebos change the patient's brain. *Neuropsychopharmacology, 36*(1), 339–354.

Benedetti, F., Mayberg, H. S., Wager, T. D., Stohler, C. S., & Zubieta, J. K. (2005). Neurobiological mechanisms of the placebo effect. *Journal of Neuroscience, 25*(45), 10390–10402.

Benowitz, N. L. (2008). Clinical pharmacology of nicotine: Implications for understanding, preventing, and treating tobacco addiction. *Clinical Pharmacology and Therapeutics, 83*(4), 531–541.

Berk, L., Hallam, K. T., Colom, F., Vieta, E., Hasty, M., Macneil, C., & Berk, M. (2010). Enhancing medication adherence in patients with bipolar disorder. *Human Psychopharmacology, 25*(1), 1–16.

Berman, S. M., Kuczenski, R., McCracken, J. T., & London, E. D. (2009). Potential adverse effects of amphetamine treatment on brain and behavior: A review. *Molecular Psychiatry, 14*(2), 123–142.

Bernardy, N. C., Lund, B. C., Alexander, B., & Friedman, M. J. (2012). Prescribing trends in veterans with posttraumatic stress disorder. *Journal of Clinical Psychiatry, 73*(3), 297–303.

Berrendero, F., Robledo, P., Trigo, J. M., Martin-Garcia, E., & Maldonado, R. (2010). Neurobiological mechanisms involved in nicotine dependence and reward: Participation of the endogenous opioid system. *Neuroscience and Biobehavioral Reviews, 35*(2), 220–231.

Berton, O., Hahn, C. G., & Thase, M. E. (2012). Are we getting closer to valid translational models for major depression? *Science, 338*(6103), 75–79.

Buelow, G., Hebert, S., & Buelow, S. (2000). *Psychotherapist's resource on psychiatric medications: Issues of treatment and referral* (2nd ed.). Stamford, CT: Brooks/Cole.

Biederman, J., Melmed, R. D., Patel, A., McBurnett, K., Konow, J., Lyne, A., . . . SPD503 Study Group. (2008a). A randomized, double-blind, placebo-controlled study of guanfacine extended release in children and adolescents with attention-deficit/hyperactivity disorder. *Pediatrics, 121*(1), e73–e84.

Biederman, J., Monuteaux, M. C., Spencer, T., Wilens, T. E., Macpherson, H. A., & Faraone, S. V. (2008b). Stimulant therapy and risk for subsequent substance use disorders in male adults with ADHD: A naturalistic controlled 10-year follow-up study. *American Journal of Psychiatry, 165*(5), 597–603.

Biederman, J., & Spencer, T. J. (2008). Psychopharmacological interventions. *Child and Adolescent Psychiatric Clinics of North America, 17*(2), 439–458, xi.

Bies, R. R., Bigos, K. L., & Pollock, B. G. (2003). Gender differences in the pharmacokinetics and pharmacodynamics of antidepressants. *Journal of Gender-Specific Medicine, 6*(3), 12–20.

Bigos, K. L., Pollock, B. G., Coley, K. C., Miller, D. D., Marder, S. R., Aravagiri, M., . . . Bies, R. R. (2008). Sex, race, and smoking impact olanzapine exposure. *Journal of Clinical Pharmacology, 48*(2), 157–165.

Bizot, J. C., David, S., & Trovero, F. (2011). Effects of atomoxetine, desipramine, d-amphetamine and methylphenidate on impulsivity in juvenile rats, measured in a T-maze procedure. *Neuroscience Letters, 489*(1), 20–24.

Blanco, C., Bragdon, L. B., Schneier, F. R., & Liebowitz, M. R. (2012). Evidence-based pharmacotherapy of social anxiety disorder. In D. J. Stein, B. Lerer, & S. M. Stahl (Eds.), *Essential evidence-based psychopharmacology* (2nd ed., pp. 90–109). New York, NY: Cambridge University Press.

Blanco, C., Bragdon, L. B., Schneier, F. R., & Liebowitz, M. R. (2013). The evidence-based pharmacotherapy of social anxiety disorder. *International Journal of Neuropsychopharmacology, 16*(1), 235–249.

Blanco, C., Heimberg, R. G., Schneier, F. R., Fresco, D. M., Chen, H., Turk, C. L., . . . Liebowitz, M. R. (2010). A placebo-controlled trial of phenelzine, cognitive behavioral group therapy, and their combination for social anxiety disorder. *Archives of General Psychiatry, 67*(3), 286–295.

Block, D. R., Yonkers, K. A., & Carpenter, L. L. (2009). Sertraline. In A. F. Schatzberg & C. B. Nemeroff (Eds.), *Textbook of psychopharmacology* (4th ed., pp. 307–320). Washington, DC: American Psychiatric Publishing.

Blom, M. B., Jonker, K., Dusseldorp, E., Spinhoven, P., Hoencamp, E., Haffmans, J., & van Dyck, R. (2007). Combination treatment for acute depression is superior only when psychotherapy is added to medication. *Psychotherapy and Psychosomatics, 76*(5), 289–297.

Bondolfi, G., Morel, F., Crettol, S., Rachid, F., Baumann, P., & Eap, C. B. (2005). Increased clozapine plasma concentrations and side effects induced by smoking cessation in 2 CYP1A2 genotyped patients. *Therapeutic Drug Monitoring, 27*(4), 539–543.

Bottino, C. M., Barcelos-Ferreira, R., & Ribeiz, S. R. (2012). Treatment of depression in older adults. *Current Psychiatry Reports, 14*(4), 289–297.

Bouet, V., Klomp, A., Freret, T., Wylezinska-Arridge, M., Lopez-Tremoleda, J., Dauphin, F., . . . Reneman, L. (2012). Age-dependent effects of chronic fluoxetine treatment on the serotonergic system one week following treatment. *Psychopharmacology, 221*(2), 329–339.

Bowers, W. A., & Anderson, A. E. (2007). Cognitive-behavior therapy with eating disorders: The role of medications in treatment. *Journal of Cognitive Psychotherapy, 21*(1), 16–27.

Boyer, W. F., & Feighner, J. P. (1994). Clinical significance of early non-response in depressed patients. *Depression, 2,* 32–35.

Bradley, C. (1950). Benzedrine and dexedrine in the treatment of children's behavior disorders. *Pediatrics, 5*(1), 24–37.

Bray, G. A. (2011). Medications for weight reduction. *Medical Clinics of North America, 95*(5), 989–1008.

Bresee, C. B., Gotto, J., & Z. Rapaport, M. H. (2009). Treatment of depression. In A. F. Schatzberg & C. B. Nemeroff (Eds.), *Textbook of psychopharmacology* (4th ed., pp. 1081–1111). Washington, DC: American Psychiatric Publishing.

Brody, A. L., Saxena, S., Stoessel, P., Gillies, L. A., Fairbanks, L. A., Alborzian, S., . . . Baxter, L. R., Jr. (2001). Regional brain metabolic changes in patients with major depression treated with either paroxetine or interpersonal therapy: Preliminary findings. *Archives of General Psychiatry, 58*(7), 631–640.

Brody, H. (1982). The lie that heals: The ethics of giving placebos. *Annals of Internal Medicine, 97*(1), 112–118.

Bushe, C. J., & Savill, N. C. (2013). Systematic review of atomoxetine data in childhood and adolescent attention-deficit hyperactivity disorder 2009–2011: Focus on clinical efficacy and safety. *Journal of Psychopharmacology.* doi:10.1177/0269881113478475

Camarini, R., Marcourakis, T., Teodorov, E., Yonamine, M., & Calil, H. M. (2011). Ethanol-induced sensitization depends preferentially on D1 rather than D2 dopamine receptors. *Pharmacology, Biochemistry, and Behavior, 98*(2), 173–180.

Campbell, M. L., & Mathys, M. L. (2001). Pharmacologic options for the treatment of obesity. *American Journal of Health-System Pharmacy, 58*(14), 1301–1308.

Canuso, C. M., & Pandina, G. (2007). Gender and schizophrenia. *Psychopharmacology Bulletin, 40*(4), 178–190.

Cao, A. H., Yu, L., Wang, Y. W., Wang, J. M., Yang, L. J., & Lei, G. F. (2012). Effects of methylphenidate on attentional set-shifting in a genetic model of attention-deficit/hyperactivity disorder. *Behavioral and Brain Functions, 8*(1), 10–9081–8–10.

Capone, C., Kahler, C. W., Swift, R. M., & O'Malley, S. S. (2011). Does family history of alcoholism moderate naltrexone's effects on alcohol use? *Journal of Studies on Alcohol and Drugs, 72*(1), 135–140.

Caprioli, D., Celentano, M., Dubla, A., Lucantonio, F., Nencini, P., & Badiani, A. (2009). Ambience and drug choice: Cocaine- and heroin-taking as a function of environmental context in humans and rats. *Biological Psychiatry, 65*(10), 893–899.

Carlsson, A., & Lindqvist, M. (1963). Effect of chlorpromazine or haloperidol on formation of 3-methoxytyramine and normetanephrine in mouse brain. *Acta Pharmacologica et Toxicologica, 20*, 140–144.

Caroff, S. N., Hurford, I., Lybrand, J., & Campbell, E. C. (2011). Movement disorders induced by antipsychotic drugs: Implications of the CATIE schizophrenia trial. *Neurologic Clinics, 29*(1), 127–148, viii.

Carpenter, D. J. (2011). St. John's wort and S-adenosyl methionine as "natural" alternatives to conventional antidepressants in the era of the suicidality boxed warning: What is the evidence for clinically relevant benefit? *Alternative Medicine Review, 16*(1), 17–39.

Carroll, K. M., & Onken, L. S. (2005). Behavioral therapies for drug abuse. *American Journal of Psychiatry, 162*(8), 1452–1460.

Casey, D. E. (2000). Tardive dyskinesia: Pathophysiology and animal models. *Journal of Clinical Psychiatry, 61*(Suppl. 4), 5–9.

Casey, D. E. (2004). Pathophysiology of antipsychotic drug-induced movement disorders. *Journal of Clinical Psychiatry, 65*(Suppl. 9), 25–28.

Castle, L., Aubert, R. E., Verbrugge, R. R., Khalid, M., & Epstein, R. S. (2007). Trends in medication treatment for ADHD. *Journal of Attention Disorders, 10*(4), 335–342.

Cerullo, M. A. (2006). Cosmetic psychopharmacology and the president's council on bioethics. *Perspectives in Biology and Medicine, 49*(4), 515–523.

Chang, L., & Chronicle, E. P. (2007). Functional imaging studies in cannabis users. *Neuroscientist, 13*(5), 422–432.

Chansky, T. E. (2001). *Freeing your child from obsessive-compulsive disorder: A powerful, practical program for parents of children and adolescents.* New York, NY: Crown Publishing.

Chaudhry, I., Neelam, K., Duddu, V., & Husain, N. (2008). Ethnicity and psychopharmacology. *Journal of Psychopharmacology, 22*(6), 673–680.

Chen, C. Y., Gerhard, T., & Winterstein, A. G. (2009a). Determinants of initial pharmacological treatment for youths with attention-deficit/hyperactivity disorder. *Journal of Child and Adolescent Psychopharmacology, 19*(2), 187–195.

Chen, C. Y., Storr, C. L., & Anthony, J. C. (2009b). Early-onset drug use and risk for drug dependence problems. *Addictive Behaviors, 34*(3), 319–322.

Chen, J., Lipska, B. K., & Weinberger, D. R. (2006). Genetic mouse models of schizophrenia: From hypothesis-based to susceptibility gene-based models. *Biological Psychiatry, 59*(12), 1180–1188.

Chen, M. L. (2006). Ethnic or racial differences revisited: Impact of dosage regimen and dosage form on pharmacokinetics and pharmacodynamics. *Clinical Pharmacokinetics, 45*(10), 957–964.

Chenhall, R., & Senior, K. (2009). "Those young people all crankybella": Indigenous youth mental health and globalization. *International Journal of Mental Health, 38*(3), 28–43.

Cherniack, E. P. (2010). Would the elderly be better off if they were given more placebos? *Geriatrics and Gerontology International, 10*(2), 131–137.

Chisolm, M. S. (2011). Prescribing psychotherapy. *Perspectives in Biology and Medicine, 54*(2), 168–175.

Christensen, R., Kristensen, P. K., Bartels, E. M., Bliddal, H., & Astrup, A. (2007). Efficacy and safety of the weight-loss drug rimonabant: A meta-analysis of randomised trials. *Lancet, 370*(9600), 1706–1713.

Chugh, P. K., & Sharma, S. (2012). Recent advances in the pathophysiology and pharmacological treatment of obesity. *Journal of Clinical Pharmacy and Therapeutics, 37*(5), 525–535.

Clayton, A. H., & Gillespie, E. H. (2009). Bupropion. In A. F. Schatzberg & C. B. Nemeroff (Eds.), *Textbook of psychopharmacology* (4th ed., pp. 415–427). Washington, DC: American Psychiatric Publishing.

Cleland, K., Peipert, J. F., Westhoff, C., Spear, S., & Trussell, J. (2012). Plan B, one step not taken: Politics trumps science yet again. *Contraception, 85*(4), 340–341.

Colman, E., Golden, J., Roberts, M., Egan, A., Weaver, J., & Rosebraugh, C. (2012). The FDA's assessment of two drugs for chronic weight management. *New England Journal of Medicine, 367*(17), 1577–1579.

Comas-Diaz, L. (2012). *Multicultural care: A clinician's guide to cultural competence.* Washington, DC: American Psychological Association.

Comer, J. S., Olfson, M., & Mojtabai, R. (2010). National trends in child and adolescent psychotropic polypharmacy in office-based practice, 1996–2007. *Journal of the American Academy of Child and Adolescent Psychiatry, 49*(10), 1001–1010.

Connolly, H. M., Crary, J. L., McGoon, M. D., Hensrud, D. D., Edwards, B. S., Edwards, W. D., & Schaff, H. V. (1997). Valvular heart disease associated with fenfluramine-phentermine. *New England Journal of Medicine, 337*(9), 581–588.

Connolly, K. R., & Thase, M. E. (2011). If at first you don't succeed: A review of the evidence for antidepressant augmentation, combination and switching strategies. *Drugs, 71*(1), 43–64.

Connolly, K. R., & Thase, M. E. (2012). Emerging drugs for major depressive disorder. *Expert Opinion on Emerging Drugs, 17*(1), 105–126.

Cooper, L. A., Gonzales, J. J., Gallo, J. J., Rost, K. M., Meredith, L. S., Rubenstein, L. V., . . . Ford, D. E. (2003). The acceptability of treatment for depression among African-American, Hispanic, and white primary care patients. *Medical Care, 41*(4), 479–489.

Cooper, Z. D., & Haney, M. (2008). Cannabis reinforcement and dependence: Role of the cannabinoid CB1 receptor. *Addiction Biology, 13*(2), 188–195.

Cox, G. R., Callahan, P., Churchill, R., Hunot, V., Merry, S. N., Parker, A. G., & Hetrick, S. E. (2012). Psychological therapies versus antidepressant medication, alone and in combination for depression in children and adolescents. *Cochrane Database of Systematic Reviews, 11,* CD008324.

Craighead, W. E., Sheets, E. S., Brosse, A. L., & Ilardi, S. S. (2007). Psychosocial treatments for major depressive disorder. In P. E. Nathan & J. M. Gorman (Eds.), *A guide to treatments that work* (3rd ed., pp. 289–307). New York, NY: Oxford University Press.

Cryan, J. F., & Sweeney, F. F. (2011). The age of anxiety: Role of animal models of anxiolytic action in drug discovery. *British Journal of Pharmacology, 164*(4), 1129–1161.

Dago, P. L., & Quitkin, F. M. (1995). Role of the placebo response in the treatment of depressive disorders. *CNS Drugs, 4*(5), 335–340.

Daitch, C. (2011). *Anxiety disorders: The go-to guide for clients and therapists.* New York, NY: Norton.

Danzinger, P. R., & Welfel, E. R. (2001). The impact of managed care on mental health counselors: A survey of perceptions, practices, and compliance with ethical standards. *Journal of Mental Health Counseling, 23*(2), 137–150.

Dave, D., & Mukerjee, S. (2011). Mental health parity legislation, cost-sharing and substance-abuse treatment admissions. *Health Economics, 20*(2), 161–183.

Davids, E., Zhang, K., Tarazi, F. I., & Baldessarini, R. J. (2002). Stereoselective effects of methylphenidate on motor hyperactivity in juvenile rats induced by neonatal 6-hydroxydopamine lesioning. *Psychopharmacology, 160*(1), 92–98.

Davidson, J. R. T., Connor, K. M., & Zhang, W. (2009). Treatment of anxiety disorders. In A. F. Schatzberg & C. B. Nemeroff (Eds.), *Textbook of psychopharmacology* (4th ed., pp. 1171–1199). Washington, DC: American Psychiatric Publishing.

Deligiannidis, K. M., & Freeman, M. P. (2010). Complementary and alternative medicine for the treatment of depressive disorders in women. *Psychiatric Clinics of North America, 33*(2), 441–463.

Demjaha, A., Murray, R. M., McGuire, P. K., Kapur, S., & Howes, O. D. (2012). Dopamine synthesis capacity in patients with treatment-resistant schizophrenia. *American Journal of Psychiatry, 169*(11), 1203–1210.

Derosa, G., & Maffioli, P. (2012). Anti-obesity drugs: A review about their effects and their safety. *Expert Opinion on Drug Safety, 11*(3), 459–471.

De Sousa, A., & Kalra, G. (2012). Drug therapy of attention deficit hyperactivity disorder: Current trends. *Mens Sana Monographs, 10*(1), 45–69.

Devlin, M. J., Yanovski, S. Z., & Wilson, G. T. (2000). Obesity: What mental health professionals need to know. *American Journal of Psychiatry, 157*(6), 854–866.

Deyo, R. A. (2004). Gaps, tensions, and conflicts in the FDA approval process: Implications for clinical practice. *Journal of the American Board of Family Practice/American Board of Family Practice, 17*(2), 142–149.

Diamond, R. J. (2011). *The medication question: weighing your mental health treatment options.* New York, NY: Norton.

Diaz, E., Woods, S. W., & Rosenheck, R. A. (2005). Effects of ethnicity on psychotropic medications adherence. *Community Mental Health Journal, 41*(5), 521–537.

Dietz, D. M., Dietz, K. C., Nestler, E. J., & Russo, S. J. (2009). Molecular mechanisms of psychostimulant-induced structural plasticity. *Pharmacopsychiatry, 42*(Suppl. 1), S69–S78.

Dohmen, K., Baraona, E., Ishibashi, H., Pozzato, G., Moretti, M., Matsunaga, C., . . . Lieber, C. S. (1996). Ethnic differences in gastric sigma-alcohol dehydrogenase activity and ethanol first-pass metabolism. *Alcoholism, Clinical and Experimental Research, 20*(9), 1569–1576.

Donohue, J. M., Berndt, E. R., Rosenthal, M., Epstein, A. M., & Frank, R. G. (2004). Effects of pharmaceutical promotion on adherence to the treatment guidelines for depression. *Medical Care, 42*(12), 1176–1185.

Donohue, J. M., Cevasco, M., & Rosenthal, M. B. (2007). A decade of direct-to-consumer advertising of prescription drugs. *New England Journal of Medicine, 357*(7), 673–681.

Dougherty, D. D., Rauch, S. L., & Jenike, M. A. (2007). Pharmacological treatments for obsessive-compulsive disorder. In P. E. Nathan & J. M. Gorman (Eds.), *A guide to treatments that work* (3rd ed., pp. 447–473). New York, NY: Oxford University Press.

Downing, N. S., Aminawung, J. A., Shah, N. D., Braunstein, J. B., Krumholz, H. M., & Ross, J. S. (2012). Regulatory review of novel therapeutics—comparison of three regulatory agencies. *New England Journal of Medicine, 366*(24), 2284–2293.

Dubovsky, S. L. (2005). *Clinical guide to psychotropic medications.* New York, NY: Norton.

Dubovsky, S. L., & Dubovsky, A. N. (2007). *Psychotropic drug prescriber's survival guide: Ethical mental health treatment in the age of big pharma.* New York, NY: Norton.

Duman, R. S. (2009). Neurochemical theories of depression: Preclinical studies. In D. S. Charney & E. J. Nestler (Eds.), *Neurobiology of mental illness* (3rd ed., pp. 413–434). New York, NY: Oxford University Press.

Dunlop, B. W., Garlow, S. J., & Nemeroff, C. B. (2009). The neurochemistry of depressive disorders: Clinical studies. In D. S. Charney & E. J. Nestler (Eds.), *Neurobiology of mental illness* (3rd ed., pp. 435–460). New York, NY: Oxford University Press.

DuPont, R. L. (2010). Prescription drug abuse: An epidemic dilemma. *Journal of Psychoactive Drugs, 42*(2), 127–132.

Dupuy, J. M., Ostacher, M. J., Huffman, J., Perlis, R. H., & Nierenberg, A. A. (2012). Evidence-based pharmacotherapy of major depressive disorder. In D. J. Stein, B. Lerer, & S. M. Stahl (Eds.), *Essential evidence-based psychopharmacology* (2nd ed., pp. 53–72). New York, NY: Cambridge University Press.

Dziegielewski, S. F. (2006). *Psychopharmacology handbook for the non-medically trained.* New York, NY: Norton.

Eddy, K. T., Dutra, L., Bradley, R., & Westen, D. (2004). A multidimensional meta-analysis of psychotherapy and pharmacotherapy for obsessive-compulsive disorder. *Clinical Psychology Review, 24*(8), 1011–1030.

Edwards, S., & Koob, G. F. (2012). Experimental psychiatric illness and drug abuse models: From human to animal, an overview. *Methods in Molecular Biology (Clifton, NJ), 829*, 31–48.

Ellgren, M., Artmann, A., Tkalych, O., Gupta, A., Hansen, H. S., Hansen, S. H., . . . Hurd, Y. L. (2008). Dynamic changes of the endogenous cannabinoid and opioid mesocorticolimbic systems during adolescence: THC effects. *European Neuropsychopharmacology: Journal of the European College of Neuropsychopharmacology, 18*(11), 826–834.

Ellgren, M., Spano, S. M., & Hurd, Y. L. (2007). Adolescent cannabis exposure alters opiate intake and opioid limbic neuronal populations in adult rats. *Neuropsychopharmacology, 32*(3), 607–615.

Emanuele, E. (2011). Generic versus brand name drugs in psychopharmacology: A pharmacoeconomic perspective. *Southern Medical Journal, 104*(10), 715–716.

Engel, G. L. (1977). The need for a new medical model: A challenge for biomedicine. *Science, 196*(4286), 129–136.

Epping-Jordan, M. P., Watkins, S. S., Koob, G. F., & Markou, A. (1998). Dramatic decreases in brain reward function during nicotine withdrawal. *Nature, 393*(6680), 76–79.

Ernst, E. (2007). Placebo: New insights into an old enigma. *Drug Discovery Today, 12*(9–10), 413–418.

Eyding, D., Lelgemann, M., Grouven, U., Harter, M., Kromp, M., Kaiser, T., . . . Wieseler, M. (2010). Reboxetine for acute treatment of major depression: Systematic review and meta-analysis of published and unpublished placebo and selective serotonin reuptake inhibitor controlled trials. *British Medical Journal, 341*:c4737.

Fang, Q., Li, F. Q., Li, Y. Q., Xue, Y. X., He, Y. Y., Liu, J. F., . . . Wang, J. S. (2011). Cannabinoid CB1 receptor antagonist rimonabant disrupts nicotine reward-associated memory in rats. *Pharmacology, Biochemistry, and Behavior, 99*(4), 738–742.

Fava, G. A., Grandi, S., Zielezny, M., Rafanelli, C., & Canestrari, R. (1996). Four-year outcome for cognitive behavioral treatment of residual symptoms in major depression. *American Journal of Psychiatry, 153*(7), 945–947.

Fedoroff, I. C., & Taylor, S. (2001). Psychological and pharmacological treatments of social phobia: A meta-analysis. *Journal of Clinical Psychopharmacology, 21*(3), 311–324.

Ferguson, J. M., Khan, A., Mangano, R., Entsuah, R., & Tzanis, E. (2007). Relapse prevention of panic disorder in adult outpatient responders to treatment with venlafaxine extended release. *Journal of Clinical Psychiatry, 68*(1), 58–68.

Fernando, A. B., & Robbins, T. W. (2011). Animal models of neuropsychiatric disorders. *Annual Review of Clinical Psychology, 7*, 39–61.

Fidler, M. C., Sanchez, M., Raether, B., Weissman, N. J., Smith, S. R., Shanahan, W. R., . . . BLOSSOM Clinical Trial Group. (2011). A one-year randomized trial of lorcaserin for weight loss in obese and overweight adults: The BLOSSOM trial. *Journal of Clinical Endocrinology and Metabolism, 96*(10), 3067–3077.

Field, M. J., Oles, R. J., & Singh, L. (2001). Pregabalin may represent a novel class of anxiolytic agents with a broad spectrum of activity. *British Journal of Pharmacology, 132*(1), 1–4.

Fineberg, N. A., Brown, A., & Pampaloni, I. (2012a). Evidence-based pharmacotherapy of obsessive-compulsive disorder. In D. J. Stein, B. Lerer, & S. M. Stahl (Eds.), *Essential evidence-based psychopharmacology* (2nd ed., pp. 128–170). New York, NY: Cambridge University Press.

Fineberg, N. A., Brown, A., Reghunandanan, S., & Pampaloni, I. (2012b). Evidence-based pharmacotherapy of obsessive-compulsive disorder. *International Journal of Neuropsychopharmacology, 15*(8), 1173–1191.

Fineberg, N. A., Chamberlain, S. R., Hollander, E., Boulougouris, V., & Robbins, T. W. (2011). Translational approaches to obsessive-compulsive disorder: From animal models to clinical treatment. *British Journal of Pharmacology, 164*(4), 1044–1061.

Fineberg, N. A., Reghunandanan, S., Brown, A., & Pampaloni, I. (2013). Pharmacotherapy of obsessive-compulsive disorder: Evidence-based treatment and beyond. *Australian and New Zealand Journal of Psychiatry, 47*(2), 121–141.

Finney, J. W., Wilbourne, P. L., & Moos, R. H. (2007). Psychosocial treatments for substance use disorders. In P. E. Nathan & J. M. Gorman (Eds.), *A guide to treatments that work* (3rd ed., pp. 179–202). New York, NY: Oxford University Press.

Finniss, D. G., Kaptchuk, T. J., Miller, F., & Benedetti, F. (2010). Biological, clinical, and ethical advances of placebo effects. *Lancet, 375*(9715), 686–695.

Foa, E., & Andrews, L. W. (2006). *If your adolescent has an anxiety disorder: An essential resource for parents*. New York, NY: Oxford University Press.

Fowler, J. S., & Volkow, N. D. (2009). PET and SPECT imaging in substance abuse research. In D. S. Charney & E. J. Nestler (Eds.), *Neurobiology of mental illness* (3rd ed., pp. 828–845). New York, NY: Oxford University Press.

Frank, R. G., Conti, R. M., & Goldman, H. H. (2005). Mental health policy and psychotropic drugs. *Milbank Quarterly, 83*(2), 271–298.

Frank, R. G., & McGuire, T. G. (1986). A review of studies of the impact of insurance on the demand and utilization of specialty mental health services. *Health Services Research, 21*(2 Pt 2), 241–265.

Franklin, M. E., & Foa, E. B. (2007). Cognitive behavioral treatment of obsessive-compulsive disorder. In P. E. Nathan & J. M. Gorman (Eds.), *A guide to treatments that work* (3rd ed., pp. 431–473). New York, NY: Oxford University Press.

Freeman, M. P., Fava, M., Lake, J., Trivedi, M. H., Wisner, K. L., & Mischoulon, D. (2010). Complementary and alternative medicine in major depressive disorder: The American Psychiatric Association Task Force report. *Journal of Clinical Psychiatry, 71*(6), 669–681.

Freeman, M. P., Wiegand, C. B., & Gelenberg, A. J. (2009). Lithium. In A. F. Schatzberg

& C. B. Nemeroff (Eds.), *Textbook of psychopharmacology* (4th ed., pp. 697–717). Washington, DC: American Psychiatric Publishing.

Frezza, M., di Padova, C., Pozzato, G., Terpin, M., Baraona, E., & Lieber, C. S. (1990). High blood alcohol levels in women. The role of decreased gastric alcohol dehydrogenase activity and first-pass metabolism. *New England Journal of Medicine, 322*(2), 95–99.

Fucito, L. M., Park, A., Gulliver, S. B., Mattson, M. E., Gueorguieva, R. V., & O'Malley, S. S. (2012). Cigarette smoking predicts differential benefit from naltrexone for alcohol dependence. *Biological Psychiatry, 72*(10), 832–838.

Fullerton, C. A., Epstein, A. M., Frank, R. G., Normand, S. L., Fu, C. X., & McGuire, T. G. (2012). Medication use and spending trends among children with ADHD in Florida's Medicaid program, 1996–2005. *Psychiatric Services, 63*(2), 115–121.

Gadde, K. M., Allison, D. B., Ryan, D. H., Peterson, C. A., Troupin, B., Schwiers, M. L., & Day, W. W. (2011). Effects of low-dose, controlled-release, phentermine plus topiramate combination on weight and associated comorbidities in overweight and obese adults (CONQUER): A randomised, placebo-controlled, phase 3 trial. *Lancet, 377*(9774), 1341–1352.

Gardner, E. L., & Wise, R. A. (2009). Animal models of addiction. In D. S. Charney & E. J. Nestler (Eds.), *Neurobiology of mental illness* (3rd ed., pp. 757–774). New York, NY: Oxford University Press.

Garfield, C. F., Dorsey, E. R., Zhu, S., Huskamp, H. A., Conti, R., Dusetzina, S. B., . . . Alexander, G. C. (2012). Trends in attention deficit hyperactivity disorder ambulatory diagnosis and medical treatment in the United States, 2000–2010. *Academic Pediatrics, 12*(2), 110–116.

Garnock-Jones, K. P., & Keating, G. M. (2010). Spotlight on atomoxetine in attention-deficit hyperactivity disorder in children and adolescents. *CNS Drugs, 24*(1), 85–88.

Garvey, W. T., Ryan, D. H., Look, M., Gadde, K. M., Allison, D. B., Peterson, C. A., . . . Bowden, C. H. (2012). Two-year sustained weight loss and metabolic benefits with controlled-release phentermine/topiramate in obese and overweight adults (SEQUEL): A randomized, placebo-controlled, phase 3 extension study. *American Journal of Clinical Nutrition, 95*(2), 297–308.

Gerard, R. W. (1957). Drugs for the soul; the rise of psychopharmacology. *Science, 125*, 201–203.

Getahun, D., Jacobsen, S. J., Fassett, M. J., Chen, W., Demissie, K., & Rhoads, G. G. (2013). Recent trends in childhood attention-deficit/hyperactivity disorder. *JAMA Pediatrics, 167*(3), 282–288.

Ghafari, E., Fararouie, M., Shirazi, H. G., Farhangfar, A., Ghaderi, F., & Mohammadi, A. (2013). Combination of estrogen and antipsychotics in the treatment of women with chronic schizophrenia: A double-blind, randomized, placebo-controlled clinical trial. *Clinical Schizophrenia and Related Psychoses, 6*(4), 172–176.

Gillespie, C. F., Garlow, S. J., Binder, E. B., Schatzberg, A. F., & Nemeroff, C. B. (2009). Neurobiology of mood disorders. In A. F. Schatzberg & C. B. Nemeroff (Eds.), *Textbook of psychopharmacology* (4th ed., pp. 903–944). Washington, DC: American Psychiatric Publishing.

Gilpin, N. W., & Koob, G. F. (2010). Effects of beta-adrenoceptor antagonists on alcohol drinking by alcohol-dependent rats. *Psychopharmacology, 212*(3), 431–439.

Ginsburg, G. S., Kendall, P. C., Sakolsky, D., Compton, S. N., Piacentini, J., Albano,

A. M., . . . March, J. (2011). Remission after acute treatment in children and adolescents with anxiety disorders: Findings from the CAMS. *Journal of Consulting and Clinical Psychology, 79*(6), 806–813.

Givens, J. L., Katz, I. R., Bellamy, S., & Holmes, W. C. (2007). Stigma and the acceptability of depression treatments among African Americans and whites. *Journal of General Internal Medicine, 22*(9), 1292–1297.

Gleason, M. M., Egger, H. L., Emslie, G. J., Greenhill, L. L., Kowatch, R. A., Lieberman, A. F., . . . Zeanah, C. H. (2007). Psychopharmacological treatment for very young children: Contexts and guidelines. *Journal of the American Academy of Child and Adolescent Psychiatry, 46*(12), 1532–1572.

Goldapple, K., Segal, Z., Garson, C., Lau, M., Bieling, P., Kennedy, S., & Mayberg, H. (2004). Modulation of cortical-limbic pathways in major depression: Treatment-specific effects of cognitive behavior therapy. *Archives of General Psychiatry, 61*(1), 34–41.

Goldstein, A. (1976). Naltrexone in the management of heroin addiction: Critique of the rationale. *NIDA Research Monograph,* (9), 158–161.

Goldstein, A. (2001). *Addiction: From biology to drug policy* (2nd ed.). New York, NY: Oxford University Press.

Goldstein, J. M., Cohen, L. S., Horton, N. J., Lee, H., Andersen, S., Tohen, M., . . . Tollefson, G. (2002a). Sex differences in clinical response to olanzapine compared with haloperidol. *Psychiatry Research, 110*(1), 27–37.

Goldstein, J. M., Seidman, L. J., O'Brien, L. M., Horton, N. J., Kennedy, D. N., Makris, N., . . . Tsuang, M. T. (2002b). Impact of normal sexual dimorphisms on sex differences in structural brain abnormalities in schizophrenia assessed by magnetic resonance imaging. *Archives of General Psychiatry, 59*(2), 154–164.

Gonzales, R. A., & Weiss, F. (1998). Suppression of ethanol-reinforced behavior by naltrexone is associated with attenuation of the ethanol-induced increase in dialysate dopamine levels in the nucleus accumbens. *Journal of Neuroscience, 18*(24), 10663–10671.

Gonzalez, R., & Swanson, J. M. (2012). Long-term effects of adolescent-onset and persistent use of cannabis. *Proceedings of the National Academy of Sciences of the United States of America, 109*(40), 15970–15971.

Grant, P. M., Huh, G. A., Perivoliotis, D., Stolar, N. M., & Beck, A. T. (2012). Randomized trial to evaluate the efficacy of cognitive therapy for low-functioning patients with schizophrenia. *Archives of General Psychiatry, 69*(2), 121–127.

Greenway, F. L., & Bray, G. A. (2010). Combination drugs for treating obesity. *Current Diabetes Reports, 10*(2), 108–115.

Haller, J., & Alicki, M. (2012). Current animal models of anxiety, anxiety disorders, and anxiolytic drugs. *Current Opinion in Psychiatry, 25*(1), 59–64.

Halmi, K. A. (2005). The multimodal treatment of eating disorders. *World Psychiatry: Official Journal of the World Psychiatric Association (WPA), 4*(2), 69–73.

Hamrosi, K., Taylor, S. J., & Aslani, P. (2006). Issues with prescribed medications in aboriginal communities: Aboriginal health workers' perspectives. *Rural and Remote Health, 6*(2), 557.

Hanson, K. L., Winward, J. L., Schweinsburg, A. D., Medina, K. L., Brown, S. A., & Tapert, S. F. (2010). Longitudinal study of cognition among adolescent marijuana users over three weeks of abstinence. *Addictive Behaviors, 35*(11), 970–976.

Harris, C. S., & Raz, A. (2012). Deliberate use of placebos in clinical practice: What we really know. *Journal of Medical Ethics, 38*(7), 406–407.

Hasani-Ranjbar, S., Nayebi, N., Larijani, B., & Abdollahi, M. (2009). A systematic review of the efficacy and safety of herbal medicines used in the treatment of obesity. *World Journal of Gastroenterology: WJG, 15*(25), 3073–3085.

Haslemo, T., Eikeseth, P. H., Tanum, L., Molden, E., & Refsum, H. (2006). The effect of variable cigarette consumption on the interaction with clozapine and olanzapine. *European Journal of Clinical Pharmacology, 62*(12), 1049–1053.

Hawkins, E. J., Malte, C. A., Imel, Z. E., Saxon, A. J., & Kivlahan, D. R. (2012). Prevalence and trends of benzodiazepine use among veterans affairs patients with posttraumatic stress disorder, 2003–2010. *Drug and Alcohol Dependence, 124*(1–2), 154–161.

Heal, D. J., Gosden, J., & Smith, S. L. (2009). Regulatory challenges for new drugs to treat obesity and comorbid metabolic disorders. *British Journal of Clinical Pharmacology, 68*(6), 861–874.

Heal, D. J., Gosden, J., & Smith, S. L. (2012). What is the prognosis for new centrally-acting anti-obesity drugs? *Neuropharmacology, 63*(1), 132–146.

Heal, D. J., Smith, S. L., Gosden, J., & Nutt, D. J. (2013). Amphetamine, past and present—a pharmacological and clinical perspective. *Journal of Psychopharmacology, 27*(6), 479–496.

Hemo, B., Endevelt, R., Porath, A., Stampfer, M. J., & Shai, I. (2011). Adherence to weight loss medications; post-marketing study from HMO pharmacy data of one million individuals. *Diabetes Research and Clinical Practice, 94*(2), 269–275.

Hernandez, S. H., & Nelson, L. S. (2010). Prescription drug abuse: Insight into the epidemic. *Clinical Pharmacology and Therapeutics, 88*(3), 307–317.

Hilmer, S. N., McLachlan, A. J., & Le Couteur, D. G. (2007). Clinical pharmacology in the geriatric patient. *Fundamental and Clinical Pharmacology, 21*(3), 217–230.

Hilts, P. J. (2003). *Protecting America's Health: The FDA, business, and one hundred years of regulation.* New York, NY: Knopf.

Hinshaw, S. P., Klein, R. G., & Abikoff, H. B. (2007). Childhood attention-deficit/hyperactivity disorder: Nonpharmacological treatments and their combination with medication. In P. E. Nathan & J. M. Gorman (Eds.), *A guide to treatments that work* (3rd ed., pp. 3–27). New York, NY: Oxford University Press.

Hirsch, J. (1998). Magic bullet for obesity. *British Medical Journal, 317*, 1136–1138.

Hirvonen, J., Goodwin, R. S., Li, C. T., Terry, G. E., Zoghbi, S. S., Morse, C., . . . Innis, R. B. (2012). Reversible and regionally selective downregulation of brain cannabinoid CB1 receptors in chronic daily cannabis smokers. *Molecular Psychiatry, 17*(6), 642–649.

Hodgkin, D., Horgan, C. M., Garnick, D. W., & Merrick, E. L. (2009). Benefit limits for behavioral health care in private health plans. *Administration and Policy in Mental Health, 36*(1), 15–23.

Hodgkin, D., Merrick, E. L., & Hiatt, D. (2012). The relationship of antidepressant prescribing concentration to treatment duration and cost. *Journal of Mental Health Policy and Economics, 15*(1), 3–11.

Hodgson, K., Hutchinson, A. D., & Denson, L. (2012). Nonpharmacological treatments for ADHD: A meta-analytic review. *Journal of Attention Disorders.* doi:10.1177/1087054712444732

Hoffman, K. L. (2011). Animal models of obsessive compulsive disorder: Recent findings and future directions. *Expert Opinion on Drug Discovery, 6*(7), 725–737.

Holsboer, F. (2009). Putative new-generation antidepressants. In A. F. Schatzberg & C. B. Nemeroff (Eds.), *Textbook of psychopharmacology* (4th ed., pp. 503–529). Washington, DC: American Psychiatric Publishing.

Holmes, D. (2012). Prescription drug addiction: The treatment challenge. *Lancet, 379*(9810), 17–18.

Horgan, C. M., Garnick, D. W., Merrick, E. L., & Hodgkin, D. (2009). Changes in how health plans provide behavioral health services. *Journal of Behavioral Health Services and Research, 36*(1), 11–24.

Howland, R. H. (2008a). How are drugs approved? Part 1: The evolution of the Food and Drug Administration. *Journal of Psychosocial Nursing and Mental Health Services, 46*(1), 15–19.

Howland, R. H. (2008b). How are drugs approved? Part 2: Ethical foundations of clinical research. *Journal of Psychosocial Nursing and Mental Health Services, 46*(2), 15–20.

Howland, R. H. (2008c). How are drugs approved? Part 3. the stages of drug development. *Journal of Psychosocial Nursing and Mental Health Services, 46*(3), 17–20.

Howland, R. H. (2012a). Dietary supplement drug therapies for depression. *Journal of Psychosocial Nursing and Mental Health Services, 50*(6), 13–16.

Howland, R. H. (2012b). Off-label medication use. *Journal of Psychosocial Nursing and Mental Health Services, 50*(9), 11–13.

Huebner, D. (2007). *What to do when your brain gets stuck: A kid's guide for overcoming OCD.* Washington, DC: American Psychological Association.

Hunt, J., Sullivan, G., Chavira, D. A., Stein, M. B., Craske, M. G., Golinelli, D., . . . Sherbourne, C. D. (2013). Race and beliefs about mental health treatment among anxious primary care patients. *Journal of Nervous and Mental Disease, 201*(3), 188–195.

Hunter, A. M., Leuchter, A. F., Morgan, M. L., & Cook, I. A. (2006). Changes in brain function (quantitative EEG cordance) during placebo lead-in and treatment outcomes in clinical trials for major depression. *American Journal of Psychiatry, 163*(8), 1426–1432.

Hurt, R. D., Sachs, D. P., Glover, E. D., Offord, K. P., Johnston, J. A., Dale, L. C., . . . Sullivan, P. M. (1997). A comparison of sustained-release bupropion and placebo for smoking cessation. *New England Journal of Medicine, 337*(17), 1195–1202.

Huskamp, H. A., Deverka, P. A., Epstein, A. M., Epstein, R. S., McGuigan, K. A., Muriel, A. C., & Frank, R. G. (2005). Impact of 3-tier formularies on drug treatment of attention-deficit/hyperactivity disorder in children. *Archives of General Psychiatry, 62*(4), 435–441.

Ioannides-Demos, L. L., Piccenna, L., & McNeil, J. J. (2011). Pharmacotherapies for obesity: Past, current, and future therapies. *Journal of Obesity, 2011,* 179674.

Ioannides-Demos, L. L., Proietto, J., & McNeil, J. J. (2005). Pharmacotherapy for obesity. *Drugs, 65*(10), 1391–1418.

Ipser, J. C., & Stein, D. J. (2012). Evidence-based pharmacotherapy of post-traumatic stress disorder (PTSD). *International Journal of Neuropsychopharmacology, 15*(6), 825–840.

Isaacs, A. N., Pyett, P., Oakley-Browne, M. A., Gruis, H., & Waples-Crowe, P. (2010). Barriers and facilitators to the utilization of adult mental health services by Australia's indigenous people: Seeking a way forward. *International Journal of Mental Health Nursing, 19*(2), 75–82.

Iversen, L. L., Iversen, S. D., Bloom, F. E., & Roth, R. H. (2009). *Introduction to neuropsychopharmacology.* New York, NY: Oxford.

Jacobsen, E. (1986). The early history of psychotherapeutic drugs. *Psychopharmacology, 89*(2), 138–144.

Jeffreys, M., Capehart, B., & Friedman, M. J. (2012). Pharmacotherapy for posttraumatic stress disorder: Review with clinical applications. *Journal of Rehabilitation Research and Development, 49*(5), 703–715.

Jenike, M. A., Baer, L., Summergrad, P., Minichiello, W. E., Holland, A., & Seymour, R. (1990). Sertraline in obsessive-compulsive disorder: A double-blind comparison with placebo. *American Journal of Psychiatry, 147*(7), 923–928.

Jensen, P. S., Bhatara, V. S., Vitiello, B., Hoagwood, K., Feil, M., & Burke, L. B. (1999). Psychoactive medication prescribing practices for U.S. children: Gaps between research and clinical practice. *Journal of the American Academy of Child and Adolescent Psychiatry, 38*(5), 557–565.

Jeste, D. V. (2004). Tardive dyskinesia rates with atypical antipsychotics in older adults. *Journal of Clinical Psychiatry, 65*(Suppl. 9), 21–24.

Johansson, K., Neovius, K., DeSantis, S. M., Rossner, S., & Neovius, M. (2009). Discontinuation due to adverse events in randomized trials of orlistat, sibutramine and rimonabant: A meta-analysis. *Obesity Reviews, 10*(5), 564–575.]

Johnson, J. A. (1997). Influence of race or ethnicity on pharmacokinetics of drugs. *Journal of Pharmaceutical Sciences, 86*(12), 1328–1333.

Johnstone, E. C., Cunningham Owens, D. G., Firth, C. D., McPherson, K., Dowie, C., Riley, G., & Gold, A. (1980). Neurotic illness and its response to anxiolytic and antidepressant treatment. *Psychological medicine, 10,* 321–328.

Julien, R. M., Advocat, C. D., & Comaty, J. E. (2010). *A primer of drug action* (12th ed.). New York, NY: Worth.

Kaffman, A., & Krystal, J. H. (2012). New frontiers in animal research of psychiatric illness. *Methods in Molecular Biology (Clifton, NJ), 829,* 3–30.

Kahende, J. W., Malarcher, A. M., Teplinskaya, A., & Asman, K. J. (2011). Quit attempt correlates among smokers by race/ethnicity. *International Journal of Environmental Research and Public Health, 8*(10), 3871–3888.

Kalivas, P. W., & Volkow, N. D. (2005). The neural basis of addiction: A pathology of motivation and choice. *American Journal of Psychiatry, 162*(8), 1403–1413.

Kane, J. M. (2004). Tardive dyskinesia rates with atypical antipsychotics in adults: Prevalence and incidence. *Journal of Clinical Psychiatry, 65*(Suppl. 9), 16–20.

Kang, J. G., & Park, C. Y. (2012). Anti-obesity drugs: A review about their effects and safety. *Diabetes and Metabolism Journal, 36*(1), 13–25.

Kaplan, L. M. (2005). Pharmacological therapies for obesity. *Gastroenterology Clinics of North America, 34*(1), 91–104.

Kaptchuk, T. J., Friedlander, E., Kelley, J. M., Sanchez, M. N., Kokkotou, E., Singer, J. P., . . . Lembo, A. J. (2010). Placebos without deception: A randomized controlled trial in irritable bowel syndrome. *PLoS One, 5*(12), e15591.

Katzman, M. A., Brawman-Mintzer, O., Reyes, E. B., Olausson, B., Liu, S., & Eriksson, H. (2011). Extended release quetiapine fumarate (quetiapine XR) monotherapy as maintenance treatment for generalized anxiety disorder: A long-term, randomized, placebo-controlled trial. *International Clinical Psychopharmacology, 26*(1), 11–24.

Kaye, W., Strober, M., & Jimerson, D. (2009). The neurobiology of eating disorders. In D. S. Charney & E. J. Nestler (Eds.), *Neurobiology of mental illness* (3rd ed., pp. 1349–1369). New York, NY: Oxford University Press.

Keck, P. E., & McElroy, S. L. (2007). Pharmacological treatments for bipolar disorder. In P. E. Nathan & J. M. Gorman (Eds.), *A guide to treatments that work* (3rd ed., pp. 323–350). New York, NY: Oxford University Press.

Keck, P. E., & McElroy, S. L. (2009). Treatment of bipolar disorder. In A. F. Schatzberg & C. B. Nemeroff (Eds.), *Textbook of psychopharmacology* (4th ed., pp. 1113–1133). Washington, DC: American Psychiatric Publishing.

Keck, P. E., Jr., McElroy, S. L., Strakowski, S. M., & Soutullo, C. A. (2000). Antipsychotics in the treatment of mood disorders and risk of tardive dyskinesia. *Journal of Clinical Psychiatry, 61*(Suppl. 4), 33–38.

Keers, R., & Aitchison, K. J. (2010). Gender differences in antidepressant drug response. *International Review of Psychiatry, 22*(5), 485–500.

Keller, M. B., McCullough, J. P., Klein, D. N., Arnow, B., Dunner, D. L., Gelenberg, A. J., . . . Zajecka, J. (2000). A comparison of nefazodone, the cognitive behavioral-analysis system of psychotherapy, and their combination for the treatment of chronic depression. *New England Journal of Medicine, 342*(20), 1462–1470.

Kennedy, S. H., Evans, K. R., Kruger, S., Mayberg, H. S., Meyer, J. H., McCann, S., . . . Vaccarino, F. J. (2001). Changes in regional brain glucose metabolism measured with positron emission tomography after paroxetine treatment of major depression. *American Journal of Psychiatry, 158*(6), 899–905.

Kennedy, S. H., Konarski, J. Z., Segal, Z. V., Lau, M. A., Bieling, P. J., McIntyre, R. S., & Mayberg, H. S. (2007). Differences in brain glucose metabolism between responders to CBT and venlafaxine in a 16-week randomized controlled trial. *American Journal of Psychiatry, 164*(5), 778–788.

Kennett, G. A., & Clifton, P. G. (2010). New approaches to the pharmacological treatment of obesity: Can they break through the efficacy barrier? *Pharmacology, Biochemistry, and Behavior, 97*(1), 63–83.

Kessler, D. A., Hass, A. E., Feiden, K. L., Lumpkin, M., & Temple, R. (1996). Approval of new drugs in the United States. Comparison with the United Kingdom, Germany, and Japan. *Journal of the American Medical Association, 276*(22), 1826–1831.

Kessler, R. C., Berglund, P., Demler, O., Jin, R., Koretz, D., Merikangas, K. R., . . . National Comorbidity Survey Replication. (2003). The epidemiology of major depressive disorder: Results from the national comorbidity survey replication (NCS-R). *Journal of the American Medical Association, 289*(23), 3095–3105.

Kessler, R. C., Chiu, W. T., Demler, O., Merikangas, K. R., & Walters, E. E. (2005). Prevalence, severity, and comorbidity of 12-month DSM-IV disorders in the national comorbidity survey replication. *Archives of General Psychiatry, 62*(6), 617–627.

Kiecolt-Glaser, J. K., Belury, M. A., Andridge, R., Malarkey, W. B., & Glaser, R. (2011). Omega-3 supplementation lowers inflammation and anxiety in medical students: A randomized controlled trial. *Brain, Behavior, and Immunity, 25*(8), 1725–1734.

King, A., de Wit, H., Riley, R. C., Cao, D., Niaura, R., & Hatsukami, D. (2006). Efficacy of naltrexone in smoking cessation: A preliminary study and an examination of sex differences. *Nicotine and Tobacco Research, 8*(5), 671–682.

King, A. C., Cao, D., O'Malley, S. S., Kranzler, H. R., Cai, X., deWit, H., . . . Stachoviak, R. J. (2012). Effects of naltrexone on smoking cessation outcomes and weight gain in nicotine-dependent men and women. *Journal of Clinical Psychopharmacology, 32*(5), 630–636.

Klomp, A., Tremoleda, J. L., Wylezinska, M., Nederveen, A. J., Feenstra, M., Gsell, W., & Reneman, L. (2012). Lasting effects of chronic fluoxetine treatment on the late developing rat brain: Age-dependent changes in the serotonergic neurotransmitter system assessed by pharmacological MRI. *Neuroimage, 59*(1), 218–226.

Kocsis, J. H., Gelenberg, A. J., Rothbaum, B. O., Klein, D. N., Trivedi, M. H., Manber, R., . . . REVAMP Investigators. (2009). Cognitive behavioral analysis system of psychotherapy and brief supportive psychotherapy for augmentation of antidepressant nonresponse in chronic depression: The REVAMP trial. *Archives of General Psychiatry, 66*(11), 1178–1188.

Kocsis, J. H., Rush, A. J., Markowitz, J. C., Borian, F. E., Dunner, D. L., Koran, L. M., . . . Keller, M. B. (2003). Continuation treatment of chronic depression: A comparison of nefazodone, cognitive behavioral analysis system of psychotherapy, and their combination. *Psychopharmacology Bulletin, 37*(4), 73–87.

Kohn, R., Saxena, S., Levav, I., & Saraceno, B. (2004). The treatment gap in mental health care. *Bulletin of the World Health Organization, 82*(11), 858–866.

Kolanowski, J. (1999). A risk-benefit assessment of anti-obesity drugs. *Drug Safety: An International Journal of Medical Toxicology and Drug Experience, 20*(2), 119–131.

Koob, G. F., Kenneth Lloyd, G., & Mason, B. J. (2009). Development of pharmacotherapies for drug addiction: A Rosetta stone approach. *Nature Reviews. Drug Discovery, 8*(6), 500–515.

Koob, G. F., Roberts, A. J., Schulteis, G., Parsons, L. H., Heyser, C. J., Hyytia, P., . . . Weiss, F. (1998). Neurocircuitry targets in ethanol reward and dependence. *Alcoholism, Clinical and Experimental Research, 22*(1), 3–9.

Kopelowicz, A., Liberman, R. P., & Zarate, R. (2007). Psychosocial treatments for schizophrenia. In P. E. Nathan & J. M. Gorman (Eds.), *A guide to treatments that work* (3rd ed., pp. 243–269). New York, NY: Oxford University Press.

Koran, L. M., Hanna, G. L., Hollander, E., Nestadt, G., Simpson, H. B., & American Psychiatric Association. (2007). Practice guideline for the treatment of patients with obsessive-compulsive disorder. *American Journal of Psychiatry, 164*(7 Suppl.), 5–53.

Kornstein, S. G., Schatzberg, A. F., Thase, M. E., Yonkers, K. A., McCullough, J. P., Keitner, G. I., . . . Keller, M. B. (2000). Gender differences in treatment response to sertraline versus imipramine in chronic depression. *American Journal of Psychiatry, 157*(9), 1445–1452.

Koshi, E. B., & Short, C. A. (2007). Placebo theory and its implications for research and clinical practice: A review of the recent literature. *Pain Practice: The Official Journal of World Institute of Pain, 7*(1), 4–20.

Kostrzewa, R. M., Kostrzewa, J. P., Kostrzewa, R. A., Nowak, P., & Brus, R. (2008). Pharmacological models of ADHD. *Journal of Neural Transmission (Vienna, Austria: 1996), 115*(2), 287–298.

Kraly, F. S. (2009). *The unwell brain: Understanding the psychobiology of mental health.* New York, NY: Norton.

Kratochvil, C. J., Lake, M., Pliszka, S. R., & Walkup, J. T. (2005). Pharmacological management of treatment-induced insomnia in ADHD. *Journal of the American Academy of Child and Adolescent Psychiatry, 44*(5), 499–501.

Kreek, M. J., Nielsen, D. A., Butelman, E. R., & LaForge, K. S. (2005). Genetic influences on impulsivity, risk taking, stress responsivity and vulnerability to drug abuse and addiction. *Nature Neuroscience, 8*(11), 1450–1457.

Krishnan-Sarin, S., Krystal, J. H., Shi, J., Pittman, B., & O'Malley, S. S. (2007). Family history of alcoholism influences naltrexone-induced reduction in alcohol drinking. *Biological Psychiatry, 62*(6), 694–697.

Kroon, L. A. (2007). Drug interactions with smoking. *American Journal of Health-System Pharmacy, 64*(18), 1917–1921.

Kulkarni, J., Gavrilidis, E., Worsley, R., & Hayes, E. (2012). Role of estrogen treatment in the management of schizophrenia. *CNS Drugs, 26*(7), 549–557.

Ladue, L. (2011). Generic psychotropic medications: Issues of cost-effectiveness and patient benefit. *Southern Medical Journal, 104*(10), 711–714.

Lagerros, Y. T., & Rossner, S. (2013). Obesity management: What brings success? *Therapeutic Advances in Gastroenterology, 6*(1), 77–88.

Landi, F., Onder, G., Cesari, M., Barillaro, C., Russo, A., Bernabei, R., & Silver Network Home Care Study Group. (2005). Psychotropic medications and risk for falls among community-dwelling frail older people: An observational study. *Journals of Gerontology. Series A, Biological Sciences and Medical Sciences, 60*(5), 622–626.

Langer, S. Z. (2008). Therapeutic use of release-modifying drugs. *Handbook of Experimental Pharmacology,* (184), 561–573.

Laniado-Laborin, R. (2010). Smoking cessation intervention: An evidence-based approach. *Postgraduate Medicine, 122*(2), 74–82.

Lariscy, J. T., Hummer, R. A., Rath, J. M., Villanti, A. C., Hayward, M. D., & Vallone, D. M. (2013). Race/Ethnicity, nativity, and tobacco use among U.S. young adults: Results from a nationally representative survey. *Nicotine and Tobacco Research, 15*(8): 1417–1426.

Laufer, M. W., Denhoff, E., & Solomons, G. (1957). Hyperkinetic impulse disorder in children's behavior problems. *Psychosomatic Medicine, 19*(1), 38–49.

Le Couteur, D. G., Hilmer, S. N., Glasgow, N., Naganathan, V., & Cumming, R. G. (2004). Prescribing in older people. *Australian Family Physician, 33*(10), 777–781.

Lehmann, H. E., & Ban, T. A. (1997). The history of the psychopharmacology of schizophrenia. *Canadian Journal of Psychiatry. Revue Canadienne De Psychiatrie, 42*(2), 152–162.

Leipzig, R. M., Cumming, R. G., & Tinetti, M. E. (1999). Drugs and falls in older people: A systematic review and meta-analysis: I. Psychotropic drugs. *Journal of the American Geriatrics Society, 47*(1), 30–39.

Leshner, A. I. (1997). Addiction is a brain disease, and it matters. *Science, 278*(5335), 45–47.

Leucht, S., Heres, S., Kissling, W., & Davis, J. M. (2012). Evidence-based pharmacotherapy of schizophrenia. In D. J. Stein, B. Lerer, & S. M. Stahl (Eds.), *Essential evidence-based psychopharmacology* (2nd ed., pp. 18–38). New York, NY: Cambridge University Press.

Leuchter, A. F., Cook, I. A., Witte, E. A., Morgan, M., & Abrams, M. (2002). Changes in brain function of depressed subjects during treatment with placebo. *American Journal of Psychiatry, 159*(1), 122–129.

LeVine, E. S., & Foster, E. O. (2010). Integration of psychotherapy and pharmacotherapy by prescribing-medical psychologists: A psychobiosocial model of care. In R. E. McGrath & B. A. Moore (Eds.), *Pharmacotherapy for psychologists: Prescribing and collaborative roles* (pp. 105–131). Washington, DC: American Psychological Association.

Levitan, M. N., Papelbaum, M., & Nardi, A. E. (2012). A review of preliminary observations on agomelatine in the treatment of anxiety disorders. *Experimental and Clinical Psychopharmacology, 20*(6), 504–509.

Levy, N. (2013). Addiction is not a brain disease (and it matters). *Frontiers in Psychiatry, 4*, 1–7.

Leweke, F. M., & Schneider, M. (2011). Chronic pubertal cannabinoid treatment as a behavioural model for aspects of schizophrenia: Effects of the atypical antipsychotic quetiapine. *International Journal of Neuropsychopharmacology, 14*(1), 43–51.

Lin, K. M., Anderson, D., & Poland, R. E. (1995). Ethnicity and psychopharmacology. bridging the gap. *Psychiatric Clinics of North America, 18*(3), 635–647.

Lin, K. M., & Cheung, F. (1999). Mental health issues for Asian Americans. *Psychiatric Services, 50*(6), 774–780.

Lin, K. M., Poland, R. E., Nuccio, I., Matsuda, K., Hathuc, N., Su, T. P., & Fu, P. (1989). A longitudinal assessment of haloperidol doses and serum concentrations in Asian and Caucasian schizophrenic patients. *American Journal of Psychiatry, 146*(10), 1307–1311.

Lin, K. M., Smith, M. W., & Ortiz, V. (2001). Culture and psychopharmacology. *The Psychiatric Clinics of North America, 24*(3), 523–538.

Linden, M., Pyrkosch, L., & Hundemer, H. P. (2008). Frequency and effects of psychosocial interventions additional to olanzapine treatment in routine care of schizophrenic patients. *Social Psychiatry and Psychiatric Epidemiology, 43*(5), 373–379.

Lindenmayer, J. P. (2000). Treatment refractory schizophrenia. *Psychiatric Quarterly, 71*(4), 373–384.

Lindsey, P. L. (2009). Psychotropic medication use among older adults: What all nurses need to know. *Journal of Gerontological Nursing, 35*(9), 28–38.

Lipsky, M. S., & Sharp, L. K. (2001). From idea to market: The drug approval process. *Journal of the American Board of Family Practice / American Board of Family Practice, 14*(5), 362–367.

Liu, Q., Lawrence, A. J., & Liang, J. H. (2011). Traditional Chinese medicine for treatment of alcoholism: From ancient to modern. *American Journal of Chinese Medicine, 39*(1), 1–13.

Liu, X., & Weiss, F. (2002). Additive effect of stress and drug cues on reinstatement of ethanol seeking: Exacerbation by history of dependence and role of concurrent activation of corticotropin-releasing factor and opioid mechanisms. *Journal of Neuroscience, 22*(18), 7856–7861.

Liu, Y., von Deneen, K. M., Kobeissy, F. H., & Gold, M. S. (2010). Food addiction and obesity: Evidence from bench to bedside. *Journal of Psychoactive Drugs, 42*(2), 133–145.

Loebel, A. D., Lieberman, J. A., Alvir, J. M., Mayerhoff, D. I., Geisler, S. H., & Szymanski, S. R. (1992). Duration of psychosis and outcome in first-episode schizophrenia. *American Journal of Psychiatry, 149*(9), 1183–1188.

Lubman, D. I., King, J. A., & Castle, D. J. (2010). Treating comorbid substance use disorders in schizophrenia. *International Review of Psychiatry, 22*(2), 191–201.

Lund, B. C., Bernardy, N. C., Alexander, B., & Friedman, M. J. (2012). Declining benzodiazepine use in veterans with posttraumatic stress disorder. *Journal of Clinical Psychiatry, 73*(3), 292–296.

Luscher, C., & Malenka, R. C. (2011). Drug-evoked synaptic plasticity in addiction: From molecular changes to circuit remodeling. *Neuron, 69*(4), 650–663.

Lydiard, R. B. (1994). Obsessive-compulsive disorder: A new perspective in diagnosis and treatment. *International Clinical Psychopharmacology, 9*(Suppl. 3), 33–37.

Lynch, F. L., Dickerson, J. F., Clarke, G., Vitiello, B., Porta, G., Wagner, K. D., . . . Brent, D. (2011). Incremental cost-effectiveness of combined therapy vs medication only for youth with selective serotonin reuptake inhibitor-resistant depression: Treatment of SSRI-resistant depression in adolescents trial findings. *Archives of General Psychiatry, 68*(3), 253–262.

Machado-Vieira, R., Ibrahim, L., Henter, I. D., & Zarate, C. A., Jr. (2012). Novel glutamatergic agents for major depressive disorder and bipolar disorder. *Pharmacology, Biochemistry, and Behavior, 100*(4), 678–687.

Maher, A. R., & Theodore, G. (2012). Summary of the comparative effectiveness review on off-label use of atypical antipsychotics. *Journal of Managed Care Pharmacy, 18*(5 Suppl. B), S1–S20.

March, J. S., & Vitiello, B. (2009). Clinical messages from the treatment for adolescents with depression study (TADS). *American Journal of Psychiatry, 166*(10), 1118–1123.

Marco, E. M., Adriani, W., Ruocco, L. A., Canese, R., Sadile, A. G., & Laviola, G. (2011). Neurobehavioral adaptations to methylphenidate: The issue of early adolescent exposure. *Neuroscience and Biobehavioral Reviews, 35*(8), 1722–1739.

Marcus, S. C., & Olfson, M. (2010). National trends in the treatment for depression from 1998 to 2007. *Archives of General Psychiatry, 67*(12), 1265–1273.

Marder, S. R. (2000). Integrating pharmacological and psychosocial treatments for schizophrenia. *Acta Psychiatrica Scandinavica Supplementum,* (407), 87–90.

Marder, S. R., & Wirshing, D. A. (2009). Clozapine. In A. F. Schatzberg & C. B. Nemeroff (Eds.), *Textbook of psychopharmacology* (4th ed., pp. 555–571). Washington, DC: American Psychiatric Publishing.

Mark, T. L., Kassed, C., Levit, K., & Vandivort-Warren, R. (2012). An analysis of the slowdown in growth of spending for psychiatric drugs, 1986–2008. *Psychiatric Services, 63*(1), 13–18.

Markou, A., Kosten, T. R., & Koob, G. F. (1998). Neurobiological similarities in depression and drug dependence: A self-medication hypothesis. *Neuropsychopharmacology, 18*(3), 135–174.

Martin, S. D., Martin, E., Rai, S. S., Richardson, M. A., & Royall, R. (2001). Brain blood flow changes in depressed patients treated with interpersonal psychotherapy or venlafaxine hydrochloride: Preliminary findings. *Archives of General Psychiatry, 58*(7), 641–648.

Martin-Latry, K., Ricard, C., & Verdoux, H. (2007). A one-day survey of characteristics of off-label hospital prescription of psychotropic drugs. *Pharmacopsychiatry, 40*(3), 116–120.

Mathew, S. J., Hoffman, E. J., & Charney, D. S. (2009). Pharmacotherapy of anxiety disorders. In D. S. Charney & E. J. Nestler (Eds.), *Neurobiology of mental illness* (3rd ed., pp. 731–754). New York, NY: Oxford University Press.

Mathew, S. J., Manji, H. K., & Charney, D. S. (2008). Novel drugs and therapeutic targets for severe mood disorders. *Neuropsychopharmacology, 33*(9), 2080–2092.

Mavissakalian, M. R., Jones, B., & Olson, S. (1990). Absence of placebo response in obsessive-compulsive disorder. *Journal of Nervous and Mental Disease, 178*(4), 268–270.

Mayberg, H. S., Silva, J. A., Brannan, S. K., Tekell, J. L., Mahurin, R. K., McGinnis, S., & Jerabek, P. A. (2002). The functional neuroanatomy of the placebo effect. *American Journal of Psychiatry, 159*(5), 728–737.

McDonald, W. M., Meeks, T. W., McCall, W. V., & Zorumski, C. F. (2009). Electroconvulsive therapy. In A. F. Schatzberg & C. B. Nemeroff (Eds.), *Textbook of psychopharmacology* (4th ed., pp. 861–897). Washington, DC: American Psychiatric Publishing.

McGrath, R. E. (2010). Evaluating drug research. In R. E. McGrath & B. A. Moore (Eds.), *Pharmacotherapy for psychologists: Prescribing and collaborative roles* (pp. 133–150). Washington, DC: American Psychological Association.

McGrath, R. E. (2012). Research in clinical psychopharmacology. In M. Muse & R. A. Moore (Eds.), *Handbook of clinical psychopharmacology for psychologists* (pp. 431–456). Hoboken, NJ: John Wiley & Sons.

McGrath, R. E., & Moore, B. A. (Eds.). (2010). *Pharmacotherapy for psychologists: Prescribing and collaborative roles.* Washington, DC: American Psychological Association.

McIntosh, A. L., Ballard, T. M., Steward, L. J., Moran, P. M., & Fone, K. C. (2013). The atypical antipsychotic risperidone reverses the recognition memory deficits induced by post-weaning social isolation in rats. *Psychopharmacology, 228*(1), 31–42.

McKusick, D. R., Mark, T. L., King, E. C., Coffey, R. M., & Genuardi, J. (2002). Trends in mental health insurance benefits and out-of-pocket spending. *Journal of Mental Health Policy and Economics, 5*(2), 71–78.

McLean, A. J., & Le Couteur, D. G. (2004). Aging biology and geriatric clinical pharmacology. *Pharmacological Reviews, 56*(2), 163–184.

Meier, M. H., Caspi, A., Ambler, A., Harrington, H., Houts, R., Keefe, R. S., . . . Moffitt, T. E. (2012). Persistent cannabis users show neuropsychological decline from childhood to midlife. *Proceedings of the National Academy of Sciences of the United States of America, 109*(40), E2657–E2664.

Meltzer, C. C., Becker, J. T., Price, J. C., & Moses-Kolko, E. (2003). Positron emission tomography imaging of the aging brain. *Neuroimaging Clinics of North America, 13*(4), 759–767.

Meltzer, H. Y. (2013). Update on typical and atypical antipsychotic drugs. *Annual Review of Medicine, 64*, 393–406.

Meye, F. J., Trezza, V., Vanderschuren, L. J., Ramakers, G. M., & Adan, R. A. (2012). Neutral antagonism at the cannabinoid 1 receptor: A safer treatment for obesity. *Molecular Psychiatry.* doi:10.1038/mp.2012.145

Meyer, J. S., & Quenzer, L. F. (2013). *Psychopharmacology: Drugs, the brain, and behavior* (2nd ed.). Sunderland, MA: Sinauer.

Michelson, D., Allen, A. J., Busner, J., Casat, C., Dunn, D., Kratochvil, C., . . . Harder, D. (2002). Once-daily atomoxetine treatment for children and adolescents with attention deficit hyperactivity disorder: A randomized, placebo-controlled study. *American Journal of Psychiatry, 159*(11), 1896–1901.

Miklowitz, D. J., & Craighead, W. E. (2007). Psychosocial treatments for bipolar disorder. In P. E. Nathan & J. M. Gorman (Eds.), *A guide to treatments that work* (3rd ed., pp. 309–322). New York, NY: Oxford University Press.

Millan, M. J., Girardon, S., Mullot, J., Brocco, M., & Dekeyne, A. (2002). Stereospecific blockade of marble-burying behaviour in mice by selective, non-peptidergic neurokinin1 (NK1) receptor antagonists. *Neuropharmacology, 42*(5), 677–684.

Miller, D. D., McEvoy, J. P., Davis, S. M., Caroff, S. N., Saltz, B. L., Chakos, M. H., . . .

Lieberman, J. A. (2005). Clinical correlates of tardive dyskinesia in schizophrenia: Baseline data from the CATIE schizophrenia trial. *Schizophrenia Research, 80*(1), 33–43.

Miller, M. C. (2005). What is the significance of the new warnings about suicide risk with Strattera? *Harvard Mental Health Letter, 22*(6), 8.

Mischoulon, D. (2009). Update and critique of natural remedies as antidepressant treatments. *Obstetrics and Gynecology Clinics of North America, 36*(4), 789–807, x.

Moerman, D. E. (2000). Cultural variations in the placebo effect: Ulcers, anxiety, and blood pressure. *Medical Anthropology Quarterly, 14*(1), 51–72.

Mojtabai, R., & Olfson, M. (2008). National trends in psychotherapy by office-based psychiatrists. *Archives of General Psychiatry, 65*(8), 962–970.

Mojtabai, R., & Olfson, M. (2010). National trends in psychotropic medication polypharmacy in office-based psychiatry. *Archives of General Psychiatry, 67*(1), 26–36.

Moore, H. (2010). The role of rodent models in the discovery of new treatments for schizophrenia: Updating our strategy. *Schizophrenia Bulletin, 36*(6), 1066–1072.

Morton, G. J., Cummings, D. E., Baskin, D. G., Barsh, G. S., & Schwartz, M. W. (2006). Central nervous system control of food intake and body weight. *Nature, 443*(7109), 289–295.

Munro, J. F., & Ford, M. J. (1982). Drug treatment of obesity. In T. Silverstone (Ed.), *Drugs and appetite* (pp. 125–157). London: Academic Press.

Murphy, G. M., Jr., Hollander, S. B., Rodrigues, H. E., Kremer, C., & Schatzberg, A. F. (2004). Effects of the serotonin transporter gene promoter polymorphism on mirtazapine and paroxetine efficacy and adverse events in geriatric major depression. *Archives of General Psychiatry, 61*(11), 1163–1169.

Nagel, T., Robinson, G., Condon, J., & Trauer, T. (2009). Approach to treatment of mental illness and substance dependence in remote indigenous communities: Results of a mixed methods study. *Australian Journal of Rural Health, 17*(4), 174–182.

Nasrallah, H. A., & Tandon, R. (2009). Classic antipsychotic medications. In A. F. Schatzberg & C. B. Nemeroff (Eds.), *Textbook of psychopharmacology* (4th ed., pp. 533–554). Washington, DC: American Psychiatric Publishing.

Nathan, P. E., & Gorman, J. M. (Eds.). (2007). *A guide to treatments that work* (3rd ed.). New York, NY: Oxford University Press.

Navarra, R., Graf, R., Huang, Y., Logue, S., Comery, T., Hughes, Z., & Day, M. (2008). Effects of atomoxetine and methylphenidate on attention and impulsivity in the 5-choice serial reaction time test. *Progress in Neuro-psychopharmacology and Biological Psychiatry, 32*(1), 34–41.

Nemeroff, C. B., & Schatzberg, A. F. (2007). Pharmacological treatments for unipolar depression. In P. E. Nathan & J. M. Gorman (Eds.), *A guide to treatments that work* (3rd ed., pp. 271–287). New York, NY: Oxford University Press.

Nestler, E. J. (2009). Epigenetic mechanisms in psychiatry. *Biological Psychiatry, 65*(3), 189–190.

Newcorn, J. H., Kratochvil, C. J., Allen, A. J., Casat, C. D., Ruff, D. D., Moore, R. J., . . . Atomoxetine/Methylphenidate Comparative Study Group. (2008). Atomoxetine and osmotically released methylphenidate for the treatment of attention deficit hyperactivity disorder: Acute comparison and differential response. *American Journal of Psychiatry, 165*(6), 721–730.

Nierenberg, A. A., McLean, N. E., Alpert, J. E., Worthington, J. J., Rosenbaum, J. F., &

Fava, M. (1995). Early nonresponse to fluoxetine as a predictor of poor 8-week outcome. *American Journal of Psychiatry, 152*(10), 1500–1503.

Novak, E., & Allen, P. J. (2007). Prescribing medications in pediatrics: Concerns regarding FDA approval and pharmacokinetics. *Pediatric Nursing, 33*(1), 64–70.

Nowakowska, E., Kus, K., & Chodera, A. (2003). Comparison of behavioural effects of venlafaxine and imipramine in rats. *Arzneimittel-Forschung, 53*(4), 237–242.

Nutt, D. J., King, L. A., Phillips, L. D., & Independent Scientific Committee on Drugs. (2010). Drug harms in the UK: A multicriteria decision analysis. *Lancet, 376*(9752), 1558–1565.

O'Brien, C. P. (2005). Anticraving medications for relapse prevention: A possible new class of psychoactive medications. *American Journal of Psychiatry, 162*(8), 1423–1431.

O'Brien, C. P., & Dackis, C. A. (2009). Treatment of substance-related disorders. In A. F. Schatzberg & C. B. Nemeroff (Eds.), *Textbook of psychopharmacology* (4th ed., pp. 1213–1229). Washington, DC: American Psychiatric Publishing.

O'Brien, C. P., & McKay, J. (2007). Psychopharmacological treatments for substance use disorders. In P. E. Nathan & J. M. Gorman (Eds.), *A guide to treatments that work* (3rd ed., pp. 145–177). New York, NY: Oxford University Press.

O'Brien, C. P., Volkow, N., & Li, T. K. (2006). What's in a word? Addiction versus dependence in *DSM-V*. *American Journal of Psychiatry, 163*(5), 764–765.

O'Connell, G., Lawrie, S. M., McIntosh, A. M., & Hall, J. (2011). Schizophrenia risk genes: Implications for future drug development and discovery. *Biochemical Pharmacology, 81*(12), 1367–1373.

Odgers, C. L., Caspi, A., Nagin, D. S., Piquero, A. R., Slutske, W. S., Milne, B. J., . . . Moffitt, T. E. (2008). Is it important to prevent early exposure to drugs and alcohol among adolescents? *Psychological Science, 19*(10), 1037–1044.

Oleson, E. B., & Cheer, J. F. (2012). A brain on cannabinoids: The role of dopamine release in reward seeking. *Cold Spring Harbor Perspectives in Medicine, 2*(8), a012229.

Olfson, M., Blanco, C., Liu, L., Moreno, C., & Laje, G. (2006a). National trends in the outpatient treatment of children and adolescents with antipsychotic drugs. *Archives of General Psychiatry, 63*(6), 679–685.

Olfson, M., Marcus, S. C., Tedeschi, M., & Wan, G. J. (2006b). Continuity of antidepressant treatment for adults with depression in the United States. *American Journal of Psychiatry, 163*(1), 101–108.

Olfson, M., Marcus, S. C., Weissman, M. M., & Jensen, P. S. (2002). National trends in the use of psychotropic medications by children. *Journal of the American Academy of Child and Adolescent Psychiatry, 41*(5), 514–521.

Oliver, J. E. (2006). The politics of pathology: How obesity became an epidemic disease. *Perspectives in Biology and Medicine, 49*(4), 611–627.

O'Malley, S. S., Cooney, J. L., Krishnan-Sarin, S., Dubin, J. A., McKee, S. A., Cooney, N. L., . . . Jatlow, P. (2006). A controlled trial of naltrexone augmentation of nicotine replacement therapy for smoking cessation. *Archives of Internal Medicine, 166*(6), 667–674.

O'Malley, S. S., Krishnan-Sarin, S., Farren, C., Sinha, R., & Kreek, M. J. (2002). Naltrexone decreases craving and alcohol self-administration in alcohol-dependent subjects and activates the hypothalamo-pituitary-adrenocortical axis. *Psychopharmacology, 160*(1), 19–29.

Owen, R. T. (2012). Glutamatergic approaches in major depressive disorder: Focus on ketamine, memantine and riluzole. *Drugs of Today, 48*(7), 469–478.

Padwal, R. S., & Majumdar, S. R. (2007). Drug treatments for obesity: Orlistat, sibutramine, and rimonabant. *Lancet, 369*(9555), 71–77.

Pampallona, S., Bollini, P., Tibaldi, G., Kupelnick, B., & Munizza, C. (2004). Combined pharmacotherapy and psychological treatment for depression: A systematic review. *Archives of General Psychiatry, 61*(7), 714–719.

Papakostas, G. I. (2009). Managing partial response or nonresponse: Switching, augmentation, and combination strategies for major depressive disorder. *Journal of Clinical Psychiatry, 70*(Suppl. 6), 16–25.

Papakostas, Y. G., & Daras, M. D. (2001). Placebos, placebo effect, and the response to the healing situation: The evolution of a concept. *Epilepsia, 42*(12), 1614–1625.

Papp, M., Litwa, E., Gruca, P., & Mocaer, E. (2006). Anxiolytic-like activity of agomelatine and melatonin in three animal models of anxiety. *Behavioural Pharmacology, 17*(1), 9–18.

Parker, R. (2010). Australia's aboriginal population and mental health. *Journal of Nervous and Mental Disease, 198*(1), 3–7.

Parlesak, A., Billinger, M. H., Bode, C., & Bode, J. C. (2002). Gastric alcohol dehydrogenase activity in man: Influence of gender, age, alcohol consumption and smoking in a Caucasian population. *Alcohol and Alcoholism, 37*(4), 388–393.

Patel, V., Chowdhary, N., Rahman, A., & Verdeli, H. (2011). Improving access to psychological treatments: Lessons from developing countries. *Behaviour Research and Therapy, 49*(9), 523–528.

Patten, S. B., Waheed, W., & Bresee, L. (2012). A review of pharmacoepidemiologic studies of antipsychotic use in children and adolescents. *Canadian Journal of Psychiatry. Revue Canadienne de Psychiatrie, 57*(12), 717–721.

Paykina, N., Greenhill, L. I., & Gorman, J. M. (2007). Pharmacological treatments for attention-deficit/hyperactivity disorder. In P. E. Nathan & J. M. Gorman (Eds.), *A guide to treatments that work* (3rd ed., pp. 29–70). New York, NY: Oxford University Press.

Peeters, F., Huibers, M., Roelofs, J., van Breukelen, G., Hollon, S. D., Markowitz, J. C., ... Arntz, A. (2013). The clinical effectiveness of evidence-based interventions for depression: A pragmatic trial in routine practice. *Journal of Affective Disorders, 145*(3), 349–355.

Pellow, J., Solomon, E. M., & Barnard, C. N. (2011). Complementary and alternative medical therapies for children with attention-deficit/hyperactivity disorder (ADHD). *Alternative Medicine Review, 16*(4), 323–337.

Pert, C. B., Pasternak, G., & Snyder, S. H. (1973). Opiate agonists and antagonists discriminated by receptor binding in brain. *Science, 182*(4119), 1359–1361.

Pierce, R. C., O'Brien, C. P., Kenny, P. J., & Vanderschuren, L. J. (2012). Rational development of addiction pharmacotherapies: Successes, failures, and prospects. *Cold Spring Harbor Perspectives in Medicine, 2*(6), a012880.

Pies, R. (2012). Are antidepressants effective in the acute and long-term treatment of depression? Sic et non. *Innovations in Clinical Neuroscience, 9*(5–6), 31–40.

Pillitteri, J. L., Shiffman, S., Rohay, J. M., Harkins, A. M., Burton, S. L., & Wadden, T. A. (2008). Use of dietary supplements for weight loss in the United States: Results of a national survey. *Obesity (Silver Spring, MD), 16*(4), 790–796.

Pinals, D. A., Malhotra, A. K., Missar, C. D., Pickar, D., & Breier, A. (1996). Lack of gender differences in neuroleptic response in patients with schizophrenia. *Schizophrenia Research, 22*(3), 215–222.

Pincus, H. A., Tanielian, T. L., Marcus, S. C., Olfson, M., Zarin, D. A., Thompson, J., & Magno Zito, J. (1998). Prescribing trends in psychotropic medications: Primary care, psychiatry, and other medical specialties. *Journal of the American Medical Association, 279*(7), 526–531.

Pi-Sunyer, F. X., Aronne, L. J., Heshmati, H. M., Devin, J., Rosenstock, J., & RIO-North America Study Group. (2006). Effect of rimonabant, a cannabinoid-1 receptor blocker, on weight and cardiometabolic risk factors in overweight or obese patients: RIO-North America: A randomized controlled trial. *Journal of the American Medical Association, 295*(7), 761–775.

Pi-Sunyer, X., Kissileff, H. R., Thornton, J., & Smith, G. P. (1982). C-terminal octapeptide of cholecystokinin decreases food intake in obese men. *Physiology and Behavior, 29*(4), 627–630.

Plessen, K. J., & Peterson, B. S. (2009). The neurobiology of impulsivity and self-regulatory control in children with attention-deficit/hyperactivity disorder. In D. S. Charney & E. J. Nestler (Eds.), *Neurobiology of mental illness* (3rd ed., pp. 1129–1152). New York, NY: Oxford University Press.

Pliszka, S., & AACAP Work Group on Quality Issues. (2007). Practice parameter for the assessment and treatment of children and adolescents with attention-deficit/hyperactivity disorder. *Journal of the American Academy of Child and Adolescent Psychiatry, 46*(7), 894–921.

Pliszka, S. R., Crismon, M. L., Hughes, C. W., Corners, C. K., Emslie, G. J., Jensen, P. S., . . . Texas Consensus Conference Panel on Pharmacotherapy of Childhood Attention Deficit Hyperactivity Disorder. (2006). The Texas Children's Medication Algorithm Project: Revision of the algorithm for pharmacotherapy of attention-deficit/hyperactivity disorder. *Journal of the American Academy of Child and Adolescent Psychiatry, 45*(6), 642–657.

Pollack, M. H., Lepola, U., Koponen, H., Simon, N. M., Worthington, J. J., Emilien, G., . . . Gao, B. (2007). A double-blind study of the efficacy of venlafaxine extended-release, paroxetine, and placebo in the treatment of panic disorder. *Depression and Anxiety, 24*(1), 1–14.

Pollo, A., & Benedetti, F. (2009). The placebo response: Neurobiological and clinical issues of neurological relevance. *Progress in Brain Research, 175*, 283–294.

Powers, R. L., Marks, D. J., Miller, C. J., Newcorn, J. H., & Halperin, J. M. (2008). Stimulant treatment in children with attention-deficit/hyperactivity disorder moderates adolescent academic outcome. *Journal of Child and Adolescent Psychopharmacology, 18*(5), 449–459.

Pratt, J., Winchester, C., Dawson, N., & Morris, B. (2012). Advancing schizophrenia drug discovery: Optimizing rodent models to bridge the translational gap. *Nature Reviews. Drug Discovery, 11*(7), 560–579.

Preston, J. D., O'Neal, J. H., & Talaga, M. C. (2013). *Handbook of clinical psychopharmacology for therapists* (7th ed.). Oakland, CA: New Harbinger.

Rasmussen, S. A., & Eisen, J. L. (1990). Epidemiology of obsessive compulsive disorder. *Journal of Clinical Psychiatry, 51*(Suppl.), 10–14.

Ravindran, L. N., & Stein, M. B. (2010). The pharmacologic treatment of anxiety disorders: A review of progress. *Journal of Clinical Psychiatry, 71*(7), 839–854.

Ray, L. A., & Hutchison, K. E. (2007). Effects of naltrexone on alcohol sensitivity and genetic moderators of medication response: A double-blind placebo-controlled study. *Archives of General Psychiatry, 64*(9), 1069–1077.

Raz, A., Campbell, N., Guindi, D., Holcroft, C., Dery, C., & Cukier, O. (2011). Placebos in clinical practice: Comparing attitudes, beliefs, and patterns of use between academic psychiatrists and nonpsychiatrists. *Canadian Journal of Psychiatry. Revue Canadienne de Psychiatrie, 56*(4), 198–208.

Reinhold, J. A., Mandos, L. A., Lohoff, F. W., & Rickels, K. (2012). Evidence for the use of vilazodone in the treatment of major depressive disorder. *Expert Opinion on Pharmacotherapy, 13*(15), 2215–2224.

Reininghaus, E. Z., Reininghaus, B., Ille, R., Fitz, W., Lassnig, R. M., Ebner, C., . . . Enzinger, C. (2013). Clinical effects of electroconvulsive therapy in severe depression and concomitant changes in cerebral glucose metabolism—an exploratory study. *Journal of Affective Disorders, 146*(2), 290–294.

Rey, J. A. (2006). The interface of multiculturalism and psychopharmacology. *Journal of Pharmacy Practice, 19*(6), 379–385.

Richelson, E. (2013). Multi-modality: A new approach for the treatment of major depressive disorder. *International Journal of Neuropsychopharmacology, 16*, 1433–1442.

Rickels, K., DeMartinis, N., Garcia-Espana, F., Greenblatt, D. J., Mandos, L. A., & Rynn, M. (2000). Imipramine and buspirone in treatment of patients with generalized anxiety disorder who are discontinuing long-term benzodiazepine therapy. *American Journal of Psychiatry, 157*(12), 1973–1979.

Rigby, C. W., Rosen, A., Berry, H. L., & Hart, C. R. (2011). If the land's sick, we're sick:* The impact of prolonged drought on the social and emotional well-being of Aboriginal communities in rural New South Wales. *Australian Journal of Rural Health, 19*(5), 249–254.

Roberts, A. J., McDonald, J. S., Heyser, C. J., Kieffer, B. L., Matthes, H. W., Koob, G. F., & Gold, L. H. (2000). Mu-opioid receptor knockout mice do not self-administer alcohol. *Journal of Pharmacology and Experimental Therapeutics, 293*(3), 1002–1008.

Robinson, D., Woerner, M. G., Alvir, J. M., Bilder, R., Goldman, R., Geisler, S., . . . Lieberman, J. A. (1999). Predictors of relapse following response from a first episode of schizophrenia or schizoaffective disorder. *Archives of General Psychiatry, 56*(3), 241–247.

Robinson, E. S., Eagle, D. M., Mar, A. C., Bari, A., Banerjee, G., Jiang, X., . . . Robbins, T. W. (2008). Similar effects of the selective noradrenaline reuptake inhibitor atomoxetine on three distinct forms of impulsivity in the rat. *Neuropsychopharmacology, 33*(5), 1028–1037.

Robst, J. (2012). Changes in antipsychotic medication use after implementation of a Medicaid mental health carve-out in the US. *Pharmacoeconomics, 30*(5), 387–396.

Rocca, P., Fonzo, V., Scotta, M., Zanalda, E., & Ravizza, L. (1997). Paroxetine efficacy in the treatment of generalized anxiety disorder. *Acta Psychiatrica Scandinavica, 95*(5), 444–450.

Rodrigues, H., Figueira, I., Goncalves, R., Mendlowicz, M., Macedo, T., & Ventura, P. (2011). CBT for pharmacotherapy non-remitters—a systematic review of a next-step strategy. *Journal of Affective Disorders, 129*(1–3), 219–228.

Rohsenow, D. J., Miranda, R., Jr., McGeary, J. E., & Monti, P. M. (2007). Family history and antisocial traits moderate naltrexone's effects on heavy drinking in alcoholics. *Experimental and Clinical Psychopharmacology, 15*(3), 272–281.

Rosenthal, M. B., Berndt, E. R., Donohue, J. M., Frank, R. G., & Epstein, A. M. (2002). Promotion of prescription drugs to consumers. *New England Journal of Medicine, 346*(7), 498–505.

Ross, S., & Peselow, E. (2009). Pharmacotherapy of addictive disorders. *Clinical Neuropharmacology, 32*(5), 277–289.

Rowland, N. E., Lo, J., & Robertson, K. (2001). Acute anorectic effect of single and combined drugs in mice using a non-deprivation protocol. *Psychopharmacology, 157*(2), 193–196.

Roy, K., & Miller, M. (2010). Parity and the medicalization of addiction treatment. *Journal of Psychoactive Drugs, 42*(2), 115–120.

Rucker, D., Padwal, R., Li, S. K., Curioni, C., & Lau, D. C. (2007). Long term pharmacotherapy for obesity and overweight: Updated meta-analysis. *British Medical Journal, 335*(7631), 1194–1199.

Rush, A. J., Trivedi, M. H., Stewart, J. W., Nierenberg, A. A., Fava, M., Kurian, B. T., . . . Wisniewski, S. R. (2011). Combining medications to enhance depression outcomes (CO-MED): Acute and long-term outcomes of a single-blind randomized study. *American Journal of Psychiatry, 168*(7), 689–701.

Rush, A. J., Trivedi, M. H., Wisniewski, S. R., Stewart, J. W., Nierenberg, A. A., Thase, M. E., . . . STAR*D Study Team. (2006). Bupropion-SR, sertraline, or venlafaxine-XR after failure of SSRIs for depression. *New England Journal of Medicine, 354*(12), 1231–1242.

Rush, A. J., Wisniewski, S. R., Warden, D., Luther, J. F., Davis, L. L., Fava, M., . . . Trivedi, M. H. (2008). Selecting among second-step antidepressant medication monotherapies: Predictive value of clinical, demographic, or first-step treatment features. *Archives of General Psychiatry, 65*(8), 870–880.

Russell, V. A. (2011). Overview of animal models of attention deficit hyperactivity disorder (ADHD). In J. N. Crawley et al. (Eds.), *Current protocols in neuroscience* (chap. 9, unit 9.35). New York, NY: Wiley. doi:10.1002/0471142301.ns0935s54

Russo, S. J., Dietz, D. M., Dumitriu, D., Morrison, J. H., Malenka, R. C., & Nestler, E. J. (2010). The addicted synapse: Mechanisms of synaptic and structural plasticity in nucleus accumbens. *Trends in Neurosciences, 33*(6), 267–276.

Rygula, R., Abumaria, N., Domenici, E., Hiemke, C., & Fuchs, E. (2006). Effects of fluoxetine on behavioral deficits evoked by chronic social stress in rats. *Behavioural Brain Research, 174*(1), 188–192.

Rygula, R., Abumaria, N., Flugge, G., Hiemke, C., Fuchs, E., Ruther, E., & Havemann-Reinecke, U. (2006). Citalopram counteracts depressive-like symptoms evoked by chronic social stress in rats. *Behavioural Pharmacology, 17*(1), 19–29.

Rygula, R., Abumaria, N., Havemann-Reinecke, U., Ruther, E., Hiemke, C., Zernig, G., . . . Flugge, G. (2008). Pharmacological validation of a chronic social stress model of depression in rats: Effects of reboxetine, haloperidol and diazepam. *Behavioural Pharmacology, 19*(3), 183–196.

Sagud, M., Mihaljevic-Peles, A., Muck-Seler, D., Pivac, N., Vuksan-Cusa, B., Brataljenovic, T., & Jakovljevic, M. (2009). Smoking and schizophrenia. *Psychiatria Danubina, 21*(3), 371–375.

Sagvolden, T., Dasbanerjee, T., Zhang-James, Y., Middleton, F., & Faraone, S. (2008). Behavioral and genetic evidence for a novel animal model of attention-deficit/hyperactivity disorder predominantly inattentive subtype. *Behavioral and Brain Functions, 4*, 56–9081-4-56.

Sagvolden, T., & Johansen, E. B. (2012). Rat models of ADHD. *Current Topics in Behavioral Neurosciences, 9*, 301–315.

Sajatovic, M., Blow, F. C., Kales, H. C., Valenstein, M., Ganoczy, D., & Ignacio, R. V. (2007). Age comparison of treatment adherence with antipsychotic medications among individuals with bipolar disorder. *International Journal of Geriatric Psychiatry, 22*(10), 992–998.

Sallee, F. R., McGough, J., Wigal, T., Donahue, J., Lyne, A., Biederman, J., & SPD503 Study Group. (2009). Guanfacine extended release in children and adolescents with attention-deficit/hyperactivity disorder: A placebo-controlled trial. *Journal of the American Academy of Child and Adolescent Psychiatry, 48*(2), 155–165.

Sandler, A. D., Glesne, C. E., & Bodfish, J. W. (2010). Conditioned placebo dose reduction: A new treatment in attention-deficit hyperactivity disorder? *Journal of Developmental and Behavioral Pediatrics, 31*(5), 369–375.

Saper, R. B., Eisenberg, D. M., & Phillips, R. S. (2004). Common dietary supplements for weight loss. *American Family Physician, 70*(9), 1731–1738.

Sari, R., Balci, M. K., Cakir, M., Altunbas, H., & Karayalcin, U. (2004). Comparison of efficacy of sibutramine or orlistat versus their combination in obese women. *Endocrine Research, 30*(2), 159–167.

Sarris, J., Lake, J., & Hoenders, R. (2011). Bipolar disorder and complementary medicine: Current evidence, safety issues, and clinical considerations. *Journal of Alternative and Complementary Medicine, 17*(10), 881–890.

Sarris, J., Mischoulon, D., & Schweitzer, I. (2011). Adjunctive nutraceuticals with standard pharmacotherapies in bipolar disorder: A systematic review of clinical trials. *Bipolar Disorders, 13*(5–6), 454–465.

Saxena, S., Thornicroft, G., Knapp, M., & Whiteford, H. (2007). Resources for mental health: Scarcity, inequity, and inefficiency. *Lancet, 370*(9590), 878–889.

Sayyah, M., Sayyah, M., Boostani, H., Ghaffari, S. M., & Hoseini, A. (2012). Effects of aripiprazole augmentation in treatment-resistant obsessive-compulsive disorder (a double blind clinical trial). *Depression and Anxiety, 29*(10), 850–854.

Schaffer, S. D., Yoon, S., & Zadezensky, I. (2009). A review of smoking cessation: Potentially risky effects on prescribed medications. *Journal of Clinical Nursing, 18*(11), 1533–1540.

Schatzberg, A. F. (2009). Mirtazapine. In A. F. Schatzberg & C. B. Nemeroff (Eds.), *Textbook of psychopharmacology* (4th ed., pp. 429–437). Washington, DC: American Psychiatric Publishing.

Schermer, M., Bolt, I., de Jongh, R., & Olivier, B. (2009). The future of psychopharmacological enhancements: Expectations and policies. *Neuroethics*, (2), 75–87.

Schimmelmann, B. G., Schmidt, S. J., Carbon, M., & Correll, C. U. (2013). Treatment of adolescents with early-onset schizophrenia spectrum disorders: In search of a rational, evidence-informed approach. *Current Opinion in Psychiatry, 26*(2), 219–230.

Schindler, C. W., Gilman, J. P., Panlilio, L. V., McCann, D. J., & Goldberg, S. R. (2011). Comparison of the effects of methamphetamine, bupropion, and methylphenidate on the self-administration of methamphetamine by rhesus monkeys. *Experimental and Clinical Psychopharmacology, 19*(1), 1–10.

Schooler, N. R. (2006). Relapse prevention and recovery in the treatment of schizophrenia. *Journal of Clinical Psychiatry, 67*(Suppl. 5), 19–23.

Schramm, E., van Calker, D., Dykierek, P., Lieb, K., Kech, S., Zobel, I., . . . Berger, M. (2007). An intensive treatment program of interpersonal psychotherapy plus pharmacotherapy for depressed inpatients: Acute and long-term results. *American Journal of Psychiatry, 164*(5), 768–777.

Schramm-Sapyta, N. L., Walker, Q. D., Caster, J. M., Levin, E. D., & Kuhn, C. M. (2009). Are adolescents more vulnerable to drug addiction than adults? Evidence from animal models. *Psychopharmacology, 206*(1), 1–21.

Schweinsburg, A. D., Brown, S. A., & Tapert, S. F. (2008). The influence of marijuana use on neurocognitive functioning in adolescents. *Current Drug Abuse Reviews, 1*(1), 99–111.

Sclafani, A. (1984). Animal models of obesity: Classification and characterization. *International Journal of Obesity, 8*(5), 491–508.

Sclar, D. A., Robison, L. M., Schmidt, J. M., Bowen, K. A., Castillo, L. V., & Oganov, A. M. (2012). Diagnosis of depression and use of antidepressant pharmacotherapy among adults in the United States: Does a disparity persist by ethnicity/race? *Clinical Drug Investigation, 32*(2), 139–144.

Seeman, P. (2002). Atypical antipsychotics: Mechanism of action. *Canadian Journal of Psychiatry. Revue Canadienne de Psychiatrie, 47*(1), 27–38.

Seeman, P. (2011). All roads to schizophrenia lead to dopamine supersensitivity and elevated dopamine D2(high) receptors. *CNS Neuroscience and Therapeutics, 17*(2), 118–132.

Seger, D. (2010). Cocaine, metamfetamine, and MDMA abuse: The role and clinical importance of neuroadaptation. *Clinical Toxicology, 48*(7), 695–708.

Seitz, H. K., Egerer, G., Simanowski, U. A., Waldherr, R., Eckey, R., Agarwal, D. P., ... von Wartburg, J. P. (1993). Human gastric alcohol dehydrogenase activity: Effect of age, sex, and alcoholism. *Gut, 34*(10), 1433–1437.

Shalev, A. Y. (2009). Posttraumatic stress disorder and stress-related disorders. *Psychiatric Clinics of North America, 32*(3), 687–704.

Sharif, Z., Bradford, D., Stroup, S., & Lieberman, J. (2007). Pharmacological treatment of schizophrenia. In P. E. Nathan & J. M. Gorman (Eds.), *A guide to treatments that work* (3rd ed., pp. 203–241). New York, NY: Oxford University Press.

Sharif, Z. A., & Lieberman, J. A. (2009). Aripiprazole. In A. F. Schatzberg & C. B. Nemeroff (Eds.), *Textbook of psychopharmacology* (4th ed., pp. 613–625). Washington, DC: American Psychiatric Publishing.

Shaw, M., Hodgkins, P., Caci, H., Young, S., Kahle, J., Woods, A. G., & Arnold, L. E. (2012). A systematic review and analysis of long-term outcomes in attention deficit hyperactivity disorder: Effects of treatment and non-treatment. *BMC Medicine, 10,* 99–7015-10–99.

Shelton, R. C., Tollefson, G. D., Tohen, M., Stahl, S., Gannon, K. S., Jacobs, T. G., ... Meltzer, H. Y. (2001). A novel augmentation strategy for treating resistant major depression. *American Journal of Psychiatry, 158*(1), 131–134.

Shen, X. Y., Orson, F. M., & Kosten, T. R. (2012). Vaccines against drug abuse. *Clinical Pharmacology and Therapeutics, 91*(1), 60–70.

Sherafat-Kazemzadeh, R., Yanovski, S. Z., & Yanovski, J. A. (2013). Pharmacotherapy for childhood obesity: Present and future prospects. *International Journal of Obesity (2005), 37*(1), 1–15.

Shoptaw, S., Yang, X., Rotheram-Fuller, E. J., Hsieh, Y. C., Kintaudi, P. C., Charuvastra, V. C., & Ling, W. (2003). Randomized placebo-controlled trial of baclofen for cocaine dependence: Preliminary effects for individuals with chronic patterns of cocaine use. *Journal of Clinical Psychiatry, 64*(12), 1440–1448.

Shorter, E. (2011). A brief history of placebos and clinical trials in psychiatry. *Canadian Journal of Psychiatry. Revue Canadienne de Psychiatrie, 56*(4), 193–197.

Sillaber, I., Holsboer, F., & Wotjak, C. T. (2009). Animal models of mood disorders. In D. S. Charney & E. J. Nestler (Eds.), *Neurobiology of mental illness* (3rd ed., pp. 378–391). New York, NY: Oxford University Press.

Silverstone, T. (1972). The anorectic effect of a long-acting preparation of phentermine (Duromine). *Psychopharmacologia, 25*(4), 315–320.

Silverstone, T., & Kyriakides, M. (1982). Clinical pharmacology of appetite. In T. Silverstone (Ed.), *Drugs and appetite* (pp. 93–123). London: Academic Press.

Simon, G. E., Grothaus, L., Durham, M. L., VonKorff, M., & Pabiniak, C. (1996). Impact of visit copayments on outpatient mental health utilization by members of a health maintenance organization. *American Journal of Psychiatry, 153*(3), 331–338.

Simon, N. M., Otto, M. W., Worthington, J. J., Hoge, E. A., Thompson, E. H., Lebeau, R. T., . . . Pollack, M. H. (2009). Next-step strategies for panic disorder refractory to initial pharmacotherapy: A 3-phase randomized clinical trial. *Journal of Clinical Psychiatry, 70*(11), 1563–1570.

Sim-Selley, L. J. (2003). Regulation of cannabinoid CB1 receptors in the central nervous system by chronic cannabinoids. *Critical Reviews in Neurobiology, 15*(2), 91–119.

Sim-Selley, L. J., Schechter, N. S., Rorrer, W. K., Dalton, G. D., Hernandez, J., Martin, B. R., & Selley, D. E. (2006). Prolonged recovery rate of CB1 receptor adaptation after cessation of long-term cannabinoid administration. *Molecular Pharmacology, 70*(3), 986–996.

Singh, M. K., & Chang, K. D. (2012). The neural effects of psychotropic medications in children and adolescents. *Child and Adolescent Psychiatric Clinics of North America, 21*(4), 753–771.

Smith, S. (2010). Gender differences in antipsychotic prescribing. *International Review of Psychiatry, 22*(5), 472–484.

Smith, S. R., Weissman, N. J., Anderson, C. M., Sanchez, M., Chuang, E., Stubbe, S., . . . Behavioral Modification and Lorcaserin for Overweight and Obesity Management (BLOOM) Study Group. (2010). Multicenter, placebo-controlled trial of lorcaserin for weight management. *New England Journal of Medicine, 363*(3), 245–256.

Sobel, S. V. (2012). *Successful psychopharmacology: Evidence-based treatment solutions for achieving remission.* New York, NY: Norton.

Sonawalla, S. B., & Rosenbaum, J. F. (2002). Placebo response in depression. *Dialogues in Clinical Neuroscience, 4*(1), 105–113.

Sood, A., Ebbert, J. O., Prasad, K., Croghan, I. T., Bauer, B., & Schroeder, D. R. (2010). A randomized clinical trial of St. John's wort for smoking cessation. *Journal of Alternative and Complementary Medicine, 16*(7), 761–767.

Spear, L. P. (2011). Adolescent neurobehavioral characteristics, alcohol sensitivities, and intake: Setting the stage for alcohol use disorders? *Child Development Perspectives, 5*(4), 231–238.

Stahl, S. M. (2012). Psychotherapy as an epigenetic "drug": Psychiatric therapeutics target symptoms linked to malfunctioning brain circuits with psychotherapy as well as with drugs. *Journal of Clinical Pharmacy and Therapeutics, 37*(3), 249–253.

Stein, B. D., & Zhang, W. (2003). Drug and alcohol treatment among privately insured patients: Rate of specialty substance abuse treatment and association with cost-sharing. *Drug and Alcohol Dependence, 71*(2), 153–159.

Stein, D. J., Ipser, J., & McAnda, N. (2009). Pharmacotherapy of posttraumatic stress disorder: A review of meta-analyses and treatment guidelines. *CNS Spectrums, 14*(1 Suppl. 1), 25–31.

Steinbrook, R. (2012). Science, politics, and over-the-counter emergency contraception. *Journal of the American Medical Association, 307*(4), 365–366.

Stewart, C. L., & Wrobel, T. A. (2009). Evaluation of the efficacy of pharmacotherapy and psychotherapy in treatment of combat-related post-traumatic stress disorder: A meta-analytic review of outcome studies. *Military Medicine, 174*(5), 460–469.

Stewart, J. W., Quitkin, F. M., McGrath, P. J., Amsterdam, J., Fava, M., Fawcett, J., . . . Roback, P. (1998). Use of pattern analysis to predict differential relapse of remitted patients with major depression during 1 year of treatment with fluoxetine or placebo. *Archives of General Psychiatry, 55*(4), 334–343.

Stitzer, M. L. (1999). Combined behavioral and pharmacological treatments for smoking cessation. *Nicotine and Tobacco Research, 1*(Suppl. 2), S181–S187; discussion S207–S210.

Stitzer, M. L., & Walsh, S. L. (1997). Psychostimulant abuse: The case for combined behavioral and pharmacological treatments. *Pharmacology, Biochemistry, and Behavior, 57*(3), 457–470.

Stokes, P. R., Egerton, A., Watson, B., Reid, A., Lappin, J., Howes, O. D., . . . Lingford-Hughes, A. R. (2012). History of cannabis use is not associated with alterations in striatal dopamine D2/D3 receptor availability. *Journal of Psychopharmacology, 26*(1), 144–149.

Stokes, P. R., Mehta, M. A., Curran, H. V., Breen, G., & Grasby, P. M. (2009). Can recreational doses of THC produce significant dopamine release in the human striatum? *Neuroimage, 48*(1), 186–190.

Storch, E. A., Lehmkuhl, H., Geffken, G. R., Touchton, A., & Murphy, T. K. (2008). Aripiprazole augmentation of incomplete treatment response in an adolescent male with obsessive-compulsive disorder. *Depression and Anxiety, 25*(2), 172–174.

Strawn, J. R., Sakolsky, D. J., & Rynn, M. A. (2012). Psychopharmacologic treatment of children and adolescents with anxiety disorders. *Child and Adolescent Psychiatric Clinics of North America, 21*(3), 527–539.

Strohl, M. P. (2011). Bradley's benzedrine studies on children with behavioral disorders. *Yale Journal of Biology and Medicine, 84*(1), 27–33.

Sudak, D. M. (2011). *Combining CBT and medication: An evidence-based approach.* Hoboken, NJ: John Wiley & Sons.

Sullivan, G. M., Debiec, J., Bush, D. E. A., Lyons, D. M., & LeDoux, J. E. (2009). The neurobiology of fear and anxiety: Contributions of animal models to current understanding. In D. S. Charney & E. J. Nestler (Eds.), *Neurobiology of mental illness* (3rd ed., pp. 603–626). New York, NY: Oxford University Press.

Sylvia, L. G., Peters, A. T., Deckersbach, T., & Nierenberg, A. A. (2013). Nutrient-based therapies for bipolar disorder: A systematic review. *Psychotherapy and Psychosomatics, 82*(1), 10–19.

Szechtman, H., Sulis, W., & Eilam, D. (1998). Quinpirole induces compulsive checking behavior in rats: A potential animal model of obsessive-compulsive disorder (OCD). *Behavioral Neuroscience, 112*(6), 1475–1485.

Szymanski, S., Lieberman, J. A., Alvir, J. M., Mayerhoff, D., Loebel, A., Geisler, S., . . . Kane, J. (1995). Gender differences in onset of illness, treatment response, course, and biologic indexes in first-episode schizophrenic patients. *American Journal of Psychiatry, 152*(5), 698–703.

Takeuchi, T., Owa, T., Nishino, T., & Kamei, C. (2010). Assessing anxiolytic-like effects of selective serotonin reuptake inhibitors and serotonin-noradrenaline reuptake inhibitors using the elevated plus maze in mice. *Methods and Findings in Experimental and Clinical Pharmacology, 32*(2), 113–121.

Tallett, A. J., Blundell, J. E., & Rodgers, R. J. (2010). Effects of acute low-dose combined treatment with rimonabant and sibutramine on appetite and weight gain in rats. *Pharmacology, Biochemistry, and Behavior, 97*(1), 92–100.

Tam, C. S., Lecoultre, V., & Ravussin, E. (2011). Novel strategy for the use of leptin for obesity therapy. *Expert Opinion on Biological Therapy, 11*(12), 1677–1685.

Tam, J., Cinar, R., Liu, J., Godlewski, G., Wesley, D., Jourdan, T., . . . Kunos, G. (2012). Peripheral cannabinoid-1 receptor inverse agonism reduces obesity by reversing leptin resistance. *Cell Metabolism, 16*(2), 167–179.

Tamminga, C. A. (2009). Principles of the pharmacotherapy of schizophrenia. In D. S. Charney & E. J. Nestler (Eds.), *Neurobiology of mental illness* (3rd ed., pp. 329–347). New York, NY: Oxford University Press.

Tasman, A., Riba, M. B., & Silk, K. R. (2000). *The doctor-patient relationship in pharmacotherapy.* New York, NY: Guilford Press.

Taylor, M. J., & Geddes, J. R. (2012). Evidence-based pharmacotherapy of bipolar disorder. In D. J. Stein, B. Lerer, & S. M. Stahl (Eds.), *Essential evidence-based psychopharmacology* (2nd ed., pp. 39–52). New York, NY: Cambridge University Press.

Teo, C., Borlido, C., Kennedy, J. L., & De Luca, V. (2013). The role of ethnicity in treatment refractory schizophrenia. *Comprehensive Psychiatry, 54*(2), 167–172.

Thase, M. E., Friedman, E. S., Biggs, M. M., Wisniewski, S. R., Trivedi, M. H., Luther, J. F., . . . Rush, A. J. (2007). Cognitive therapy versus medication in augmentation and switch strategies as second-step treatments: A STAR*D report. *American Journal of Psychiatry, 164*(5), 739–752.

Time for Plan B. (2013). *Nature, 496*(7444), 138.

Tollefson, G. D. (2009). Drug discovery and development methods for mental illness. (2009). In D. S. Charney & E. J. Nestler (Eds.), *Neurobiology of mental illness* (3rd ed., pp. 225–237). New York, NY: Oxford University Press.

Trevaskis, J. L., Turek, V. F., Griffin, P. S., Wittmer, C., Parkes, D. G., & Roth, J. D. (2010). Multi-hormonal weight loss combinations in diet-induced obese rats: Therapeutic potential of cholecystokinin? *Physiology and Behavior, 100*(2), 187–195.

Trifiro, G., & Spina, E. (2011). Age-related changes in pharmacodynamics: Focus on drugs acting on central nervous and cardiovascular systems. *Current Drug Metabolism, 12*(7), 611–620.

Trigo, J. M., Martin-Garcia, E., Berrendero, F., Robledo, P., & Maldonado, R. (2010). The endogenous opioid system: A common substrate in drug addiction. *Drug and Alcohol Dependence, 108*(3), 183–194.

Tripp, G., & Wickens, J. (2012). Reinforcement, dopamine and rodent models in drug development for ADHD. *Neurotherapeutics, 9*(3), 622–634.

Tseng, W.-S. (2004). Culture and psychotherapy: Asian perspectives. *Journal of Mental Health, 13*(2), 151–161.

Urban, N. B., & Martinez, D. (2012). Neurobiology of addiction: Insight from neurochemical imaging. *Psychiatric Clinics of North America, 35*(2), 521–541.

Urban, N. B., Slifstein, M., Thompson, J. L., Xu, X., Girgis, R. R., Raheja, S., . . . Abi-Dargham, A. (2012). Dopamine release in chronic cannabis users: A [11c]raclopride positron emission tomography study. *Biological Psychiatry, 71*(8), 677–683.

van den Brink, W. (2012). Evidence-based pharmacological treatment of substance use disorders and pathological gambling. *Current Drug Abuse Reviews, 5*(1), 3–31.

Van den Oever, M. C., Spijker, S., & Smit, A. B. (2012). The synaptic pathology of drug addiction. *Advances in Experimental Medicine and Biology, 970,* 469–491.

Van Gaal, L. F., Rissanen, A. M., Scheen, A. J., Ziegler, O., Rossner, S., & RIO-Europe Study Group. (2005). Effects of the cannabinoid-1 receptor blocker rimonabant on weight reduction and cardiovascular risk factors in overweight patients: 1-year experience from the RIO-Europe study. *Lancet, 365*(9468), 1389–1397.

Vaughan, B. S., March, J. S., & Kratochvil, C. J. (2012). Evidence-based pharmacotherapy of attention deficit hyperactivity disorder. In D. J. Stein, B. Lerer, & S. M. Stahl (Eds.), *Essential evidence-based psychopharmacology* (2nd ed., pp. 1–17). New York, NY: Cambridge University Press.

Vemuri, V. K., Janero, D. R., & Makriyannis, A. (2008). Pharmacotherapeutic targeting of the endocannabinoid signaling system: Drugs for obesity and the metabolic syndrome. *Physiology and Behavior, 93*(4–5), 671–686.

Vetter, M. L., Faulconbridge, L. F., Webb, V. L., & Wadden, T. A. (2010). Behavioral and pharmacologic therapies for obesity. *Nature Reviews. Endocrinology, 6*(10), 578–588.

Vicary, D., & Westerman, T. (2004). "That's just the way he is": Some implications of aboriginal mental health beliefs. *Australian e-Journal for the Advancement of Mental Health, 3*(3), 1–10.

Vickers, S. P., & Clifton, P. G. (2012). Animal models to explore the effects of CNS drugs on food intake and energy expenditure. *Neuropharmacology, 63*(1), 124–131.

Vickers, S. P., Jackson, H. C., & Cheetham, S. C. (2011). The utility of animal models to evaluate novel anti-obesity agents. *British Journal of Pharmacology, 164*(4), 1248–1262.

Volkow, N. D., Chang, L., Wang, G. J., Fowler, J. S., Ding, Y. S., Sedler, M., . . . Pappas, N. (2001). Low level of brain dopamine D2 receptors in methamphetamine abusers: Association with metabolism in the orbitofrontal cortex. *American Journal of Psychiatry, 158*(12), 2015–2021.

Volkow, N. D., & Insel, T. R. (2003). What are the long-term effects of methylphenidate treatment? *Biological Psychiatry, 54*(12), 1307–1309.

Volkow, N. D., & Swanson, J. M. (2008). Does childhood treatment of ADHD with stimulant medication affect substance abuse in adulthood? *American Journal of Psychiatry, 165*(5), 553–555.

Volkow, N. D., Wang, G. J., Begleiter, H., Porjesz, B., Fowler, J. S., Telang, F., . . . Thanos, P. K. (2006a). High levels of dopamine D2 receptors in unaffected members of alcoholic families: Possible protective factors. *Archives of General Psychiatry, 63*(9), 999–1008.

Volkow, N. D., Wang, G. J., Telang, F., Fowler, J. S., Logan, J., Childress, A. R., . . . Wong, C. (2006b). Cocaine cues and dopamine in dorsal striatum: Mechanism of craving in cocaine addiction. *Journal of Neuroscience, 26*(24), 6583–6588.

Volkow, N. D., Wang, G. J., Tomasi, D., & Baler, R. D. (2013a). The addictive dimensionality of obesity. *Biological Psychiatry, 73*(9), 811–818.

Volkow, N. D., Wang, G. J., Tomasi, D., & Baler, R. D. (2013b). Obesity and addiction: Neurobiological overlaps. *Obesity Reviews, 14*(1), 2–18.

Volkow, N. D., Wang, G. J., Tomasi, D., Kollins, S. H., Wigal, T. L., Newcorn, J. H., . . . Swanson, J. M. (2012). Methylphenidate-elicited dopamine increases in ventral striatum are associated with long-term symptom improvement in adults with attention deficit hyperactivity disorder. *Journal of Neuroscience, 32*(3), 841–849.

Volkow, N. D., & Wise, R. A. (2005). How can drug addiction help us understand obesity? *Nature Neuroscience, 8*(5), 555–560.

von Wolff, A., Holzel, L. P., Westphal, A., Harter, M., & Kriston, L. (2012). Combination of pharmacotherapy and psychotherapy in the treatment of chronic depression: A systematic review and meta-analysis. *BMC Psychiatry, 12*, 61–244X-12–61.

Wagner, A. P. (2002). *What to do when your child has obsessive-compulsive disorder: Strategies and solutions.* Apex, NC: Lighthouse Press.

Wagner, K. D., & Pliszka, S. R. (2009). Treatment of child and adolescent disorders. In A. F. Schatzberg & C. B. Nemeroff (Eds.), *Textbook of psychopharmacology* (4th ed., pp. 1309–1366). Washington, DC: American Psychiatric Publishing.

Walkup, J. T., Albano, A. M., Piacentini, J., Birmaher, B., Compton, S. N., Sherrill, J. T., . . . Kendall, P. C. (2008). Cognitive behavioral therapy, sertraline, or a combination in childhood anxiety. *New England Journal of Medicine, 359*(26), 2753–2766.

Walkup, J. T., McAlpine, D. D., Olfson, M., Labay, L. E., Boyer, C., & Hansell, S. (2000). Patients with schizophrenia at risk for excessive antipsychotic dosing. *Journal of Clinical Psychiatry, 61*(5), 344–348.

Walsh, B. T., Seidman, S. N., Sysko, R., & Gould, M. (2002). Placebo response in studies of major depression: Variable, substantial, and growing. *Journal of the American Medical Association, 287*(14), 1840–1847.

Walsh, B. T., Wilson, G. T., Loeb, K. L., Devlin, M. J., Pike, K. M., Roose, S. P., . . . Waternaux, C. (1997). Medication and psychotherapy in the treatment of bulimia nervosa. *American Journal of Psychiatry, 154*(4), 523–531.

Walton, S. M., Schumock, G. T., Lee, K. V., Alexander, G. C., Meltzer, D., & Stafford, R. S. (2008). Prioritizing future research on off-label prescribing: Results of a quantitative evaluation. *Pharmacotherapy, 28*(12), 1443–1452.

Wang, G. J., Volkow, N. D., Chang, L., Miller, E., Sedler, M., Hitzemann, R., . . . Fowler, J. S. (2004). Partial recovery of brain metabolism in methamphetamine abusers after protracted abstinence. *American Journal of Psychiatry, 161*(2), 242–248.

Watson, D. J., Marsden, C. A., Millan, M. J., & Fone, K. C. (2012). Blockade of dopamine D(3) but not D(2) receptors reverses the novel object discrimination impairment produced by post-weaning social isolation: Implications for schizophrenia and its treatment. *International Journal of Neuropsychopharmacology, 15*(4), 471–484.

Wehrenberg, M., & Prinz, S. (2007). *The anxious brain: The neurobiological basis of anxiety disorders and how to effectively treat them.* New York, NY: Norton.

Weintraub, M. (1992). Long-term weight control: The national heart, lung, and blood institute funded multimodal intervention study. *Clinical Pharmacology and Therapeutics, 51*(5), 581–585.

Weintraub, M., Hasday, J. D., Mushlin, A. I., & Lockwood, D. H. (1984). A double-blind clinical trial in weight control. use of fenfluramine and phentermine alone and in combination. *Archives of Internal Medicine, 144*(6), 1143–1148.

Weisler, R. H., Pandina, G. J., Daly, E. J., Cooper, K., Gassmann-Mayer, C., & 31001074-ATT2001 Study Investigators. (2012). Randomized clinical study of a histamine H3 receptor antagonist for the treatment of adults with attention-deficit hyperactivity disorder. *CNS Drugs, 26*(5), 421–434.

Weiss, R. D., O'malley, S. S., Hosking, J. D., Locastro, J. S., Swift, R., & COMBINE Study Research Group. (2008). Do patients with alcohol dependence respond to placebo? results from the COMBINE study. *Journal of Studies on Alcohol and Drugs, 69*(6), 878–884.

Wickens, J. R., Hyland, B. I., & Tripp, G. (2011). Animal models to guide clinical drug development in ADHD: Lost in translation? *British Journal of Pharmacology, 164*(4), 1107–1128.

Wigal, S. B. (2009). Efficacy and safety limitations of attention-deficit hyperactivity disorder pharmacotherapy in children and adults. *CNS Drugs, 23*(Suppl. 1), 21–31.

Wilding, J. (2000). The future of obesity treatment. *Exs, 89*, 181–191.

Wilens, T. E., Faraone, S. V., Biederman, J., & Gunawardene, S. (2003). Does stimulant therapy of attention-deficit/hyperactivity disorder beget later substance abuse? A meta-analytic review of the literature. *Pediatrics, 111*(1), 179–185.

Winterstein, A. G., Gerhard, T., Shuster, J., Zito, J., Johnson, M., Liu, H., & Saidi, A. (2008). Utilization of pharmacologic treatment in youths with attention deficit/hyperactivity disorder in Medicaid database. *Annals of Pharmacotherapy, 42*(1), 24–31.

Wise, R. A. (1997). Drug self-administration viewed as ingestive behaviour. *Appetite, 28*(1), 1–5.

Wise, R. A. (1998). Drug-activation of brain reward pathways. *Drug and Alcohol Dependence, 51*(1–2), 13–22.

Wise, R. A. (2013). Dual roles of dopamine in food and drug seeking: The drive-reward paradox. *Biological Psychiatry, 73*(9), 819–826.

Witkamp, R. F. (2011). Current and future drug targets in weight management. *Pharmaceutical Research, 28*(8), 1792–1818.

Woo, T.-U. W., Canuso, C. M., Wojcik. J. D., Brunette, M. F., & Green, A. I. (2009). Treatment of Schizophrenia. In A. F. Schatzberg & C. B. Nemeroff (Eds.), *Textbook of psychopharmacology* (4th ed., pp. 1135–1169). Washington, DC: American Psychiatric Publishing.

Wood, A. J., Drazen, J. M., & Greene, M. F. (2005). A sad day for science at the FDA. *New England Journal of Medicine, 353*(12), 1197–1199.

Wood, J. G., Crager, J. L., Delap, C. M., & Heiskell, K. D. (2007). Beyond methylphenidate: Nonstimulant medications for youth with ADHD. *Journal of Attention Disorders, 11*(3), 341–350.

Woods, A., Smith, C., Szewczak, M., Dunn, R. W., Cornfeldt, M., & Corbett, R. (1993). Selective serotonin re-uptake inhibitors decrease schedule-induced polydipsia in rats: A potential model for obsessive compulsive disorder. *Psychopharmacology, 112*(2–3), 195–198.

Wooltorton, E. (2005). Suicidal ideation among children taking atomoxetine (Strattera). *Canadian Medical Association Journal / Journal de l'Association Medicale Canadienne, 173*(12), 1447.

Wu, E. Q., Hodgkins, P., Ben-Hamadi, R., Setyawan, J., Xie, J., Sikirica, V., . . . Erder, M. H. (2012). Cost effectiveness of pharmacotherapies for attention-deficit hyperactivity disorder: A systematic literature review. *CNS Drugs, 26*(7), 581–600.

Yonkers, K. A., & Brawman-Mintzer, O. (2002). The pharmacologic treatment of depression: Is gender a critical factor? *Journal of Clinical Psychiatry, 63*(7), 610–615.

Yonkers, K. A., Kando, J. C., Cole, J. O., & Blumenthal, S. (1992). Gender differences in pharmacokinetics and pharmacodynamics of psychotropic medication. *American Journal of Psychiatry, 149*(5), 587–595.

Yucel, M., Solowij, N., Respondek, C., Whittle, S., Fornito, A., Pantelis, C., & Lubman,

D. I. (2008). Regional brain abnormalities associated with long-term heavy cannabis use. *Archives of General Psychiatry, 65*(6), 694–701.

Zahm, D. S. (2010). Pharmacotherapeutic approach to the treatment of addiction: Persistent challenges. *Missouri Medicine, 107*(4), 276–280.

Zhaoping, L., Maglione, M., Tu, W., Mojica, W., Arterburn, D., Shugarman, L. R., . . . Morton, S. C. (2005). Meta-analysis: Pharmacologic treatment of obesity. *Annals of Internal Medicine, 142*(7), 532–546.

Zuvekas, S. H. (2005). Prescription drugs and the changing patterns of treatment for mental disorders, 1996–2001. *Health Affairs (Project Hope), 24*(1), 195–205.

Zuvekas, S. H., & Meyerhoefer, C. D. (2006). Coverage for mental health treatment: Do the gaps still persist? *Journal of Mental Health Policy and Economics, 9*(3), 155–163.

Index

Note: Italicized page locators indicate figures; tables are noted with *t*.

children (*cont.*)
   clinical trials and poor representation
      of, 81
   helpful steps to undertake in treatment
      of, 25–26
   off-label prescribing of psychotropic
      medications in, 82, 87
   psychotropic medications and concerns
      about, 24–25, 34, 54–55
   publicly *vs.* privately insured, prescribed
      antipsychotic medications for, 85
   sertraline + CBT for anxiety disorders
      in, 258
   see also developing brain
chlordiazepoxide, xv, 23, 238, 269t
   animal models for anxiety and, 256
   serendipitous discoveries about, 73
chlorpromazine, xiv, xv, 9, 76–77, 148,
   150, 151, 269t
   clinical experience with, 133–34
   off-label use of, for bipolar disorder,
      81
   schizophrenia and, 46
   serendipity and discovery of, 73, 131,
      132, 152
   tardive dyskinesia and, 47
cholecystokinin, 126, 127
choline, 206
citalopram, 211, 269t
clients as active participants
   addiction treatment and, 186
   ADHD treatment and, 235
   antipsychotic medications and, 153
   bipolar disorder treatment and, 214
   weight-loss drugs and, 129
Clinical Guide to Psychotropic Medications
   (Dubovsky), 95
clinical research, for drug development,
   costs of, 78
clinical trials, 58, 59
   challenge of individualized treatment
      and, 265
   cost of, 62
   effectiveness and safety issues and, 65
   elderly subjects inadequately repre-
      sented in, 23
   FDA, antidepressant medications and,
      199–200

   in humans, encouraging results of exper-
      iments in animal models and, 76
   limitations with, 61–62, 80, 81
   placebo control treatments and, 67
   placebo effect and, 71
   strengths of, 60–61
clomipramine, 196, 201, 239t, 269t
   animal models for anxiety and, 255, 256
   anxiety disorders and, 240t, 242–43
   as drug lacking only one effect, 256
   obsessive-compulsive disorder and, 252
   panic disorder and, 246
clonidine, 219t, 220, 226, 228, 269t
clozapine, 132, 135, 136, 144, 150, 151,
   269t
   advantages weighed against risks with,
      137
   threshold dose of, and improved symp-
      toms of schizophrenia, 13
   weight gain and, 136
Clozaril. *see* clozapine
cocaine, 156, 160t, 162–63, 164, 165,
   177
   craving for, 47
   dopamine and conditioned craving for,
      175
   downregulation of D2 dopamine recep-
      tors and, 49
   lack of only one effect with, 183
   rimonabant and relapse prevention for,
      46
Cochrane Reviews, website, 97
cognitive behavioral therapy (CBT), 243
   bipolar disorder treatment and, 198
   bulimia nervosa and, 45
   glucose metabolism alterations and, 70
   major depression treatment and, 192,
      208, 212
   obsessive-compulsive disorder and, 242,
      252
   panic disorder and, 245, 246
   pharmacotherapy combined with, 70,
      71
   social anxiety and, 248
cognitive impairment
   animal models and, 149
   schizophrenia and, 133
cognitive therapy, for schizophrenia, 141.

FDA and removal of, from marketplace, 79, 106, 111

neurotransmitters or hormones altered by, 107*t*

weight loss and, 105*t*, 115

first-generation antipsychotic drugs, 135*t*, 140, 149

clinical experience with, 133–34

clinical utility of, generalizations related to, 134

gender and, 143

smoking and nicotine ingestion and, 145

five-choice serial reaction time (5-CSRT), animal models for ADHD and, 232

5HT-1A serotonin receptors

aripiprazole and, 43

second-generation antipsychotics and, 136

vilazodone and, 44

5HT-2A serotonin receptors

MDMA and downregulation of, 49

second-generation antipsychotics and, 136

5HT-2C serotonin receptors, lorcaserin and, 43

fluoxetine, 9, 11, 35, 60, 68, 83, 188, 190, 199, 207, 211, 269*t*

animal models for anxiety and, 256

bulimia nervosa and, 45

CBT combined with, for major depression in adolescents, 212

developing brain and, 258

neuroadaptations, animal research findings and, 55

obsessive-compulsive disorder and, 252

social anxiety and, 247

fluoxetine + olanzapine, major depression and, 212

flurazepam, 23, 269*t*

fluvoxamine, 269*t*

animal models for anxiety and, 255, 256

obsessive-compulsive disorder and, 252

social anxiety and, 247

folic acid, 206

food

additives, advice regarding, 65–66

craving for, 102

Food and Drug Administration (FDA), 24, 152, 214

antidepressant drugs and, 198–203

black box warnings and, 201–2, 213, 224–25

clinical trials and, 62

cocaine vaccine explored by, 185

imperfect nature of approval of effective, safe new drugs by, 80–81

new and better drugs approved by, 78–81, 86

OCD-related website, 253

pediatric market and incentives offered by, 83

staff and budgetary resources at, 78, 79

subcontracting issues, review process, and, 79–80

user fees and drug approval process by, 79

website for, 97

weight loss drugs approved by, 108, 129

Freeing Your Child from Obsessive-Compulsive Disorder (Chansky), 253

frontal cortex, 38

full agonist drugs, 42

functional neuroanatomy, of brain, 38, 38

GABA. *see* gamma-aminobutyric acid (GABA)

GABA-A receptor subtype

alcohol and, 161

sedative-hypnotic drugs and, 156

GABA-B receptor subtype, baclofen and, 43

Gabitril. *see* tiagabine

GAD. *see* generalized anxiety disorder

gamma-aminobutyric acid (GABA)

alcohol and neurotransmission of, 161

benzodiazepines, ethanol, and, 14

gastric alcohol dehydrogenase

age, gender, genetics, and, 21–22

chronic alcohol consumption and, 26–27

gastrointestinal tract, hunger control and, 104

gender, 18

antidepressant medications and, 193, 194, 212–13